MW00713573

# VIOLENCE PREVENTION IN LOW- AND MIDDLE-INCOME COUNTRIES

## Finding a Place on the Global Agenda

### WORKSHOP SUMMARY

Kimberly A. Scott, *Rapporteur*

Board on Global Health

INSTITUTE OF MEDICINE
*OF THE NATIONAL ACADEMIES*

THE NATIONAL ACADEMIES PRESS
Washington, D.C.
**www.nap.edu**

THE NATIONAL ACADEMIES PRESS   500 Fifth Street, N.W.   Washington, DC 20001

NOTICE: The project that is the subject of this report was approved by the Governing Board of the National Research Council, whose members are drawn from the councils of the National Academy of Sciences, the National Academy of Engineering, and the Institute of Medicine.

This study was supported by a grant from the F. Felix Foundation to the National Academy of Sciences. Any opinions, findings, conclusions, or recommendations expressed in this publication are those of the author and do not necessarily reflect the view of the organizations or agencies that provided support for this project.

International Standard Book Number-13:   978-0-309-11205-5
International Standard Book Number-10:   0-309-11205-2

Additional copies of this report are available from the National Academies Press, 500 Fifth Street, N.W., Lockbox 285, Washington, DC 20055; (800) 624-6242 or (202) 334-3313 (in the Washington metropolitan area); Internet, http://www.nap.edu.

For more information about the Institute of Medicine, visit the IOM home page at: **www.iom.edu.**

Suggested citation: Institute of Medicine (IOM). 2008. *Violence prevention in low- and middle-income countries: Finding a place on the global agenda.* Washington, DC: The National Academies Press.

Cover design by Van Nguyen. Photos by Fran Henry (copyright 2007).

*"Knowing is not enough; we must apply.*
*Willing is not enough; we must do."*
—Goethe

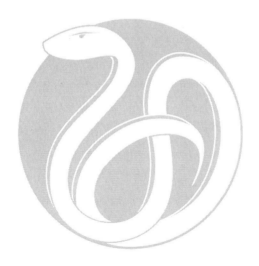

# INSTITUTE OF MEDICINE
*OF THE NATIONAL ACADEMIES*

**Advising the Nation. Improving Health.**

# THE NATIONAL ACADEMIES
*Advisers to the Nation on Science, Engineering, and Medicine*

The **National Academy of Sciences** is a private, nonprofit, self-perpetuating society of distinguished scholars engaged in scientific and engineering research, dedicated to the furtherance of science and technology and to their use for the general welfare. Upon the authority of the charter granted to it by the Congress in 1863, the Academy has a mandate that requires it to advise the federal government on scientific and technical matters. Dr. Ralph J. Cicerone is president of the National Academy of Sciences.

The **National Academy of Engineering** was established in 1964, under the charter of the National Academy of Sciences, as a parallel organization of outstanding engineers. It is autonomous in its administration and in the selection of its members, sharing with the National Academy of Sciences the responsibility for advising the federal government. The National Academy of Engineering also sponsors engineering programs aimed at meeting national needs, encourages education and research, and recognizes the superior achievements of engineers. Dr. Charles M. Vest is president of the National Academy of Engineering.

The **Institute of Medicine** was established in 1970 by the National Academy of Sciences to secure the services of eminent members of appropriate professions in the examination of policy matters pertaining to the health of the public. The Institute acts under the responsibility given to the National Academy of Sciences by its congressional charter to be an adviser to the federal government and, upon its own initiative, to identify issues of medical care, research, and education. Dr. Harvey V. Fineberg is president of the Institute of Medicine.

The **National Research Council** was organized by the National Academy of Sciences in 1916 to associate the broad community of science and technology with the Academy's purposes of furthering knowledge and advising the federal government. Functioning in accordance with general policies determined by the Academy, the Council has become the principal operating agency of both the National Academy of Sciences and the National Academy of Engineering in providing services to the government, the public, and the scientific and engineering communities. The Council is administered jointly by both Academies and the Institute of Medicine. Dr. Ralph J. Cicerone and Dr. Charles M. Vest are chair and vice chair, respectively, of the National Research Council.

**www.national-academies.org**

## PLANNING COMMITTEE FOR A WORKSHOP ON VIOLENCE PREVENTION IN LOW- AND MIDDLE-INCOME COUNTRIES

**Mark L. Rosenberg** (*Chair*), Executive Director, The Task Force for Child Survival and Development, Decatur, Georgia

**James A. Mercy** (*Vice-Chair*), Special Advisor for Strategic Directions, Division of Violence Prevention, National Center for Injury Control and Prevention at the Centers for Disease Control and Prevention, Atlanta, Georgia

**Sir George Alleyne,** Director Emeritus, Pan American Health Organization, Washington, D.C.

**Alexander Butchart,** Coordinator, Prevention of Violence in the Department of Injuries and Violence Prevention, World Health Organisation, Geneva, Switzerland

**Jacquelyn Campbell,** Anna D. Wolf Chair and Professor, The Johns Hopkins University School of Nursing, Baltimore, Maryland

**Darnell Hawkins,** Professor Emeritus, Departments of African-American Studies and Department of Sociology, University of Illinois, Chicago

*IOM Staff*

**Kimberly Scott,** Senior Program Officer and Rapporteur
**Allison Brantley,** Senior Program Assistant
**Megan Ginivan,** Intern
**Julie Wiltshire,** Financial Associate
**Patrick Kelley,** Board Director

# Reviewers

This report has been reviewed in draft form by individuals chosen for their diverse perspectives and technical expertise, in accordance with procedures approved by the National Research Council's Report Review Committee. The purpose of this independent review is to provide candid and critical comments that will assist the institution in making its published report as sound as possible and to ensure that the report meets institutional standards for objectivity, evidence, and responsiveness to the study charge. The review comments and draft manuscript remain confidential to protect the integrity of the deliberative process. We wish to thank the following individuals for their review of this report:

**Stephen W. Hargarten,** Department of Emergency Medicine, Medical College of Wisconsin
**Adetokunbo O. Lucas,** Harvard University
**James A. Mercy,** Division of Violence Prevention, National Center for Injury Control and Prevention, Centers for Disease Control and Prevention
**Susan C. Scrimshaw,** Simmons College, Boston, Massachusetts

Although the reviewers listed above have provided many constructive comments and suggestions, they were not asked to endorse the final draft of the report before its release. The review of this report was overseen by **Dr. Elena Nightingale,** Scholar-in-Residence, Institute of Medicine. Appointed by the Institute of Medicine, she was responsible for making certain that an independent examination of this report was carried out in accordance with institutional procedures and that all review comments were carefully considered. Responsibility for the final content of this report rests entirely with the author and the institution.

# Contents

# Preface

This report summarizes a two-day workshop convened in June 2007 that reviewed the state of the science related to the application of a public health approach to violence prevention in low- and middle-income countries—with an emphasis on what is known to be effective to prevent interpersonal violence. It highlights some of the views expressed by workshop speakers and participants. Although the time frame for the workshop did not allow a comprehensive review of this topic (e.g., violence in video games; the use of the Internet for sexually predatory behavior against young people, or gang violence), the workshop itself provided a unique and timely opportunity for researchers, practitioners, and advocates from different disciplines and areas to come together for scientific discourse. Participants were also asked to make suggestions about how to elevate the issue of violence prevention on the global public health agenda based on the evidence presented, as well as their own policy, research, programmatic, and clinical experiences; but these should not be construed as recommendations from the Institute of Medicine. This report does not contain a comprehensive review of the literature that exists on this topic but rather, like the workshop, is intended to spur further action by others who can play a pivotal role in increasing human, technical, and fiscal resources for global violence prevention. The report appendixes do, however, contain papers commissioned for this report that have reviewed the existing literature for different aspects of violence and its consequences (see Appendix C). The content and views expressed in the papers do not necessarily represent the views of the Institute of Medicine (IOM).

As occurs for many other topics of interest in public health, violence prevention has historically been approached in an insular way with researchers from a variety of fields working in "silos." In these silos, researchers and practitioners are often without the benefit of major findings or funding from other disciplines that are truly necessary for an interdisciplinary approach to address the commonalities among not only the risk factors for different types of violence, but also the consequences for its victims and communities. Thus the workshop was intended and structured as a forum for researchers and practitioners addressing the seven types of violence (child maltreatment and other violence directed at children; youth violence; intimate partner violence; sexual violence; abuse of the elderly; self-directed violence; and collective violence) to come together to discuss cross-cutting risk factors and synergistic approaches to violence prevention (see Appendix A for the workshop agenda). Additionally, these synergistic approaches and linkages among disciplines and types of violence could be another step to help facilitate the translation of emerging and innovative research findings into domestic and international policy and practice. Other participants in the workshop included those with a wide array of expertise in fields related to health, criminal justice, and economic development, as well as representatives from U.S. government agencies, private philanthropic foundations, nonprofit organizations in the private sector, the Department of State, and bilateral and multilateral organizations (see Appendix B for participant list).

The overarching goals of the workshop were to illuminate the issue of global violence prevention and to identify and mobilize specific actions for the U.S. government and other leaders with resources to more effectively support programming for prevention of the many forms of violence. We greatly appreciate the support of the F Felix Foundation, as well as the collaboration with Global Violence Prevention Advocacy, in convening this workshop. Special appreciation is extended to Rosemary Chalk, director of the Board on Children, Youth, and Families, for her expertise and guidance during the organization of this meeting. We are also grateful for the contributions of our expert presenters and moderators, as well as the participants who contributed to the discussions. Many were eager to see and be a part of additional activities that might result from the meeting, and all of their contributions enriched the process of open dialogue that may result in new research, programmatic, and advocacy collaborations beyond the traditional confines of the silo approach.

Several members of the planning committee met once in person, with the rest connected by teleconference, and 13 international teleconferences were held over three months to plan and convene the workshop. Deep appreciation goes to the committee members for the amount of time they volunteered to this project. The workshop rapporteur and IOM Senior

Program Officer, Kimberly Scott, deserves special recognition for coordinating the entire effort over a rather short time frame. Her dedication and responsiveness were notable. Special appreciation also goes to members of the project staff including Allison Brantley, senior program assistant; Megan Ginivan, student intern; and Julie Wiltshire, financial associate, for their able assistance in the organization of this meeting. Additional thanks go to Sarah Bronko for research and logistic support during the meeting, as well as to Tia Carter, Angela Mensah, and Rachel Passman for support during the meeting.

Patrick Kelley
Board on Global Health

# Summary

## INTRODUCTION

In June of 2007, the Institute of Medicine, in collaboration with Global Violence Prevention Advocacy and with support from the F Felix Foundation, held a workshop in Washington, D.C., on violence prevention in low- and middle-income countries (for definition, see Appendix C, Sidel and Levy, 2007, p. 173). Many of the participants were domestic and international researchers, clinicians, and advocacy organizations from different disciplines focusing on violence prevention. Other participants in the workshop included those with a wide array of expertise in fields related to health, criminal justice, and economic development, as well as representatives from U.S. government agencies, private philanthropic foundations, nonprofit organizations in the private sector, the U.S. Department of State, and bilateral and multilateral organizations.

The overarching goals of the two-day workshop were to illuminate the issue of global violence prevention and to articulate specific opportunities for the U.S. government and other leaders with resources to more effectively support programming for prevention of the many forms of violence. While this workshop report does not contain formal recommendations from the Institute of Medicine, several important messages and participants' suggestions emerged that could help facilitate new dialogue

---

The planning committee's role was limited to planning the workshop, and the workshop summary has been prepared by the workshop rapporteur as a factual summary of what occurred at the workshop.

among those who will play critical roles in elevating violence as a priority issue for increased global attention. Increased support for global violence prevention could have far-reaching impact since violence occurs in different settings and affects different populations, with many of the different types of violence often sharing underlying risk factors and occurring in similar contexts.

There is scant scientific literature available that comprehensively reviews the harmful impact of different types of violence on a range of health outcomes in developed or developing countries. The first report to successfully attempt this was the 2002 World Health Organization (WHO) *Report on Violence and Health*. Despite this pioneering effort by WHO and the synergism between violence and other factors that hinder the health and well-being of populations, violence prevention has lagged behind other issues on global agendas for public health, economic development, politics, and governance in terms of the priority and resources it receives. For example, statistics show that collective violence and armed conflicts represent approximately 11 percent of deaths due to violence globally, compared to the nearly 54 percent attributed to suicide (WHO, 2002a); yet collective violence often receives a disproportionate level of attention, especially from the media.

## WORKSHOP MESSAGES

One of the overarching messages from the workshop is that violence is costly in both human and monetary costs. In 2000, more than 1.5 million deaths globally were attributed to violence compared to other public health priorities. Of those deaths, more than half were due to suicide (about 800,000 deaths annually); 35 percent to interpersonal violence; and 11 percent to collective violence, which can include organized violence, forms of war, and gang violence (WHO, 2002a). The global distribution of deaths due to violence shows that 91 percent of this burden is disproportionately shouldered by low- and middle-income countries, compared to 9 percent by developed countries:

• The overall economic direct and indirect costs associated with the short and the long-term consequences of violence (other than physical injury and death) are difficult to assess accurately. There is a paucity of studies on the economic costs of interpersonal and other types of violence, especially in low- and middle-income countries (WHO, 2004). Innovative research, advocacy, and policy analyses are beginning to examine the critical issue of costing and economic effects to define areas in need of greater research and programmatic focus or needed advances or changes in health, public, and economic policy. It was also suggested that the inclusion of economic indicators and cost-effectiveness in intervention design and outcome evaluations of interventions may help bridge the gap between the official economic development community and the public health community.

• There is an increasingly recognized and documented intersection of violence with other health conditions, such as linkages to longer-term health conditions and disability and the synergism of violence and increased HIV/AIDS exposure and infection, especially for women. Child maltreatment has been shown to contribute to high-risk behaviors in adulthood such as alcohol and substance use—making an argument for increased investment and urgent focus on its prevention for lifelong benefits.

## THE VALUE OF VIOLENCE PREVENTION

Violence also has collateral effects on education and schooling, commerce and business, criminal justice and law enforcement, the environment, leadership and capacity for governance, and societal productivity and cohesion in general. The second workshop message is that emerging evidence shows that many types of violence are not only predictable but also preventable. Heightened interest and investment in prevention would confer beneficial returns not only to the places and people most affected by violence but also the world in general—by saving lives, improving health outcomes, and facilitating economic growth that could encourage foreign investments. This in turn may contribute to political, civil, and economic stability in low- and middle-income countries.

Various players in violence prevention are using different methodologies to address violence and the mitigation of its consequences. However, disciplines beyond those traditionally associated with health and health care are also advocating for an increased use of science-based approaches to better understand the patterns of violence, its risk and protective factors, and the needs of its victims, as well as to build evidence and apply best practices to pathways for intervention. It was also acknowledged that using public health science to help understand the variance in rates and types of violence can lead to risk identification and prevention in much the same way public health has exploited such variations in cancer and other diseases to identify prevention strategies. A public health approach would also include multisectoral and multidisciplinary collaboration in which public health would be only one of many partners.

## THE PROMISE OF RESEARCH

The phenomenon known as the "10/90 gap" states that less than 10 percent of funds invested in global health research ($73 billion annually) is devoted to the health problems that account for 90 percent of the global disease burden (see Appendix C, Matzopoulos et al., 2007). Growing evidence points to violence being a part of that 90 percent burden. Despite limited funding however, the current state of science in violence prevention reveals progress, promise, and a number of remaining challenges. Most of what is known about effective violence prevention comes from studies in developed countries but improved integration and collaboration could accelerate application of what is known to developing countries for appropriate adaptation. Promising, effective interventions are currently being implemented in and by developing countries, but they have not been rigorously evaluated for scaling up to regional and national levels. This is where it was thought contributions from private and corporate philanthropy could effectively bridge science with practice. Historical and emerging pathways to violence have been identified, suggesting that greater understanding of them will provide critical input for programmatic and methodological design. Some examples include efforts to improve social, emotional, and behavioral competencies, to improve family functioning and parenting practices to affect and change social norms, and to reduce access to lethal means.

## WHAT PARTICANTS THINK IS NEEDED
## TO MOVE VIOLENCE PREVENTION FORWARD

Participants highlighted the need for the timely development of an integrated, science-based approach and agenda to support research, clinical practice, program development, policy analysis, and advocacy for violence prevention. It was suggested that the agenda be based on realistic estimates of the resources and funding necessary for effectiveness—not simply what is believed "reasonable" in order to garner short-term political or financial support. Other suggestions for progressive action steps included

- learning from and linking to other economic development or health initiatives (such as HIV/AIDS or maternal and child health) as platforms from which the nascent violence prevention efforts can be launched, but continuing to build a coalition to promote widespread formal financial and programmatic support for violence prevention;
- developing collaborative relationships with reporters to influence how violence is covered in local and global news to examine the root causes of violence and pathways of prevention versus coverage of the consequences;
- conveying the critical message to organized philanthropy and government to continue funding and program implementation when true positive effects are seen. Educating funders about the time required for successful relationship building for community participatory research or collaborations to maximize comparative advantage might help explain why

multiyear funding requests are not only reasonable and appropriate, but also more likely in the future;

• developing a national plan and lead agency; enhancing capacity for data collection; increasing collaboration and exchange of information; implementing and evaluating specific actions to prevent violence, and strengthening care and support systems for victims were identified for building a strong, national foundation for violence prevention. These functional elements could provide governments with increased knowledge and confidence in workable interventions, while having alternatives to policing and public security to address violence; and

• building collaborative relationships via international initiatives to attempt breaking the cycles of interdependence between violence and underdevelopment and elevating the issue of violence prevention on the agendas of official development agencies. There are also calls for an array of violence prevention interventions for country adoption according to what is known about their effectiveness, the challenges and opportunities in implementing them, and the crosscutting interventions that are likely to deal with multiple types of violence simultaneously.

## OPPORTUNITIES FOR GREATER INVESTMENT FROM THE UNITED STATES

Presentations from representatives from U.S. government agencies and the private sector detailed their programmatic involvement in domestic and global violence prevention. Many U.S. government agencies are already involved in domestic research on pathways for violence prevention—from neurobiology to criminal justice. Of these government entities, the U.S. Centers for Disease Control and Prevention, the U.S. Agency for International Development, and the National Institute of Mental Health, as well as the multilateral organization—the United Nations Children's Fund—had the most extensive research and programmatic portfolios in international violence prevention, though they were often limited either by funding or scope. It was suggested that government agencies could bring additional resources and expertise to this area if they were statutorily directed to think and act globally for violence prevention.

From the private sector, the InterAmerican Development Bank and the International Justice Mission face different challenges than government agencies when involved in violence prevention because they are permitted by their organizational charters to engage in global activities; but they share challenges that stem from a reliance on the country governments and civil societies in which they work to prioritize violence for action, provide leadership, allocate resources, or request additional assistance to increase their attention to violence prevention.

Despite the repeated call for multidisciplinary collaborations, several presenters acknowledged that the participation of invited government agencies on the workshop panel represented the first time that many of them had ever been in the same room together to talk about violence prevention. While information could be exchanged and a common agenda developed among the agencies for violence prevention, it was also acknowledged that respect for differences in agencies would have to be maintained to facilitate effective collaboration. One important message from this panel was that, while additional research is necessary to build the evidence base for violence prevention, enough is currently known to adapt programs and polices in developing countries to increase gains in violence prevention.

Workshop participants met in small groups to brainstorm ideas for how to move violence prevention forward, with an emphasis on increasing investment or involvement from the U.S. public and private sectors, which can be found in the last chapter. The most often cited were

- integrating violence prevention with economic development and corporate interests;
- using the evidence base and precise language to tailor arguments for violence prevention to potential partners;
- building capacity in developing countries to contribute to the evidence base for violence prevention, while advocating for administrative, policy, or legislative changes that increase the ability of U.S. agencies to engage in international activities for violence prevention; and
- developing strategic alliances with professional, political, and civil associations and organizations.

Given the evidence presented during the workshop, an effective coalescence among researchers, policy makers, advocacy organizations, funders, and communities around a common framework and agenda that utilizes a public health approach could transform isolated efforts into an international, violence prevention movement—a movement from which everyone on the planet could reap immediate and future benefits.

# 1

# Introduction

Violence is among the leading causes of death and disability worldwide for people aged 15-59. In fact, suicidal behavior and interpersonal violence together rank as the third leading cause of death and disability adjusted life years in this age group. In 2000, violence claimed the lives of an estimated 1.6 million people (WHO, 2002a). That number was equal to one-half the deaths from HIV/AIDS and 1.5 times the number of deaths from malaria (WHO, 2002b). Also, while deaths constitute the easiest measure of violence, the devastating impact of violence extends far beyond immediate death—with resultant injuries that are often lifelong, hospitalizations, political instability, and stagnation of economic growth for families, communities, and nations. Violence has also been linked to myriad non-injury health consequences including alcohol and substance abuse, smoking, and high-risk sexual behavior. In turn, these high-risk behaviors contribute to other chronic health conditions with high rates of morbidity and mortality: cardiovascular disease, cancer, depression, and HIV/AIDS. Furthermore, each year, violence costs the world many billions of U.S. dollars in health care, lost productivity and investment, and criminal justice system costs (WHO, 2002a).

Although violence is not always isolated and containable, it overwhelmingly and disproportionately affects low- and middle-income countries. Less than 10 percent of violence-related deaths occur in high-income countries. Low- and middle-income countries often lack the resources to invest in prevention and to respond to the consequences of violence, which are far more severe and pervasive than in developed countries—hindering economic growth, security, and social development. The modern world is permeated by violence; as Nelson Mandela said, "No country, no city, no community is immune." We are not, however, Mandela goes on to say, "powerless against it" (WHO, 2002a, p. ix). Eleven years ago, the World Health Assembly (WHA) adopted Resolution 49.25, which declared violence to constitute a major, escalating public health crisis. In identifying violence as a public health concern, the WHA said several things about the nature of violence—most importantly, that violence is not an inevitable part of the human condition to which the world must be resigned, but rather that it is a preventable phenomenon (WHO, 2002a). While no country may be immune to violence, several of the workshop presentations identified rationales for developed countries, which are also political powers of the world, to be more invested in global violence prevention. Of the more than $70 billion invested annually toward global public health research, less than 10 percent is devoted to research into the health problems that account for 90 percent of the global disease burden. This phenomenon is known as the "10/90" gap and violence has been identified as one of those health problems constituting the 90 percent burden (see Appendix C, Matzopoulos et al., 2007). Beyond the moral imperative is the recognition that economic strength and stability of nations are tied to a global economy. Data were presented at the workshop indentifying economic stagnation and the wealth of a nation as examples of predictive factors for future conflict. In addition to affecting economies, violence can also play a role in the devastation of societal infrastructure including food and water supply systems; public health services and health care facilities; transportation, power, and communication systems; and ultimately national leadership and governance (see Appendix C, Sidel and Levy, 2007). Destruction of this infrastructure can lead to decreased quality of life, increased mortality and morbidity, disruption of people's lives, and displacement of people to other nations—possibility across the globe—that do not always have the capacity to absorb the needs of those displaced or affected.

A public health approach to violence prevention necessitates collective and collaborative action, drawing upon fields as diverse as epidemiology, medicine, nursing, psychology, sociology, anthropology, criminology, policy analysis, education, and economics. As identified in several presentations and the commissioned papers that propose and describe frameworks for applying the public health approach to violence prevention (see Appendix C), the input and inclusion of providers for violence prevention and recovery are critical partners in this approach. Primary strategies for prevention in "Preventing Violence in Developing Countries: A Framework for Action" include addressing behavioral and social drivers of violence, emphasizing building capacity for criminal justice and social welfare systems; as well as specific strategies for secondary and tertiary prevention such as engaging professionals from the health sector in efforts to monitor, identify, treat, and intervene in cases of interpersonal and self-directed violence; building and enhancing capacity for provision of social and health services to victims;

improving emergency responses to violence; and reducing recidivism among perpetrators. The "Logical Framework for Preventing Interpersonal and Self-Directed Violence in Developing Countries" also include these providers and activities in several of the domains for violence prevention activities.

The details of the public health approach are discussed in greater detail in Chapter 2, but a brief description of the role and importance of epidemiology is important. Studying the distribution of a disease within given or similar populations (i.e., within similarly economically developed countries), public health looks to identify risk factors and high-risk groups within the community, which can then direct preventive efforts toward those most likely to benefit, thereby achieving its principal goal—primary prevention. Building upon the results of these evaluations, epidemiology looks to establish a foundation for public policy and regulatory decision making regarding a disease (Gordis, 2000). The steps of this public health approach that utilize epidemiology are proactive rather than reactive and are aimed not at punishing perpetrators and treating victims, but rather at preventing the consequences of violence altogether. There is a heterogeneity with respect to both the types (operationally defined by the planning committee—see Box 1-1) and the prevalence of violence. These differences imply that, like an infectious disease, violence is a product of the interactions between people and the world around them. Thus applying an interdisciplinary, science-based, public health approach offers the prospect of successfully intervening before violence can ravage a community's physical, mental, social, and economic well-being.

In 2002, the World Health Organisation (WHO) published the *World Report on Violence and Health* (WHO, 2002a), which has been heralded as the first comprehensive review of violence on a global scale. That report looked to define violence, identify those it affects, and explore the ways in which public health can offer solutions. Despite the findings and recommendations of both the WHA and the WHO however, violence prevention, especially in developing countries, is just beginning to take hold as a global issue. Previous studies and reports of the Institute of Medicine (IOM) have focused primarily on the domestic context of different types of violence in a number of different settings and among a variety of populations—interpersonal and self-directed violence, violence in society at large and in urban settings, violence in the family, and violence against women and children, among others.[1] To build on its previous work and on the concepts presented in the *World Report*, the IOM hosted a two-day

---

[1]Select report titles include *Understanding and Preventing Violence, Volumes 1-4* (NRC, 1993, 1994); *Understanding Violence Against Women* (NRC, 1996); *Understanding Child Abuse and Neglect* (NRC, 1993); and *Violence in Families: Assessing Prevention and Treatment Programs* (NRC-IOM, 1998). These reports and others are available at www.nap.edu.

---

**BOX 1-1**
**Defining and Classifying Violence**

**Violence:** The intentional use of physical force or power, threatened or actual, against oneself, another person, or against a group or community, that either results in or has a high likelihood of resulting in injury, death, psychological harm, maldevelopment, or deprivation. Classified by three general types (WHO, 2002a):

**1. Interpersonal Violence:**

• *Child maltreatment:* any act or series of acts of commission or omission by a parent or other caregiver (i.e., in the context of a relationship of responsibility, trust, or power) that results in harm, potential for harm, or threat of harm to a child's health, survival, development, or dignity. This definition encompasses physical, emotional, and sexual abuse; neglect or negligent treatment; and commercial or other forms of exploitation (adapted from WHO, 1999, and CDC, 2007).
• *Youth violence:* the intentional use of physical force or power, threatened or actual, against another person, group or community, that either results in or has a high likelihood of resulting in injury, death, psychological harm, maldevelopment, or deprivation in which the perpetrator or victim is between 10 and 29 years of age (adapted from WHO, 2002a).
• *Intimate partner violence:* the intentional use of physical force or power, threatened or actual, against an intimate partner (e.g., spouse, cohabiting partner, date) that either results in or has a high likelihood of resulting in injury, death, psychological harm, maldevelopment, or deprivation. This definition encompasses physical, sexual, and emotional or psychological abuse (adapted from WHO, 2002a).

---

workshop in Washington, D.C., on June 26-27, 2007. The task to the planning committee was to plan a workshop that would promote discussion of the unmet need for high-income countries to invest in violence prevention in developing nations; to articulate feasible strategies and opportunities in both public and private sectors to increase U.S. interest and support for violence prevention in developing countries; and to review the state of science and explore the issue of elevating violence prevention on the global public health agenda. The sessions were organized to review data to identify and describe the costs of violence; how and why violence is preventable; what is known to be effective in developing countries and what might be translated from effective intervention in developed countries; the gaps in research, funding, and programmatic agendas that need to be addressed to scale up

- *Sexual violence:* nonconsensual completed or attempted sexual contact, nonconsensual non-contact acts of a sexual nature such as voyeurism and verbal or behavioral sexual harassment, or acts of sexual trafficking committed against someone who is unable to consent or refuse (adapted from CDC, 2002).
- *Elder abuse:* intentional actions that cause harm or create a serious risk of harm (whether or not harm is intended) to a vulnerable elder by a caregiver or other person who stands in a trust relationship to the elder, or failure by a caregiver to satisfy the elder's basic needs or to protect the elder from harm. This definition includes the following types of elder abuse: physical abuse, psychological abuse, sexual assault, material exploitation, and neglect (adapted from NRC, 2002).

**2. Self-Directed Violence:** fatal or non-fatal self-inflicted destructive acts that include both those with an explicit or inferred intent to die (e.g., suicide, suicide attempts) and those that cause self-harm, but without conscious suicidal intent (e.g., self-mutilation) (adapted from IOM, 2002).

**3. Collective Violence:** the instrumental use of violence by people who identify themselves as members of a group—whether this group is transitory or has a more permanent identity—against another group or set of individuals, in order to achieve political, economic, ideological, or social objectives. Collective violence includes armed conflict or social objectives. Collective violence includes armed conflict (e.g., war, genocide), state-sponsored violence (e.g., genocide, repression, disappearances, torture), and organized violent crimes (e.g., gang warfare, banditry) (WHO 2002a).

violence prevention; and how the public and private sectors in the United States might support global violence prevention with increased financial, human resources, and technical assistance investments.

Although presentations were made or data presented about the seven different types of violence defined in Box 1-1, an important objective of the workshop was to dialogue about how these types of violence can be examined in the context of the three categories that are globally recognized in violence prevention—interpersonal violence, self-directed violence, and collective violence. More importantly, the examination and discussions emphasized their shared risk factors and consequences to victims and societies; suggesting that greater and more timely progress can be made if there were a transition to cross-cutting research and interventions focused on multiple risk factors. As a result, there would potentially be simultaneous and collateral positive effects on several types of violence; as was demonstrated in research on self-directed violence with the United States Air Force. Overall, the presentations effectively achieved this objective to foster dialogue about cross-cutting research and intervention design.

With the escalating monetary, human, and political costs associated with violence; researchers, clinicians, policymakers, advocates, and others from many disciplines have been discussing and attempting to use different methodologies to address the prevention of violence and the mitigation of its consequences. One of the consistent suggestions made during the workshop was the need for a common framework, language, tools, and agenda for violence prevention around which a multidisciplinary and international coalition could be built to elevate violence prevention on the global agendas of public health and possibly, the corporate sector and official economic development agencies or initiatives.

## ORGANIZATION OF THE REPORT

This report summarizes the major themes and data discussed at the workshop.[2] The nine chapters of this report correspond to the organizational themes and resulting sessions of the workshop. This first chapter briefly describes the magnitude of global violence; some of its consequences for the physical, social, and economic health of the people it affects; and how a public health approach might yield substantive returns on investing in violence prevention. Chapter 2 sets the contextual stage for the research findings and presentations during the course of the workshop. Chapter 3 explores violence from health, criminal justice, economic, and human development perspectives. Chapter 4 identifies the intersections between violence and health by examining the impact of violence on varied health conditions. Chapter 5 examines existing interventions around the globe that are proving to be effective in preventing violence in developing countries and identifies other potentially effective interventions for these countries. Chapter 6 details suggestions for developing relationships with the media and linkages with nongovernmental organizations. Chapter 7 identifies the steps needed for international scale-up of violence prevention activities. Chapter 8 explores the challenges and opportunities that exist for U.S. agencies and other organizations that are involved in global violence

---

[2]The themes have been shaped to produce a readable narrative and do not necessarily follow the order of presentations at the workshop. With the exception of brief background statements, this summary is limited to what was discussed at the meeting, the PowerPoint presentations used by speakers, and the background papers commissioned for this report.

prevention. Chapter 9, the final chapter, provides participants' suggestions and ideas for the next steps in global violence prevention. The appendixes of the report contain the workshop agenda (A); a list of workshop participants (B); commissioned background papers (C); and planning committee and workshop speaker biographies (D).

# 2

# Setting the Stage

## WELCOMING REMARKS

To open the workshop, Dr. Patrick Kelley noted that, as the subtitle of the workshop suggests, the problem of violence has not yet obtained its proper place on the global public health agenda. The Institute of Medicine (IOM) seeks to establish a firm scientific foundation for policy deliberations and holds many events that bring together the most expert minds in the world. In this instance, the workshop provided a unique opportunity for researchers and practitioners from multiple disciplines, working to prevent all types of violence (child abuse, elder abuse, self-directed violence, intimate partner violence, violence against sexual partners, and collective violence) to come together in one forum to present the most up-to-date research and engage in dialogue to identify common, crosscutting risk factors and synergistic approaches to prevention.

Dr. Kelley also noted that in his own travels to Peru, he has observed firsthand the very violence represented by the statistics in the World Health Organization (WHO, 2005) *Multi-Country Study on Women's Health and Domestic Violence Against Women*. That study identified an Andean province in Peru as having one of the highest rates of violence against women, with approximately 70 percent reporting the experience of physical or sexual violence or both in their lifetimes by intimate partners. Lower rates for these types of violence were reported in other countries in the study: the rates were 46 percent lower in Brazil and 76 percent lower in a city in Japan (WHO, 2005). He noted that using public health science to help understand the variance in these rates can lead to risk identification and prevention in much the same way as public health has exploited such variations in cancer and other diseases to identify prevention strategies. He also noted that the interrelationship between sexual violence and sexually transmitted diseases, coupled with approximately 5 million new cases of HIV reported each year, dramatically highlights the important interconnection between HIV and violence prevention.

As director of the IOM Board on Global Health, Dr. Kelley expanded on the board's growing awareness that global health, and America's vital interest in it, must be seen in a larger context than infectious disease prevention and management. The consequences of violence are transnational and transgenerational; they emphasize the need for America's increased interest in and support for alleviating the burdensome toll and costs that pervasive violence disproportionately exacts on developing countries and their people. These consequences affect the political and economic stability of societies and their institutions; the ability of children to grow into productive adults capable of community and family leadership; and the ability of women to protect themselves from HIV/AIDS and other reproductive health problems. In conclusion, he identified the important role for workshop participants to disseminate its messages to those who can use the tools of public health and policy making, not only to elevate violence prevention to the center of the global public health agenda, but also to help identify how the U.S. government and other leaders with resources can more effectively support violence prevention programming.

## THE PUBLIC HEALTH APPROACH TO VIOLENCE PREVENTION

Dr. Mark Rosenberg, the chair of the workshop planning committee, focused his opening remarks on differentiating the public health approach from that of health care; providing a brief, selective history of violence and public health; explaining the tenets of a public health approach; and lastly, exploring the relationships among different types of violence to help lay the foundation for the ensuing discussions. To begin, the major difference between approaches is that health care is focused on providing help to those who present to its facilities, while public health is focused on the health of *everyone*—regardless of whether they are known to us, where they may live, the families to whom they belong, or whether they have yet to be born. The public health focus also takes into account what the 90 percent of people who bear the burden of interpersonal and self-directed violence in developing countries have faced for their survival and what they may face in the future. While many recognize the importance of treating the major epidemics that are ravaging the world to facilitate economic and social development, more must come to believe that these efforts must include violence prevention.

The history of violence and public health begins with the domestic violence movement started by women in the United States 35 years ago. Lessons from this movement taught that women in wealthy countries were also affected by violence and that partnerships with the victims affected by violence, their advocates, law enforcement, social services, public policy experts, psychologists, and experts from other sectors needed to be established as part of prevention efforts. Today, these partnerships must be with our neighbors to the global south and those from developing countries. Around 1982, the director of the U.S. Centers for Disease Control (CDC; now the Centers for Disease Control and Prevention) realized that the burden of disease, disability, and injury in this country was no longer dominantly attributable to infectious diseases and that the organization's programming needed reorientation.[1] In its exploration of the causes of the burden of disease and disability, the CDC decided that violence would somehow have to be addressed. Thus the CDC Violence Epidemiology Branch was formed and, as a result, developed the public health approach. The three tenets of the approach were (1) a focus on prevention; (2) a focus on scientific methodology that would enable identifying the risk factors and patterns, and answering the questions of where violence occurred, who it affected and how, what could be done to prevent it, and how prevention efforts could be implemented; and (3) a focus on multisectoral collaboration in which public health would be only one of many partners. When the statement is made that violence is a public health problem, it is not one of sole ownership, but rather one that indicates that public health must be part of the solution by bringing to bear all of its tools and knowledge.

Subsequently, in Dr. Rosenberg's historical review, an advocate named Fran Henry, working to prevent child sexual abuse, approached the CDC and asked whether the newly developed public health approach could be used to prevent such abuse. At that time, she stated that the country's method to address the issue was to intervene *after* the abuse had occurred and then put the child in therapy and incarcerate the perpetrators. She tested the public health approach by applying it to the work of an organization she started, Stop It Now! Its collaborative success changed the paradigm of addressing child sexual abuse by "going upstream" and identifying those at risk for perpetration and offering services to prevent the abuse. Next in the historic evolution, Etienne Krug, a young medical officer working in Angola and in Latin and Central America, in the course of his daily work, witnessed

---

[1]As early as 1979, the U.S. Surgeon General issued a report *Healthy People: The Surgeon General's Report on Health Promotion and Disease Prevention*, in which injury control and violence were identified as a priority to improve the nation's health, despite the Surgeon General's recognition that health programs did not generally address the lifestyle and social risk factors associated with increasing rates of intentional injury (DHEW, 1979).

countless bodies of the victims of violence. He was also spurred to action by the thoughts of going upstream to focus on preventing the violence—staunching the rivers of bloodshed from violence and reducing the numbers of its victims. He arrived at the CDC to study the public health approach for several years and later went on to apply it on an international level by spearheading the violence and injury prevention work at the World Health Organization (WHO). In 2002, he and several international colleagues authored the *World Report on Violence and Health*, which presented data to examine the magnitude of the problem, provided definitions for the different types of violence, and made recommendations for multisectoral and collaborative action to address the multifaceted nature of violence. "While individual initiative and leadership are invaluable in overcoming apathy and resistance, a key requirement for tackling violence in a comprehensive manner is for people to work together in partnerships of all kinds, and at all levels, to develop effective responses" (WHO, 2002a, pp. 1-2).

In 2006, the Disease Control Priorities Project[2] published its second edition of *Disease Control Priorities in Developing Countries (DCP2)*.[3] For the first time, a chapter was focused on interpersonal violence and how a public health approach can be used for its prevention.

The last event in this time line is this workshop in 2007 to accelerate the prevention of self-directed (suicide) and interpersonal violence in low- and middle-income countries (LMICs) by advocating the described public health approach from discovery to delivery. The focus is on these types of violence because they are the ones about which we know the most. However, collective violence and armed violence cannot be ignored in their importance, but Dr. Rosenberg pointed out that the relationship among them requires further study. For example, child soldiers can return from war and often wreak havoc in their families via intimate partner violence and child abuse, while some forms of interpersonal and self-directed vio-

---

[2]The Disease Control Priorities Project is "an alliance of organizations designed to review, generate, and disseminate information on how to improve population health in developing countries." The project also produced a number of major publications. Each product "marries economic approaches with those of epidemiology, public health, and clinical medicine" (Jamison et al., 2006, p. xvii).

[3]The first edition of *Disease Control Priorities in Developing Countries or DCP1* (Jamison et al., 1993), published in 1993, "aimed to provide systematic guidance on the selection of interventions to achieve rapid health improvements in an environment of highly constrained public sector budgets through the use of costs-effectiveness analysis." It was a result of the World Bank's review of priorities for the control of specific diseases as inputs for comparative cost-effectiveness estimates and analyses of intervention to address the conditions most important in developing countries. The second edition sought to "update and improve guidance on the 'what to do' questions in DCP1 and to address the institutional, organizational, financial, and research capacities essential for health systems to deliver the right interventions" (Jamison et al., 2006, p. xvii).

lence create instability that can increase the likelihood of war and conflict. Armed conflict in our discussions is different from collective violence and will be referred to as violence in which some sort of weapon is used. This has important implications for other types of violence—namely, youth, intimate partner, and self-directed violence—since an important intervention for common risk factors is reducing access to lethal weapons, weapons which increase the risk of fatal outcomes for all those types of violence. There are also dividends to investing in early childhood interventions, especially if very, very young children are given the social, cognitive, emotional, and intellectual skills to help them fend off violence either as a perpetrator or as a victim later in life.

To conclude, Dr. Rosenberg detailed the organizational thought processes of the planning committee and familiarized participants with the resultant materials for the workshop. Lastly, Dr. Rosenberg introduced the workshop's keynote speaker, Mr. Stephen Lewis, former United Nations Special Envoy for HIV/AIDS in Africa, who would help participants see the faces of those whose lives may be improved through violence prevention efforts.

## KEYNOTE ADDRESS BY STEPHEN LEWIS

Mr. Lewis began his remarks by acknowledging how much the definition of violence encompasses and how difficult a subject it is to address. Violence as a result of conflict, he observed, is palpable and insistent in the modern world and leads to horrendous, but often repetitive, consequences that are captured by the media. His initial experience in the 1990s with armed conflict involved the coordination of a two-year global study led by Graça Machel for the United Nations, to examine the impact of armed conflict on children, which he found "desperately upsetting because of the extraordinary violations of children on every front—physical, sexual, emotional, and physiological—unbearable violations of their tiny and vulnerable personae." Everywhere there were armed conflicts—from Burundi to Cambodia to Colombia—the study recommended the appointment of a special representative of the Secretary-General for the United Nations to deal precisely, and in an ongoing fashion, with the prevention of these destructive instincts of others toward children.

Lewis's experience working with a two-year panel appointed by the Organization of African Unity to investigate the genocide in Rwanda was "one of the most eviscerating emotional experiences possible," which he stated had a tremendous impact on the way in which he viewed these issues and the world around them. Gathered in a small, community-based clinic that provided networking and support for women who were victims and survivors of violent attacks and sexual assault, seven investigators were asked if they would be willing to meet with three women to hear their personal stories. Three of the investigators met with these women in an abominably hot, very tiny room with three metal cots and a tin roof. The women, who occupied the cots, ranged in age from the late teens or early twenties to the forties. Although they differed in age, their experiences were similarly horrific—being raped and assaulted—sometimes repeatedly, sometimes with blunt and sharp instruments to inflict more pain. All were left without hope. At least one contracted HIV and died two years later. One asked why women are constantly "asked to forgive and forget" when their perpetrators are allowed to remain free and unpunished; another stated that she would never be able to rid herself of the ever-present olfactory memories associated with being tied to a bed for three months and used as a "perpetual raping machine." If the definition of violence were expanded to include intimate partner violence—whether sexual, physical, psychological, or emotional—the victims mount to huge numbers, which most societies and countries in the developed world are reluctant to acknowledge according to Mr. Lewis. The WHO study of women's health and domestic violence [2005] and a study conducted by the nongovernmental organization ActionAid indicate that large numbers of women around the world report experiencing violence during their first sexual encounter. From other data, the Ministry of Health in South Africa reported more than 50,000 rapes in 2005, and extrapolations of nonreported cases would produce numbers that are "hallucinatory."

Sexual violence against women, child sexual abuse, and elder abuse meet in an intersection of alarming new trends in some areas of Kenya. In these areas, staggering numbers of rapes are being reported monthly, and in April 2006, 46 rapes were reported. Half of the victims were under the age of 18 years, and half of these were under the age of 12. In this same intersection, the newest pattern to emerge from the statistics—young men brutally raping women between the ages of 65 and 80 years—the rapists were confident they would be protecting themselves from contracting HIV. Manifestation of this pervasive violence against women in every country partially defines the "madness that grips the world," as it surely "destroys the soul and certainly the women." Mr. Lewis emphasized that the direct relationships between sexual violence and HIV/AIDS and our inability to address violence prevention—the desperation "to find a microbicide or vaccine as a preventive technology that can do what behavior change has not been able to do"—is underscored. The cascading effects of this relationship play a role in redefining the human family in parts of the world, as elderly grandmothers struggle in their attempts to parent their orphaned grandchildren; as pregnant mothers in Africa are unable to access drugs to prevent mother-to-child transmission of HIV; and as children infected with HIV have little access to lifesaving drugs and treatment.

His travels through Rwanda, Uganda, and Sierra Leone would have him bear witness to the effects of genocide and other forms of collective violence on children by viewing pages and pages of their startlingly similar art therapy drawings—men holding machetes and blood dripping down the pages; through his meetings with children in Uganda who had been abducted to become soldiers or sex slaves; and remembrance of the mutilation of 20,000 children made amputees by the Radical Force "in order to cow the population into subservience." The physical and mental effects of this kind of violence on the functional development of these children, if they indeed survived the ordeal at all, were visibly present in the scars that marred and mutilated their bodies, the anger in their eyes and faces, and the trauma-induced mutism that prevented them from even describing their ordeals. He also posited that ignoring epidemics of preventable illness in children can be seen as a form of maltreatment of children, citing data from a Save the Children publication that 28,000 children die each day and 10 million each year from preventable illness. Mr. Lewis suggested that these data contribute to the complex explanation of the declines of many of the hard-won gains in child survival around the world since the 1980s.

The horror in the slaughtering of 800,000 people in Rwanda in 1994, without international intervention, is relived now in Darfur where, within four years, there have been a quarter of a million deaths and unparalleled campaigns of sexual violence and rape. Still, in his observation, the 13-year-old promises of the international community for vigilance to prevent recurrences of such "human depravity and dementia" are unmet. He queried whether there is a "subterranean racism at work in all of this" that regards the peoples of Africa who, in his experience, have such generous spirit, intelligence, sophistication, and decency, as so "profoundly expendable over such a long period of time." Lewis stated that in many parts of the moderate and low-income world, societies feel under siege—as if coming apart at the seams with the imminent possibility of disintegration.

An underlying part of much of the violence, Stephen Lewis stated, is acute and overwhelming poverty, where nearly 2.5 billion people globally subsist on anywhere from less than $1 per day to $750 per year. Violence can be seen in the context of economic development. He pointed out that the first Millennium Development Goal of the United Nations, which seeks to reduce poverty and hunger by 50 percent by the year 2015, speaks directly to the resultant consequences of their relationship. He also reviewed how international financial aid policies of the last 20-30 years, including conditions that reduce access to health care and education, may have contributed to the disintegration of the fabric of many different societal sectors and directly or indirectly induced individual and broader society violence.

In conclusion, he enumerated a number of items that he felt are significant for elevating the issue on the global agenda. The first was the need for political leadership and increased financial support from the United States and the rest of the Group of 8 (G8)[4] countries, which must be held accountable to keep their promises, whether for foreign aid or trade, to ameliorate the human condition. Betrayal of these promises, he stated, "compels much of the world to live in a constant environment of violence." Attention must be given to addressing the relationships between poverty, violence, and disease—as much, in his opinion, as the amount of attention and resources that go to supporting wars in the Middle East. The second item is support of the recommendation for a full, international agency as part of the United Nations, with an Under-Secretary-General and reasonable fiscal resources, that would give women activists the capacity to have an impact and would diminish the violence against women.

The third item calls for organizational leadership, particularly from the United Nation's Children's Fund, to use its power on the ground and in relationships with governments to engage in the work that will prevent the violence inherent in situations in which so many children live and are found. The final item highlights the need for engaged advocacy, on all fronts, to make these issues come alive in a real and consistent way for the public, elected officials, and the media—thereby transforming them into an international movement.

---

[4]The Group of Eight (G8) is an international forum for the governments of Canada, France, Germany, Italy, Japan, Russia, the United Kingdom, and the United States. Together, these countries represent about 65 percent of the world economy and the majority of global military power (7 of the top 8 positions for military expenditure, and almost all of the world's active nuclear weapons). The group's activities include year-round conferences and policy research, culminating with an annual summit meeting attended by the heads of government of the member states. The European Commission is also represented at the meetings. Source: http://en.wikipedia.org/wiki/G8.

# 3

# Why the World Should Care About Violence Prevention

The *World Report on Violence and Health,* published by the World Health Organisation (WHO) in 2002, postulated that the lack of a clear definition of violence has been a contributor to its being ignored as a public health issue. Violence is often defined in cultural terms, which are based on prevailing notions of acceptable or harmful behaviors that change over time. In addition, prevailing definitions of violence have typically been influenced by who is providing the definition and the purposes for which it is being used. For example, a definition used in the criminal justice system for arrests and convictions may be different from that used in a social services system. An important point is that a useful definition of violence should not be so broad as to lose its meaning, but should capture the range of acts of those who engage in violence and the subjective experiences of victims. Additionally, there must be global agreement on a definition so that data can be compared among countries to contribute to building a sound, scientific evidence base with which to address the issue (WHO, 2002a). The report (WHO, 2002a, p. 5) defines violence as

> The intentional use of physical force or power, threatened or actual, against oneself, another person, or against a group or community, that either results in or has a high likelihood of resulting in injury, death, psychological harm, maldevelopment or deprivation.

For the purposes of this workshop, that definition was used. To ensure that participants and presenters were using the same terminology throughout discussions, the committee provided and referred to a handout of working definitions for this and the subtypes of violence that have been adapted from the most reliable scientific sources (see Box 1-1).

The moderator of this session, Sir George Alleyne, M.D., opened the discussion by observing a change in the session title. The title of this chapter was the original title of the session, but the version of the agenda he received titled it "Why the World Should Be More Invested in Violence Prevention." He believed that greater investment is really the thesis for discussion and one of the major themes of this workshop. If the question were asked, he said that the answer would be because of the tremendous returns on such investment. Another rationale of the workshop, he stated, was to reenergize ourselves and energize those who can invest in violence prevention by reawakening our sensitivities and sensibilities, which he stated had been "repeatedly dulled by the pictures and images of violence coming through our living rooms." From his own background in public health, he has come to believe that (1) health can be used as a platform or bridge to reduce some forms of violence, as we would see from the program in Bogotá, Colombia, and (2) tools of public health can be applied to address some aspects of both interpersonal and collective violence. Presentations by Etienne Krug, Irvin Waller, Bernice van Bronkhorst, and James Garbarino explored violence prevention from several different perspectives—health, criminal justice, economic development, and human development.

## HEALTH PERSPECTIVE

Dr. Etienne Krug began by contrasting the 1.6 million annual deaths globally attributed to violence to other public health priorities. Tuberculosis results in roughly the same number of deaths as violence, but more people die from HIV/AIDS, while fewer die from malaria. Of the 1.6 million deaths from violence, half of them are due to suicide, 35 percent to interpersonal violence, and 11 percent to collective violence, which can include organized violence, forms of war, and gang violence. He suggested that we have a counterintuitive or inverse level of attention, especially from the media, paid to collective violence when epidemiology shows us that the greater issue within types of violence is suicide. His professional experiences dealing with the consequences of collective violence, such as amputating the legs of people who have stepped on land mines, treating babies cut by machetes, and treating women who have had their breasts cut from their bodies during war, are horrific reminders of the importance of addressing collective violence, but he pointed out that other hugely important public health aspects of violence receive much less attention.

In terms of the pattern of distribution of violence globally, the disproportionate burden of death due to violence is in low- and middle-income countries (LMICs)—91 percent compared to 9 percent in high-income or developed countries. Violence is among the leading causes of death for those aged 15 to 29 years. Suicide is the fourth leading cause of death, homicide the fifth, and war-related deaths are the sixth (see Table 3-1). This has important, generational effects in LMICs, since these people are usually the breadwinners in families. When they die prematurely, the economic security of entire families often plunges for more than a generation.

Matzopoulos et al. 2007 (see Appendix C) propose that although mortality rates, especially for suicide, interpersonal violence, and war, show a substantial injury burden in LMICs, the data likely underrepresent the actual magnitude of the problem. They state that mortality rates only reflect the number of people who have died from specific causes, but ignore the significant health burden imposed on survivors. They also fail to capture the broad effects of violence on health that may contribute to premature mortality from a range of other deaths. They suggest that more sophisticated methods that include measures such as potential years of life lost and disability-adjusted life-years (DALYs)[1] are more appropriate to better describe the impact of violence.[2] Though deaths from violence are important, there are other health, social, and mental consequences, some of which were mentioned earlier by Stephen Lewis. Depending on the country and studies reported, 10-70 percent of women report being victims of intimate partner violence. Dr. Krug stated that data from other studies indicate that about 10 percent of men and 20 percent of women report having been sexually abused when they were children. While these events did not result in death, there are long-term mental health consequences including depression, anxiety, stress, and insomnia; unwanted pregnancies; exposure

---

[1]Years of potential life lost (YPLL) is a measure of premature mortality and is presented for persons under 75 years of age because the average life expectancy in the United States is over 75 years. YPLL-75 is calculated using eight age groups. The number of deaths for each age group is multiplied by the years of life lost, calculated as the difference between age 75 years and the midpoint of the age group. YPLL is derived by summing years of life lost over all age groups (National Center for Health Statistics; available at http://www.cdc.gov/nchs/datawh/nchsdefs/yearsofpotentiallifelost.htm; accessed on September 6, 2007). Disability-adjusted life-year (DALY) is a health gap measure that extends the concept of potential years of life lost (PYLL) due to premature death to include equivalent years of "healthy" life lost by virtue of being in states of poor health or disability. The DALY combines in one measure the time lived with disability and the time lost due to premature mortality. One DALY can be thought of as one lost year of "healthy" life and the burden of disease as a measurement of the gap between current health status and an ideal situation in which everyone lives into old age free of disease and disability (World Health Organization; available at http://www.who.int/healthinfo/boddaly/en/index.html; accessed on September 6, 2007).

[2]By contrast, Muenning (2002) states that while the DALY is frequently used for studies in developing countries and might serve as an international standard for cost-effectiveness analyses, it does have limitations because of the different cultural perceptions of human suffering and quality of life, which would be exaggerated when generating health-related quality-of-life scores and using them in cross-national comparisons.

**TABLE 3-1** Top 10 Causes of Death, Ages 5-44 Years, Both Sexes, 2002

| Rank | 5-14 Years | 15-29 Years | 30-44 Years |
|------|-----------|-------------|-------------|
| 1 | Childhood cluster 200,139 | HIV/AIDS 855,406 | HIV/AIDS 855,406 |
| 2 | Road traffic injuries 118,212 | Road traffic injuries 354,692 | Tuberculosis 368,501 |
| 3 | Drowning 113,614 | Tuberculosis 238,021 | Road traffic injuries 354,692 |
| 4 | Respiratory infections 112,739 | Self-inflicted injuries *216,661* | Ischemic heart disease 224,986 |
| 5 | Diarrheal diseases 88,430 | Interpersonal violence *188,451* | Self-inflicted injuries *215,263* |
| 6 | Malaria 76,257 | War injuries *95,015* | Interpersonal violence *146,751* |
| 7 | HIV/AIDS 46,022 | Drowning 78,639 | Cerebrovascular disease 145,965 |
| 8 | War injuries *43,671* | Respiratory infections 65,153 | Cirrhosis of the liver 135,072 |
| 9 | Tuberculosis 36,362 | Poisonings 61,865 | Respiratory infections 102,431 |
| 10 | Tropical diseases 31,845 | Fires 61,341 | Liver cancer 84,279 |

NOTE: Bold, italic figures highlight deaths or disability due to violence.
SOURCE: Krug (2007).

to sexually transmitted infections including HIV/AIDS; and engagement in high-risk behaviors such as smoking, alcohol, and substance use that are linked to chronic diseases, cancer, and cardiovascular disease. New research is providing more information about violence and its consequences beyond death and severe injury, including data about economic costs.

As Krug reviewed the causes of violence, an important message was that there is not a single cause and therefore there is a need to move away from a single risk factor approach. In fact, multiple risk factors for both individuals (being male, previous experience with violence, alcohol and substance use, family environment with poor parenting, or marital conflict) and communities (high concentrations of poverty; widespread violence in society; alcohol and substance use, access to weapons; and high rates of social, justice, economic, and gender inequalities) suggest that these risk factors need to be addressed simultaneously. When different types of violence such as abuse against children, the elderly, and women share multiple risk factors, this suggests that interventions to address them may result in an impact on several types of violence. These shared risk factors include parental loss, crime, alcohol and substance use, mental illness, and social isolation.

The *World Report on Violence and Health* began to look at violence prevention at the international level and from a public health perspective. Before this effort, violence had been considered a domestic issue that every country had to deal with in its own way. The report has been widely distributed, with more than 30,000 copies in more than 15 languages. A global campaign was created to help mobilize different agencies in the implementation of the report. A number of political bodies—the World Health Assembly (WHA), several of the WHO regional committees, the African Union, the Council of Europe, the World Medical Association, a number of personalities such as Nelson Mandela, and the ministers of several European countries and South Africa—have all endorsed the report and participated in political events to help place the report on the global agenda.

The primary recommendation of the WHO report called for a focus on primary prevention at all of the levels of an ecological model—working with individuals, families, communities, and societies—to address the root causes of violence versus a criminal justice focus on incarceration. Other recommendations called for countries to develop a national plan of action that emphasized increasing data collection capacity and strengthening research into the costs and causes of prevention; promoting gender and social equality; and strengthening victim care and support services. These and other recommendations serve as a basis for the programs WHO has been implementing for several years. Because a number of countries have adopted the report and developed national action plans, WHO is now developing a series of follow-up documents to assist countries in strengthening victims' services and to assist ministries of health to increase their focus and prevention activities on the different types of violence.

Krug stated that the WHO report also clearly shows that successful responses to violence require a multisectoral effort—health, justice, diplomacy, police, employment, and others. Like Rosenberg, he emphasized that public health does not have sole responsibility for the problem but can bring specific tools and knowledge such as data collection, research, prevention, services, and evaluation of prevention efforts to help shape policy, improve services, and conduct the advocacy that Stephen Lewis mentioned. In summation, he pointed out that Dr. Margaret Chan, the newly appointed Director General of WHO and the acknowledged global leader in public health, stated in her opening speech that violence and injuries must be addressed as part of the global public health agenda.

## CRIMINAL JUSTICE PERSPECTIVE

Dr. Irvin Waller reflected on the data presented by Dr. Krug as an underrepresentation of the magnitude of the problem. While he concurred that attention must be diverted from an obsession with collective violence to interventions and policies that reduce the number of people who are victimized by violence, his approach focused on the criminal justice industry (police, courts, and corrections), particularly in the United States. Here, he noted, the annual $200 billion spent on a reactive, judicial response is incongruous with public opinion, which has expressed twice as much interest in investing in programs for at-risk youth. Despite this public sentiment, he pointed out that the U.S. leadership has a long history of investing in corrections and is responsible for one out of five incarcerations in the world today. This effort apparently does little for the public perception of safety and security, he stated, since two out of three handgun owners in the U.S. claim they own guns to feel safe. While this "law-and-order" approach may have an economic benefit in wealthy countries by creating jobs, Waller believes that this is a "bankrupt solution" when it comes to safety and benefiting victims of violence by reducing the amount of harm done to them. By contrast, he noted that although similar expenditures are not affordable in LMICs for policing that is in complete chaos—complicated by issues such as corruption that affect and reduce the size of the police force due to jobs being terminated—the policing and criminal justice in these countries do need strengthening and upgrading.

For additional benefit to improve services to victims and greater epidemiological understanding of the problem (especially for sexual assault), Waller argued for the inclusion of victimization surveys as part of data collection efforts, such as those being demonstrated in Argentina. Waller proposed that lesser developed countries are better at obtaining justice for victims than more developed countries by focusing on truth and protection for victims rather than resorting to the execution of criminals. Sexual assault, he noted, is seldom reported in any country. In Canada, which is considered to have one of the best police forces in terms of payment and professionalism, only 8 percent of sexual assaults are reported to the police. He challenged the group to imagine the effect that corruption and other issues of poor policing would have on the reporting rate in LMICs. He also noted that even when violence is addressed through a criminal justice perspective, there are innovative initiatives, such as the all-female police stations in a province in Southern India with 16 million people that can help victims report crimes and increase cooperation with law enforcement. This is an example of the adaptation of strategies developed by other LMICs since the idea was conceived in Brazil.

Waller emphasized that organizations in different sectors in the United States, the United Kingdom, South Africa, and the United Nations have endorsed the use of evidence-based approaches to crime and victimization reduction and have issued reports similar to WHO's world report on violence. Building on some of the research findings of the National Academies' National Research Council, the United Nations Office on Drugs and Crime has published similar guidelines to emphasize a science-based approach to focus on prevention and collaboration. He also noted that efforts in the private sector are significantly important, citing the international nonprofit organization Habitat, which is implementing *Safer Cities*—a municipal safety and crime reduction strategy—in Africa and Latin America. Evidence of the effectiveness of the public health approach in LMICs is demonstrated by the work in Bogotá, Colombia, which used mayoral leadership to diagnose the problem, prepare a funded plan, implement the plan, evaluate its implementation and outcomes, and ensure a planning group with authority and responsibility for implementation and evaluation.

Dr. Waller proposed that the real solution for addressing violence is a term he called "second re-prevention"—focusing on addressing risk factors for more immediate, significant reductions in violence, while simultaneously addressing longer-term factors such as elimination of poverty and creating gender equity. His first recommendation called for implementation of youth-oriented programs in school curricula. He reinforced the call for evidence-based interventions and acknowledged that Canada and the United Kingdom have conducted randomized controlled trials of several interventions that were shown to be not only cost-effective, but also successful in reducing violent behavior in most high-risk youth. Some of these interventions focus on negotiation skills for young men in schools so they do not resort to bullying and sexual assault. This success can promote generational violence prevention by teaching young people how to become functional adults in society. His second recommendation called for an emphasis on prevention of violence against women and children, which he stated can result in reduction of a huge proportion of violence globally; it will have a generational impact on the problem by reducing violence against children, and women will become more effective contributors to their children's well-being and increasingly productive contributors to society at large. He identified empowering local partnerships with mothers, community agencies, and others as another necessary component of effective violence prevention. Strengthening the capacity of these partnerships to analyze the evidence on crime problems and focus on outcomes and results can make a difference in the levels of violence in communities.

Waller closed by underscoring the need not only for public health leadership in multisectoral collaborations, but also for presidential or prime ministerial leadership, such as that seen in South Africa with the Mandela administration. He stated that it is essential to institutionalize political leadership to focus on prevention and ensure the availability of adequate funds and the existence of legislation that will drive the success of the collaborations. In South Africa, the leadership balanced effective criminal justice with social and public health interventions. He warned this is particularly important because of the vulnerability of public health initiatives to address violence when leadership only criminalizes violence—enabling the police to expand their resources and power.

## ECONOMIC DEVELOPMENT PERSPECTIVE

Ms. Bernice van Bronkhorst focused her presentation on the economic costs of violence in the Caribbean as noted in a joint report of the World Bank and the United Nations Office on Drugs and Crime (UNODC-WB, 2007). She started with an overview of the region, which she identified as the most violent subregion in the world—with average homicide rates of 30 per 100,000 people and higher rates in Jamaica and Haiti (see Figure 3-1).

Crime statistics, she stated, are extremely difficult to compare internationally, but the most reliable gauge of violence in a society is its murder rate because lesser forms of violence may never come to the attention of the police. She cautioned, however, that even the murder figures can be deceptive because in countries with small populations, a small number of murders can result in very high rates. Also, murder rates are based on the number of residents, but many Caribbean countries swell to several times their normal size during the high season due to the influx of tourists. Any of these tourists could be a victim or perpetrator of murder, so the rates may appear artificially high. Finally, definitions of what constitutes murder

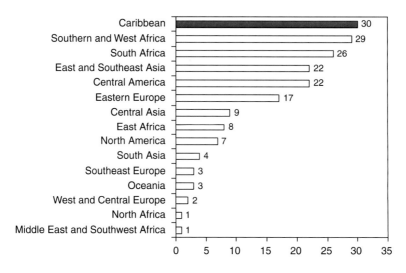

**FIGURE 3-1** Homicide rates per 100,000 people by world region, 2002.
SOURCE: Bronkhorst (2007) and UNODC-WB (2007).

vary surprisingly from country to country. Many of the countries that we might suspect to have high murder rates simply do not report them. Even with these caveats, on the basis of this figure, she asserted, it is clear that the Caribbean has a serious problem with violence. Give the prevalence of interpersonal violence around the world, including the homicide rates in Latin America—which have been steadily rising in the late 1990s and early 2000s, she reinforced earlier comments about not losing sight of the importance of interpersonal violence and not focusing extensively on collective violence. In identifying challenges for understanding what is happening in the region, Bronkhorst also underscored the issue of poor data collection and quality (particularly for sexual assault, rape, and property crimes) and reemphasized Waller's advocacy of the use of victimization surveys.

Kidnapping has emerged, particularly in Haiti, as a contributor to violence in the region. Its geographical location and the region's topography, with long shorelines that are difficult to police, also make illicit drugs and trafficking a major driver of violence and crime since the region is between drug-producing and drug-consuming countries. Drug trafficking has not only increased the quantity but also changed the type of drug used (from marijuana to cocaine). Drug trafficking promotes violence in a range of ways: drug markets are regulated by violence, which is used to collect debts, settle contract disputes, and defend or acquire turf. Drugs bring firearms into a country, resulting in their increased use for a variety of crimes and the increased lethality of injuries caused, which reinforces the need for reductions in lethality of and in access to means for violence. Perhaps more insidious, she stated, is the effect drugs have on corruption. The value of the drug flows through the Caribbean exceeds the values of the economies of many of its countries. This economic weight gives traffickers a tremendous amount of leverage in promoting corruption and undermining entire economies.

In discussing violence and its impact on economic development, she explained that the issue is often evaluated in terms of direct costs (e.g., health care, judicial costs) and indirect or nonmonetary, intangible costs (e.g., morbidity, mortality, stigma, reductions in social capital, pain). Cascading social and economic consequences of violence can include reductions in social capital and heightened fears of violence. Together, they can have a significant effect when they prevent people from either participating in social activities or engaging in activities that might facilitate a change in an individual's socioeconomic status, such as attending night classes or working a night shift that may pay a higher wage. For intimate partner violence, studies in Haiti, Peru, and Central America found that women generally earn less than non-victims, have lower productivity, have less access to neonatal services, and are more likely to be anemic.

In terms of costing methodologies for crime and violence, she reiterated the use of DALYs and identified new research focusing on estimating total costs of society's willingness to pay regardless of the methodologies used. The accounting approach—where all of the total costs in different sectors are added—is the most popular in Latin America. She mentioned that, using this approach, researchers found the cost of violence in Jamaica to be 3.7 percent of the gross domestic product (GDP),[3] including business, health, and criminal justice costs, but not private security costs. The World Bank has conducted investment climate surveys showing that the business climate is constrained by crime and violence—with issues such as cost for private security including protection of personnel and property. In Jamaica, 39 percent of businessmen indicated that violence had prevented them from expanding their businesses. She emphasized that a foreign business will examine all of these costs when considering where to locate or expand its operations and, if the costs are too high, will not consider that geographical area, so violence can seriously prevent or constrain foreign direct investments.

The World Bank has been attempting to estimate the effects on economic growth or "growth dividends" by using cross-country panel data in the Caribbean. This method attempts to distinguish between short-run economic costs (e.g., the cost imposed on an economy in a particular year by crime and violence) and long-term costs to the economy (e.g., tourism), particularly in terms of growth. In this region, she stated, the cost of tourism is a major concern and various studies have indicated that if crime and violence increase, tourism suffers. "Enclave tourism," where people stay in one resort area, increases because people are too afraid to go to other areas of the region. In their studies, econometric modeling predicted that if the current murder rate in the Caribbean were reduced by one-third, the growth rate of the region could more than double. She postulated that this example of tremendous growth through a reduction in violence represents excellent data that can be used to persuade the region's policy makers to make greater investments in violence prevention. She presented concrete examples—if the homicide rates of Jamaica and the Dominican Republic could be reduced to the levels in Costa Rica (which she reported as one of the safest, least violent countries in the region), there would be an annual increase in per capita growth of 5.4 percent. Furthermore, in Guyana, similar findings in reduction of the homicide rates predicted a growth of 1.8 percent per year. Over 20 years, this would equal a 43 percent increase in Guyana's gross domestic product. These examples demonstrate that crime and violence are economic development issues and that prevention

---

[3]The GDP is the primary indicator used to gauge the health of a country's economy. It represents the total dollar value of all goods and services produced over a specific period. It is often thought of as the size of the economy. Usually, GDP is expressed as a comparison to the previous quarter or year. For example, if the year-to-year GDP was up 3 percent, it means that the economy has grown by 3 percent over the last year (http://www.investopedia.com/ask/answers/199.asp).

is worthy of investment; yet many of the resources spent in Latin America and the United States go to the judicial system. Since we have little in the way of cost-effectiveness evidence to support prevention intervention, she advocated making systematic cost-effectiveness studies a priority. She did report that the World Bank has conducted limited cost-effectiveness studies in Brazil, where it matched a number of Brazilian crime prevention programs with similar programs that have been evaluated in North America and Europe. The preliminary findings showed that in terms of the numbers of crimes averted per *real* (monetary unit in Brazil) spent, secondary prevention was by far the most cost-effective approach. In pragmatic terms and in alignment with the research findings of Irvin Waller, if one were going to spend $5 to decrease crime and violence, it should be invested in secondary prevention.

Matzopoulos et al. (see Appendix C) note that the lack of a costing culture within many public health systems in LMICs makes the generation of reliable violence costs difficult. In such countries, rudimentary surveillance and reporting systems are still under development so costing is not viewed as a reporting priority at this time. Further empirical research is needed that takes into account the differences in treatment costs across income contexts. Moreover the calculation of the costs of other health burdens, such as HIV, has mobilized civil society to lobby for prevention. An accurate estimation of the costs of violence in LMICs is therefore imperative to the violence prevention agenda. With respect to intimate partner violence, they cite lost earnings and opportunity costs extrapolated to U.S. $1.73 billion in Chile and U.S. $32.7 million in Nicaragua from pilot study results in both countries. Intimate partner violence alone has been calculated to cost the economies of Nicaragua and Chile 1.6 and 2 percent of their GDPs, respectively. The effects of suicide on GDP appear even more difficult to measure, and figures are scarce in the literature. A study conducted in Alberta, Canada, showed that suicide significantly detracts from future GDP. The study calculated that suicide costs the equivalent of 0.3 percent of the provincial GDP.

However limited, violence costing in research has begun to clearly demonstrate the substantial economic impacts of violence in LMICs. Greater general investment in improving on and prioritizing this area of research is imperative for generating a more accurate and comprehensive profile of the costs of violence in these contexts. More specifically, such studies should disaggregate the costs of violence according to the more specific typologies of violence listed above. This would enable the identification of relative contributions of these different types to overall costs (see Appendix C, Matzopoulos et al., 2007).

## HUMAN DEVELOPMENT PERSPECTIVE

Dr. Garbarino began his presentation by explaining the ecological approach that is used in the field of human development, which concludes that there is rarely a simple cause-and-effect relationship that can be applied to everyone everywhere, but rather that development occurs contextually, which negates the universality or permanence of facts about human development. From this perspective, in terms of violence, few causal factors can be applied across the board to everyone and this creates a contextual conundrum for researchers.

Of importance and promise to those working in violence prevention, he cited research from New Zealand that explains the biological vulnerability of children to violent behavior involving the monoamine oxidase (MAO) gene that affects arousal. Garbarino explained that, in simplest terms, the gene is either turned on or turned off. Among children who are abused and had the gene turned off, nearly 85 percent developed chronic patterns of aggression with acting-out behavior and violating the rights of others—consistent with a diagnosis of conduct disorder in Version IV of the *Diagnostics and Statistical Manual.* Compared to abused children with the gene turned on, only 42 percent developed the same pattern of aggression and antisocial violence, demonstrating that biological vulnerability doubles the likelihood of abused children developing chronic patterns of aggression. Thus a compelling case can be made for preventing child abuse to counteract children's genetic vulnerability to violence. Gender, he stated, appears to play an important role with this gene since it is located on the X chromosome. Other data he presented suggest that community factors can influence whether antisocial behavior can blossom into chronic violent delinquency. Technology, he noted, is also a part of the changing context, with the evolution of current medical interventions (e.g., trauma care) to reduce the lethality of violence, as well as a decrease in access to firearms with changing laws and social norms. By the same token, the evolution of firearm technology has increased the lethality of injury when people do have access.

Garbarino identified the philosophical question at the root of the issue that has long been debated: Are we inherently violent or pacific? If one hypothesized the former, how do we learn to be nonviolent? In his discussion, he pointed to socialization as it is used to set parameters for socially acceptable aggression (e.g., horseplay between fathers and sons as a possible explanation of why fatherless boys have a disproportionate problem with violence). He also described promising research that focused on the processes that control whether innate dispositions to aggression become a coherent problem of antisocial violence and what processes can reduce this. The researchers proposed cognitive structuring (the ideas that are received about aggression) and behavior rehearsal (experience in settings where aggression is manifested or demonstrated and thus subject to the psychological processes of reinforcement, punishment, and conditioning) as the key processes for prevention. He identified cognitive structuring case studies examining the role of television violence in instigating aggressive behavior as one of the most studied areas on the influences on violence. Some recent data, he reported, indicated that the effect of TV violence on eliciting aggressive behavior is about as strong as the effect of smoking on lung cancer. Additional, older studies found that television violence elicited aggressive behavior in boys as early as the 1960s, but the same effect was not reported for girls until the 1980s. Dr. Garbarino asserted that the gender equity in this phenomenon is clearly attributable to changes in cognitive structuring. He has found cognitive structuring to be particularly important because his international research around violence and families suggests that nearly every act of violence that is committed is done so with a sense of justification; he cited the research of one of his colleagues that has examined how the dynamics of shame can lead to the validation and justification of what, to an outsider, looks like "crazy, unimaginably bizarre violence."

He noted that in behavioral rehearsal, social change can affect aggression. The issue of reducing the gender gap to increase gender equality (e.g., the increase in the number of girls playing sports) may have unintended negative consequences by environmentally exposing girls to increased violence, with validation and reinforcement of physical aggression. He explained that meta-analyses of the role of gender in explaining normal physical aggression show a progression in the United States over the last 30 years of decreasing relevance of gender. In the United States, where gender equality starts to become something approximating a reality, other factors are much more important than gender in producing and predicting normal aggressive behavior.

Dr. Garbarino closed with some thoughts on collective violence and the potentially beneficial role that peace and reconciliation efforts and the affirmative respect of human rights may have on the mental health of children exposed to and traumatized by violence. He and his colleagues conducted research on Palestinian children, and their findings supported the notion that the context in which the trauma occurred has a lot to do with the prognosis for child development. The results of the children's test responses fell into three categories: passive victimization, violent revenge, and a sort of prosocial revenge. Each of these groupings also has very different mental health scores, with passive victimization being the worst and the prosocial revenge group showing the clearest absence of debilitating mental health problems.

## QUESTIONS AND ANSWERS

Many questions were raised for the panelists, but one of note was whether there is enough evidence or scientific knowledge to move violence prevention forward. While all of the presentations focused on prevention as the necessary approach, they also acknowledged gaps in data and knowledge as they relate to cost and programmatic effectiveness, multiple risk factors or determinants of violence, the context of violence, and the environments in which interventions would be implemented. The panelists acknowledged that there are many examples of best practices and lessons learned that have already been scaled up to national levels in LMICs, as well as knowing what interventions they felt should be avoided (i.e., those that involve increased detention and incarceration, which only increase the economic costs of violence). They identified other foci including efforts to facilitate national planning, implementation, and evaluation that would call for and allow country governments to increase their investments in violence prevention. The countries would also need technical assistance from U.S. agencies such as the Centers for Disease Control and Prevention, the National Institutes of Health, the U.S. Agency for International Development, and the Department of Justice, as well as other agencies and organizations from the philanthropic and corporate sectors, to support funding for these prevention efforts. It was also pointed out that the United States has invested billions of dollars to globally support HIV/AIDS prevention, treatment, and care on a much leaner evidence base than what is currently known for violence prevention. There was also lengthy discussion about the positive and negative effects and use of television programming either to incite aggressive behavior or to educate and provide population-level messages about violence prevention.

# 4

# The Intersection of Violence and Health

The definition of violence encompasses a wide range of actions and possible deleterious health and developmental outcomes. The most common and direct ways of measuring its impact directly are in terms of the numbers and rates of deaths and injuries it causes. Although they are less easy to measure, violence also has important impacts on a range of mental and physical health problems. The paucity of accurate and detailed data, however, makes it difficult to fully measure all of these impacts in low- and middle-income countries (LMICs). Furthermore, because many of the impacts of violence present within the health sector as major risk factors for and causes of a range of other health conditions and outcomes, it could be said that violence foments a vicious cycle. For example, the adverse impacts of violence on quality of life may lead to the deterioration of mental health and well-being, which may in turn impose a direct (and measurable) burden on the health system, while at the same time driving rates of violence even higher within afflicted communities (see Appendix C, Matzopoulos et al., 2007).

This session explored how violence can worsen many health conditions and examined the impacts of violence beyond the apparent and immediate physical injuries, as well as the role of violence as a consequence of other forms of violence. Jacquelyn Campbell moderated this session and also closed with a presentation on the intersection of violence and women's health with a focus on HIV/AIDS. Presentations about collective violence and its impact on disease burden, self-directed violence and the crosscutting issues it shares with other types of violence, and the scale and consequences of child abuse and maltreatment for chronic diseases in adulthood were made by Richard Garfield, Eric Caine, and James Mercy, respectively.

## COLLECTIVE VIOLENCE

Collective violence, especially in the form of armed conflict, accounts for more death and disability than many major diseases worldwide. Collective violence destroys families, communities, and sometimes entire cultures. It directs scarce resources away from promotion and protection of health, medical care, and other health and social services. It destroys that health-supporting infrastructure of society. It limits human rights and contributes to social injustice. It leads individuals and nations to believe that violence is the only way to resolve conflicts. It contributes to destruction of the physical environment and the overuse of nonrenewable resources. In sum, collective violence threatens much of the fabric of our civilization (see Appendix C, Sidel and Levy, 2007). Self-directed violence, interpersonal violence, and collective violence in some ways overlap. Those involved in collective violence may engage in self-directed violence as a symptom of posttraumatic stress syndrome or as a result of self-hatred because of acts committed in war. Collective violence may also be associated with interpersonal violence. For example, individuals and groups engaged in collective violence may commit interpersonal violence, sometimes fueled by ethnic tensions or by conflict with superior officers or with fellow service members in the midst of war. Soldiers may return from war with a battlefield mind-set in which they commit violence to address interpersonal conflicts that could have been addressed in nonviolent ways. Children raised in the midst of war may come to believe that violence is an appropriate way to settle interpersonal conflicts (see Appendix C, Sidel and Levy, 2007).

Richard Garfield opened his presentation by providing a common operational definition of conflict, which was that at least 1,000 deaths would occur in a period of conflict, which is usually a multiyear period. The good news, he noted, is that the trend has been a long-term decline in global conflict as he defined it since the end of World War II, a short-term increase at the end of the Cold War, followed by a continued decline. Since fewer people are engaged in conflict, the resultant deaths are the lowest at any time during the last 150 years. For the first time, the prevalence of organized political violence between states or in a military fashion within states is so low that it is has become almost an exception to the political engagement between groups—a message that seldom gets out to the media or to those who work in violence prevention. These data may be indicative of two of the strategic primary prevention foci outlined by Mercy (see Appendix C, Mercy et al., 2007)—the importance of changing social norms to promote nonviolence for conflict resolution and possibly reducing the social distance between conflicting groups. The exception, Garfield noted, is Africa where most conflicts are concentrated, are often within borders, and do not come to international attention. Even here, research findings indicate that although the number of deaths as outlined by the definition is high, the proportion of the entire population in these areas is small.

Far more important is what Garfield termed the "carry-on effects" of conflict—where for every death there are likely to be 10 people injured and 100 people displaced. While there is variability in this unofficial measure, it is seen as a "rule of thumb" that the data report in terms of consistency. The context of the changing circumstances due to the disruption of people's lives during conflict affects these data since people choose one of two common coping responses to conflict. The first, he stated, is to "hunker down" and stay in the area. The other is to leave the area, which he noted is a more sincere measure internationally to understand how people are doing in areas where there is conflict. The problem he identified with these data is that once someone is registered as a displaced person or refugee, the person might have that status for 40-60 years even though his or her life circumstances may improve and the true life status may not be consistent with what is implied by those terms. As noted in discussions of earlier presentations, new forms of violence or nonpeaceful activities may occur when people return to their countries and communities, even after political peace has been attained or restored. In his opinion, changes in the life status and life chances of people are what need to be studied and measured to better understand the issues and develop appropriate interventions for aid. From his work in post-conflict Sudan, he found that in the 2.5 years of peace that followed three decades of conflict, some types of violence have increased slightly, while others have decreased. Much of the violence now happens between neighbors versus organized, armed groups; with one in five households reporting a death since peace occurred. Despite this, the Sudanese perceive their situation as much improved—neighbors now have reduced access to weapons (another strategic primary prevention focus posited by Mercy [see Appendix C, Mercy et al., 2007]) and worry less about starvation since they can now work their fields.

He observed that new measurements are emerging in the field, and his own research is examining multiple threats to well-being because violence is often associated with disasters, either preceding or following them, and geographically tends to occur in similar places and at similar times. When using these new measures, he argued, we obtain a different picture of areas of major instability in the world than when we examine death and displacement among conflicts. He stated that advocates are also moving away from the traditional use and measure of conflict deaths and are instead examining the proportion of the population whose life circumstances are radically changed for the worse in a given period. As a result, the most important lesson learned to date is that there are usually multiple ways in which a life is altered, not merely one event.

## Effects of Collective Violence on Health

Conflict has significant effects on morbidity and mortality beyond the direct deaths that occur. Along with the direct impacts of war and other military activities on health, collective violence may also cause serious health consequences through its impact on the physical, economic, social, and biological environments in which people live. The environmental damage may affect people not only in nations directly engaged in collective violence but in all nations. Much of the morbidity and mortality during war, especially among civilians, has been the result of devastation of societal infrastructure, including destruction of food and water supply systems, healthcare facilities and public health services, sewage disposal systems, power plants and electrical grids, and transportation and communication systems. Destruction of infrastructure has led to food shortages and resultant malnutrition, contamination of food and drinking water and resultant foodborne and waterborne illness, and deficiencies in health care and public health and resultant disease (see Appendix C, Sidel and Levy, 2007).

On a global scale, the areas with conflict tend to have the highest mortality rates among children. In Garfield's opinion, the two statistically strong predictors of conflict are high rates of infant mortality that do not decline and economic stagnation. Of the ten countries with the highest under-5 child mortality rates, seven have experienced recent civil conflict. In terms of economic impact, his research indicates that in low-income and middle-income countries, there are different epidemiologic conditions and solutions for the patterns of injury that are occurring, which he attributed to the continued decrease in economic growth in low-income countries as well as many forms of social decline. According to Sidel and Levy (see Appendix C), World Bank data demonstrate a striking relationship between the wealth of a nation and its chances of having a civil war. For example, a country with a gross domestic product (GDP) income per capita of U.S. $250 has a 15 percent probability of war in the next five years, and this probability drops by approximately half for a country with a GDP of $600 per person. In contrast, countries with a per capita income of more than U.S. $5,000 have less than a 1 percent chance of having a civil conflict, all else being equal. In addition to poverty, risk factors for armed conflict may be associated with poor health and poor access to quality medical care, low status of women, large gaps between the rich and the poor, weak development of a civil society within a country, people's not having the right to vote or otherwise participate in decisions that affect their lives, limited education and employment opportunities, increased access to small arms and light weapons, and failure to meet the basic needs of civilians. While other researchers might point to health conditions such as tuberculosis and infant mortality as causal factors for conflict, Garfield sees a strong and important association with poorer quality of life, which may lead to or play a role in the emergence of instability and affect the life chances or circumstances of people in the area.

Garfield has identified gaps in research and data collection that need to be addressed, including measuring the deaths that occur in relationship to conflict—not just the numbers, but also the dynamics, which are poorly understood. This is the area in which he stated there can be a reduction in mortality using a public health approach, but it is the area in which we know the least. His studies in Guatemala show that when there are excess deaths in an area, the reporting becomes worse and essentially stops. Counting numbers is not the only issue of concern; the lack of healthcare workers leads to an inability to respond to the health needs of the injured and also contributes to excess mortality, especially in Africa. These worker shortages can be due to either the explosion in mortality of local healthcare workers who work for international organizations or the reduced presence of international organizations.

As for development and humanitarian assistance, the amount of aid is increasing around the world. Yet in Garfield's estimation, only 50 percent of the Millennium Development Goals have been achieved (see Appendix C, Matzopoulos et al., 2007, for their perspective on the impact of violence in relation to the Millennium Development Goals). Garfield stated that while $10 billion of international aid per year goes for humanitarian assistance, "we are not getting much bang for this buck" because it really costs nearly three times this amount to conduct health programs in areas that are insecure. In his estimate, the more that the insecurity associated with armed conflict can be reduced, the easier it will be to address other forms of insecurity (e.g., nutritional, economic) and prevent neighboring countries from becoming less stable.

## SELF-DIRECTED VIOLENCE

Eric Caine began by detailing the central importance of a public health approach to multidisciplinary and multiorganizational suicide (self-directed violence) prevention efforts so they become more proactive and less reactive, as well as better target the high-risk people that they are missing. Many of the data he discussed were from the United States because more data are available there, but he noted that what is true in the United States is amplified greatly around the rest of the world. The interrelationship of suicide and other adverse outcomes is based on risk factors for a variety of adverse outcomes such as intimate partner violence including homicide and accidental death. The morbidity, he stated, is the suicide attempt, whereas the mortality is the suicide itself. Cultural forces, age, gender, and ethnic differences are important risk factors for understanding the epidemiology of suicide; we have little understanding of the protective cultural factors that are used to negate risk factors.

Based on data from the World Health Organisation (WHO), some places around the world have more suicides and others less, and some places do not report these statistics—which he stated may be due to lack of reporting capacity or to the strong cultural prohibition and stigmatization of the act. What is clear from these data is that suicide is underreported throughout the world—and the reported statistics of more than 50 percent of violent deaths resulting from suicide, or about 800,000 deaths annually, indicate that suicide is a major problem. In terms of years of life lost, suicide exceeds homicide and HIV/AIDS in the United States. While rates of suicide rise with age in the United States, especially for white males, the suicides accounting for the majority of years of life lost occur between the ages of 20 and 55 years—a productive workforce-related age group. These people are typically parents, have families, are employed, and are relationship filled—not "the psychiatric patient."

### Risk Factors for Suicide

Many of the data about risk factors come from psychological autopsy data and are generally not helpful in setting up prevention programs, and there are cross-national variations as well. In children and young adults, these factors include but are not limited to major psychopathology, personal or family turmoil, exposure to violence, legal problems, poor school performance, and prior suicide attempts or a family history of suicide. Factors in adulthood include comorbid depression and alcohol use or dependence; interpersonal disruptions and social isolation; poor work performance and unemployment; violence and legal problems; variable impact of marital and parental status; and prior attempts and family history of suicide. In elders, they include late-onset, comorbid depression and general medical conditions, often associated with pain and role function decline; social dependence or isolation; widowhood; inflexible personality; alcohol and prescription substance abuse; and frequent contact with primary care providers.

While their identification is important to understanding suicide, Caine suggested that what is needed is identification of risk factors as they unfold over the course of life that will enable clinicians to effectively address them in a variety of settings that relate to personal ecology and social status. He states that there is also a critical need for a developmental context, especially for people who are high risk and for whom some broad public health approaches may provide less leverage. He noted the importance of this because of the influences of socially driven policies that do not actually target the populations most in need. In the United States, most of the resources for prevention are spent on high school students. Ironically, the suicide rates in this country begin to accelerate between 18 and 22 years, where there are young people who are school dropouts, incarcerated, or subject to other circumstances that might exacerbate the risk factors. There is also a lot of attention on university students, but most suicides do not occur in this setting.

## Suicide Is Preventable

Caine's research with the U.S. Air Force showed that not only is suicide preventable, with a dose-response effect even across major commands (the intervention reduced suicide by one-third), but its prevention can also significantly reduce other forms of violence, with a 50 percent reduction in homicide rates, as well as substantial reductions in accidental deaths and moderate to severe family violence. What became very clear from the findings was that prevention is achievable, but that it is a violence prevention intervention, not just suicide prevention. He also acknowledged that addressing the symptoms of psychopathology is necessary to facilitate further efforts to address other important risk factors, but it alone is not sufficient to prevent suicide in the longer term.

As an example, he briefly explored a layered, developmental context for suicide prevention for men aged 25-54 years in which the people in this range often, but not always, have 10 to 20 years' worth of what he termed ascending alcohol abuse, ascending family turmoil, partner violence, and eventual unemployment. By and large, the typical scenario in a man's life is a dramatic life event three to six weeks before he kills himself. The turmoil-filled life situations that exacerbate psychiatric distress must be addressed for successful suicide prevention. He also noted that women in the United States attempt suicide more, but succeed less. They are less lethal in their attempts, but their attempt level far exceeds that of men. Certainly women who drink or use drugs move into another category and their statistics look much worse than their female peers and, at times, worse than their male peers. As a cascade effect of suicide among men, however, women may often become victims of homicide before the men commit suicide.

In his research in China over the past nine years, Caine has observed that the suicide rates are decreasing. Even though these rates are estimates, China still has the highest number of suicides in the world because it has the largest population. One of the cross-national differences he alluded to earlier is that young women in rural China exceed young men in actual suicides. The rates of attempt by women or men, he noted, may not necessarily be higher than in the United States—they may in fact be lower—but the methods are more lethal, such as ingestion of pesticides (58 percent). Similar to the United States, he and his colleagues noted the context of life turmoil or regular, chronic stressors that may have lasted 1-12 months prior to the time of death, even though 63 percent had a mental illness at the time of death. Nevertheless, people in rural China describe less overall stress, likely due to economic assistance from the millions of migrant workers who are sending money home.

Other examples he presented underscored the linkages between alcohol use or dependence, economic stressors, and other indicators of social turmoil, including high rates of HIV/AIDS and intimate partner violence, as drivers of suicide in Russia after the dissolution of the Soviet Union. This is another example of how these issues are linked, with common problems and risk factors at the base, but result in different adverse outcomes. Data also indicated an increase in male suicides in Hong Kong after its economic slump in the late 1990s with high rates of unemployment. Current research shows that suicide rates in Hong Kong are decreasing as the economy improves. These linkages among risk factors and outcomes are the current topic of discussion with colleagues in China to adapt interventions that may have been successful in other countries.

## CHILD MALTREATMENT AND ITS HEALTH CONSEQUENCES

James Mercy opened his presentation with his bottom line—we pay a huge price for our failure to prevent child maltreatment and we are blind to that price. By inference, the data show that the inability to address child maltreatment is a barrier to the social and economic progress of developing countries. The data on the magnitude of child maltreatment in developing countries are not robust, but we do have information that is useful in understanding the magnitude of the problem since important scientific findings that document and validate the mechanisms that lead from exposure to child maltreatment and important health outcomes have emerged in the past 30 years (see Figure 4-1).

So that we would all be talking and thinking about the same thing, he provided the following operational definition:

> Any act, or series of acts, of commission or omission by a parent or other caregiver that results in harm, the potential for harm, or threat of harm to a child's health, survival, development, or dignity. This definition encompasses physical abuse, sexual abuse, neglect or negligent treatment, abandonment, emotional or psychological abuse, and commercial or other forms of exploitation, like sexual trafficking of children.

### Magnitude of the Problem

Homicide data from around the world shows that homicides among 0-4 year olds are primarily committed by parents and caretakers and are,

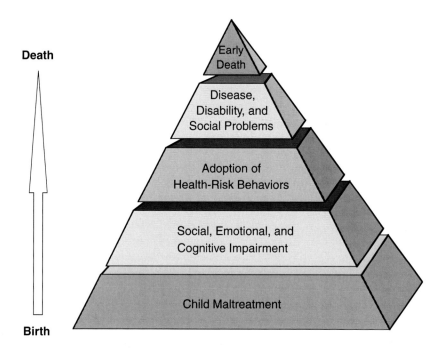

**FIGURE 4-1** The influence of child maltreatment throughout life.
SOURCE: Mercy (2007).

therefore, a good proxy for child maltreatment homicides. These homicide rates are highest in Africa and also, interestingly in North America, and represent only a small proportion of the problem. Mercy cautioned that these data were problematic because it is very difficult to get reliable estimates of child homicides, which often get buried in other causes of death, such as unintentional injury or sudden infant death syndrome in the United States. In regard to data on nonfatal child maltreatment, even though the available research uses different definitions and methodologies, a consistent picture of the seriousness of child maltreatment across nations of the world emerges. In Egypt, 37 percent of children report being beaten or tied up by parents. In Romania, nearly half the parents admit to regularly beating their children. In Ethiopia, 21 percent of urban and 65 percent of rural schoolchildren report bruises and swellings as a result of parental beatings. In Iran, in the Kurdistan province, almost 39 percent of adolescents report mild to severe injury from physical violence at home. These studies all examine physical abuse, which is highly associated with the issue of corporal punishment by parents and caretakers.

The WorldSafe study provides more reliable and comparable measures of non-fatal child maltreatment from several countries. In this study, mothers were interviewed and asked about their use of harsh physical punishments during the past 6 months. In Egypt, rural India, and the Philippines, relatively higher proportions of children were punished by being hit with an object (not on the buttocks) and by being kicked. He acknowledged this as another source that demonstrates that in many developing countries, harsh physical punishment is a day-to-day reality.

He presented data from a meta-analysis conducted by the World Health Organisation (WHO) in 2004 to estimate the fractional burden that child sexual abuse contributes to mental health problems. WHO used available studies from different regions of the world to derive estimates of the proportion of children who experience sexual abuse. He pointed out that while we must remember that the studies underlying these estimates have significant methodological weaknesses, they nevertheless show that there is a substantial prevalence of child sexual abuse across the world. Among the poorest countries of the world, the prevalence among female children varied from a low of 13 percent in Latin American/Caribbean countries to a high of 68 percent in Southeast Asian countries. With the exception of those countries in the Latin American and Caribbean region, the prevalence was consistently higher for females the males.

In addition, data from this study yielded global fractional estimates of the burden of mental disorders and suicidal behavior attributable to child sexual abuse, disaggregated by sex (see Table 4-1).

**TABLE 4-1** Fractional Estimates of Mental Disorders and Suicidal Behavior Attributable to Child Sexual Abuse, by Sex

| Behavior | Female (%) | Male (%) |
|---|---|---|
| Depression | 7-8 | 4-5 |
| Alcohol use or dependence | 7-8 | 4-5 |
| Drug use or dependence | 7-8 | 4-5 |
| Panic disorder | 13 | 7 |
| PTSD | 33 | 21 |
| Suicide attempts | 11 | 6 |

NOTE: PTSD = posttraumatic stress disorder.
SOURCE: Mercy (2007).

The study also found that based on WHO data, these estimates were greater in the poorest countries in Africa and Southeast Asia because the prevalence of child sexual abuse was also greater.

**What Science Tells Us**

The science that has emerged in the past 30 years—from neuroscience, developmental psychology, social sciences, and epidemiology—is showing a pattern that child maltreatment contributes to social, emotional, and cognitive impairments, and the adoption of health risk behaviors, which in turn lead to disease, disability, social problems, and then premature mortality (see Figure 4-1). Mercy stated that support for these findings comes from a variety of sources, many of which are documented in the NRC-IOM report *From Neurons to Neighborhoods* (NRC-IOM, 2000). Another source he mentioned was the body of research and publications from the MacArthur Research Network on early experience in brain development. There are over 50 publications on this topic from the MacArthur Research Network that are available on their website at http://www.macbrain.org/publications. htm. Translational efforts from research to policy and practice are now under way by the National Scientific Council on the Developing Child. He also pointed out a strong scientific basis that combines animal research with human research to support the kind of progression he explained in terms of the impact of child maltreatment.

One of the mechanisms being identified as contributing to this link is the damage to the brain architecture in the form of toxic stress. One critical form of toxic stress, clearly, in childhood, is exposure to child maltreatment in its various forms—which often happens repeatedly and can be severe. One example of how the brain is damaged is an altered stress-response system. He proposed an analogy between the stress-response system and a thermometer in the heating system in a house, which has a set point. If the temperature within the house goes below that set point, the heat comes on. Similarly in our brains, there are set points for the stress-response system. We inevitably deal with stress daily and our bodies have neurochemical and other responses that are activated when we experience severe stress. In many children exposed to maltreatment, however, that thermometer is damaged—such that the set point is altered. For example, it can be lowered so that the stress-response system repeatedly or constantly kicks in—as if the thermometer in the house were set at a lower point. If the heater were to kick in more frequently, it would probably burn out earlier. In the human body, this burnout could lead to premature aging.

He acknowledged that there are literally hundreds of research studies linking child maltreatment to many different types of health outcomes, specifically identifying health risk behaviors that are documented to be associated with child maltreatment—from alcohol and substance abuse to smoking, behavioral problems, and mental and social problems, including depression and anxiety. He noted that maltreatment also has an impact on cognitive development. Thus it can have a long-term impact on the development of human capital in societies with high rates of child maltreatment. These, in turn, are related to disease and injury outcomes. Going back to the analogy of the lower set point on a thermometer, he provided an example of a child who might cope with the stress by self-medicating by smoking cigarettes. Smoking, in turn, leads to cancer, heart disease, or other problems seen in our clinics and hospitals. This is the inferential mechanism and causal link that may occur in terms of child maltreatment and its relationship to health.

There are also strong epidemiological data that link child maltreatment and health—the U.S. study called the Adverse Childhood Exposure (ACE) study. Mercy provided an overview of the collaborative study between the U.S. Centers for Disease Control and Prevention (CDC) and the Kaiser Permanente Health Maintenance Organization (HMO) in California. They interviewed a sample of the participants in this HMO and asked them about their childhood exposures to maltreatment and other adverse exposures. They were also asked about their health status, their health experiences, and the health problems they have experienced in their lives.

In terms of the prevalence of the different types of adverse exposures, 28 percent reported being exposed to physical abuse as a child, along with reports of exposure to other adverse outcomes such as mental illness, parental incarceration, emotional and sexual abuse, intimate partner violence in the home, household substance abuse, and parental separation or divorce. The other point here, he noted, is that many of these adverse exposures often co-occur, so it is not always easy to look at them separately. Based on the previous review of data from developing countries, we can imagine other types of adverse exposures of children beyond just child maltreatment.

In the ACE study, researchers added those adverse exposures and each person received a score from 0 to 4+, based on the number of individual adverse exposures experienced as a child. Then they related the scores to various types of health outcomes. For example, the more adverse exposures they had experienced, the more likely were they to engage in early smoking initiation. The same trend was observed with chronic obstructive pulmonary disease, which was not as consistent, but still indicated a greater likelihood of having that disease based on the more of these adverse childhood exposures they had experienced. Examination of teen sexual behaviors (intercourse by age 15, teen pregnancy in females, teen paternity in males) revealed the same pattern of greater likelihood of engaging in these behaviors correlated with more adverse exposures. For HIV risk exposure—ever injected drugs, had 50 or more intercourse partners, or ever had a sexually transmitted disease—*the same pattern holds.* He also pointed out that these patterns held up when controlling for demographic factors and socioeconomic status.

In conclusion, Mercy stated that by all available measures—not just the studies he had described—other studies and anecdotal experience indicate that

* Child maltreatment is highly prevalent in many developing countries.
* Child maltreatment has been demonstrated by science to have a powerful influence on health and human capital, through its influence on brain architecture.
* Child maltreatment creates an enormous drag on the socioeconomic progress of developing countries; and though we may not be able to put an economic figure on the effect of this or intimate partner violence on other health outcomes, due to the paucity of economic analyses estimating the relationship of GDP to violence, these problems probably add a much greater cost than is seen in the available figures.

However, according to Mercy, it is safe to say that interventions that are effective for preventing child maltreatment in developing countries will have enormous long-term economic benefits. A lot of work is under way in the United States in terms of making investments in early childhood education because of data that show a relationship among early exposure to toxic stress, other adverse exposures, cognitive development, and an individual's ability later to contribute in economically productive ways to society.

## VIOLENCE AGAINST WOMEN AND WOMEN'S HEALTH

Violence against women can take on many forms including sexual violence that occurs during times of conflict. Although men are also victims of violence, women in low- and middle-income countries are most frequently the victims of intimate partner violence and therefore are most affected by this intersection. In the United States, approximately 1.3 million women are physically assaulted by an intimate partner compared to 835,000 men (NIJ-CDC, 2006). According to the 2005 U.S. National Violence Against Women Survey, 64 percent of the women who reported being raped, physically assaulted, or stalked since age 18 were victimized by a current or former husband, cohabitating partner, boyfriend, or date. In addition, one in six women has experienced an attempted or completed rape—defined as a forced or threatened vaginal, oral, or anal penetration—in her lifetime;

and many are raped at an early age (NIJ-CDC 2006). Of the 18 percent of all women surveyed who said they had been the victim of a completed or attempted rape at some time in their lives, 22 percent were younger than age 12 when they were first raped, and 32 percent were ages 12 to 17 years (NIJ-CDC 2006).

For a global perspective of violence against women, Jacquelyn Campbell acknowledged the value of WHO's (2005) *Multi-Country Study on Domestic Violence and Women's Health*[1] in providing reliable, comparable data about violence against women in developing and some industrialized countries, along with the ethical protocols that make the study the gold standard in terms of addressing sensitive issues of safety and confidentiality when studying interpersonal violence. In the majority of settings in the WHO study, more than 75 percent of women who had been physically or sexually abused since the age of 15 reported abuse by a partner (WHO, 2005). Lifetime prevalence estimates of physical violence by partners ranged from 13 percent in a Japanese city to 61 percent in an Andean province in Peru, with African countries such as Namibia and Tanzania reporting estimates of 31 and 47 percent, respectively. The range of reported lifetime prevalence of sexual violence by partners was between 6 percent (cities in Japan, Serbia, and Montenegro) and 59 percent (Ethiopian province). Namibia and Tanzania had lifetime sexual violence estimates of 17 and 31 percent, respectively. The Japanese sample consistently reported the lowest prevalence of all forms of violence, whereas provinces in Bangladesh, Ethiopia, Peru, Tanzania, and Namibia reported the highest estimates (WHO, 2005). Lifetime prevalence estimates of forced sex by an intimate partner varied from 4 percent in Serbia and Montenegro to 46 percent in Bangladesh and Ethiopian provinces (WHO, 2005). The high rates of forced sex are particularly alarming in light of the HIV/AIDS epidemic and the difficulty that women often face in protecting themselves from HIV infection. These data, she pointed out, showed a common, high prevalence of physical partner violence, and of sexual assault as part of intimate partner violence. In some countries, sexual assault is more common than physical violence for some women.

Nearly half of the 40 million people living with HIV/AIDS worldwide are women; and women make up the fastest growing group of persons newly infected with HIV. In sub-Saharan Africa, women represent the majority of those infected and the majority of those dying. A critical aspect of this trend is the intersection of HIV/AIDS and violence against women, which has been recognized and documented with persuasive and rigorous research. As critical as it is to address this pandemic, the issues of intimate

---

[1]This study is available at www.who.int/gener/violence/who_multicountry_study/en/index.html.

partner violence and gender inequality remain inadequately addressed by most policy, research, and prevention and intervention initiatives in the United States and globally (see Appendix C, Campbell et al., 2007).

## Other Health Effects of Violence Against Women

Other documented physical health effects include chronic pain (which may be related to previous injuries, but also has important neurological implications), mental health problems, chronic irritable bowel, smoking (which we have already heard leads to other problems), effects on stress-response systems (possible links to exacerbating hypertension in African American women), gynecological problems, sexually transmitted infections and the diseases they cause, and effects on the immune system. The latter may be linked to increased risk of STDs and HIV and may contribute to rapid reductions in Cluster of Differentiation 4 (CD4) counts in women, resulting in quicker progression to AIDS and rapid death.

Another important aspect of the health effects identified by Campbell is related to reproductive health, especially the amount of abuse during pregnancy, which exhibits cross-national variations. For now, we know that intimate partner violence around the world is significantly associated with unintended pregnancy. Other maternal health correlates mirror those identified by Mercy in his examination of child maltreatment—depression, substance abuse, low social support, smoking—with the addition of spontaneous abortion and risk of homicide. Women who are abused during pregnancy are at increased risk of being killed by their partner—if not during the pregnancy (maternal mortality), then later in that abusive relationship. Campbell identified the issue of maternal mortality as one that needs greater attention for better data collection. Anecdotal studies from India, Mozambique, and Bangladesh are beginning to consider the issue as part of their examination of intimate partner violence and homicide. In one state in India, it has been reported that 16 percent of all deaths during pregnancy were due to intimate partner violence. She noted that in India, as we also see in the United States, these deaths are often incorrectly categorized or recorded. In the United States, data from fatality reviews of intimate partner homicide cases reveal that homicide is the leading cause of maternal mortality. The CDC is initiating an approach for improved data collection by linking homicide and maternal mortality databases to improve our understanding of the magnitude of this outcome.

Related to infant outcomes, data from meta-analyses conducted by Campbell showed that infant birth weights are likely to be lower for women who are abused during pregnancy and who live in industrialized countries—which may occur through connections to smoking, substance abuse, and stress. Also, among women abused during pregnancy, there is more likely to be child abuse when the infant is born—a painful example of the interconnectedness of various types of violence.

## New Research and Promising Prevention Programs

New research is being conducted in the United States to examine the comorbidity of posttraumatic stress disorder (PTSD) and depression in women, which may have different effects on the immune system, causing a proinflammatory response that may be associated with either chronic pain or immune suppression. Similarly to the pathways described by Dr. Garbarino earlier in the day, these need to be examined not only to help understand why some women are affected the way they are, but also to guide both prevention and treatment efforts.

More proactive intimate partner violence prevention messages should be included in women's health campaigns, such as the Safer Motherhood Campaign. Campbell also stated that we need to increase health provider education and awareness about violence against women, as well as clinical initiatives for systematic, confidential, and safe assessments of intimate partner violence; appropriate referrals must be made that link health-care systems around the world with community-based nongovernmental organizations.

## Promising Prevention Programs

The Intervention with Microfinance for AIDS and Gender Equity (IMAGE) study, which used a microcredit finance mechanism to address intimate partner violence, as well as programs that promote safe dating and prevention of date rape, were offered as examples of successful community partnerships. Nurse home visitation programs have been effective in the United States, and although they may be cost-prohibitive in developing countries, she queried whether elements of the intervention for families at risk could be translated, transported, and tested in developing countries. Treatment for PTSD in adults (especially those involved in collective violence), as recommended by two previous Institute of Medicine studies, may prevent intimate partner violence and child abuse (IOM 2006, IOM-NRC, 2007). Campbell identified what she called "some good changing-the-norms kinds of campaigns" from around the world, including the "White Ribbon Campaign" that originated in Canada; "Raising Voices" in Uganda that has helped change the community norms around gender and intimate partner violence; training of new recruits in the military; and the Family Violence Prevention Fund's initiative of coaching boys into men and getting men involved in the prevention of intimate partner violence, which has translated into an international effort. While all of these efforts are promising and should be implemented on larger scales, she reinforced the need to rigorously evaluate the interventions and programs to document and facilitate the proactive translation of effective outcomes into global policy and practice.

## QUESTIONS AND ANSWERS

Key issues raised in response to questions from the audience included the need to increase the focus on resiliency of individuals, communities, societies, and systems (and the cultural and historical factors that influence resiliency) to understand their possible roles as protective factors against the types of violence and the adverse outcomes described in the presentations. Awareness of the issue of the historical trauma of oppression by colonists through time and around the globe, as well as the healing role of restorative justice programs, was also raised as worthy of consideration in global violence prevention efforts.

# 5

# What Is Working Around the World in Violence Prevention?

Linda Dahlberg, the moderator of this panel, remarked on the multiple presentations noting that violence is a global public health problem that is linked to many other health problems and disease outcomes. Before the *World Report on Violence and Health* (WHO, 2002a) and recent United Nations' studies on violence against women and children challenged the notion that violence is not predictable and preventable, many people perceived it as an inevitable part of the human condition—a fact of life to respond to rather than prevent. Part of making the case that violence is preventable, she argued, rests in demonstrating that violence prevention programs work. However, funds supporting this research are scarce. Matzopoulos et al. (see Appendix C, 2007) state that of the $73 billion invested annually toward global public health research, less than 10 percent is devoted to research into the health problems that account for 90 percent of the global disease burden. Dahlberg mentioned that this phenomenon is known as the "10/90" gap and that violence is one of those health problems. Dahlberg noted that despite limited funding, the current state of science in violence prevention reveals progress, promise, and a number of remaining challenges. Promising and effective activities include interventions in early childhood; efforts to improve social, emotional, and behavioral competencies; efforts to improve family functioning and parenting practices so as to change social norms; and some effective approaches in terms of reducing concentrated disadvantage and access to lethal means. She pointed out that the majority of the evidence base comes from high-income countries, but there are violence prevention programs in many countries throughout the world. Unfortunately, many of these programs have not been systematically and rigorously evaluated, and without this, there is the potential to actually do harm. Developing effective programs is a continuous and iterative process that requires sustained commitment and resources. It involves identifying the nature of the problem through good epidemiologic work; specifying and clarifying risk factors and, more importantly, trying to figure out how to translate those risk factors into prevention programs; and then the arduous task of testing and refining those programs and determining how best to facilitate their diffusion. This public health approach, she stated, can really make a difference in helping governments increase their knowledge of and confidence in workable interventions while providing them with alternative options to policing and public security to address violence.

From her experiences in high-income countries and in a few low- and middle-income countries, she acknowledged that the process is doable. There are, however, some challenges, including empowering stakeholders with the tools for planning, developing, implementing, and evaluating programs—building infrastructure capacity in the countries. She asserted that this is a question not only for those who are involved in prevention work, but also for donors and decision makers in terms of where their investments could and should be made. Another challenge she identified is seeking economies of scale wherever possible and whenever feasible—that is, making the most of existing prevention infrastructures and expertise. She reiterated what was said earlier in the day about the tendency to work in silos and the need for more effective methods that call for really looking at the intersection of different types of violence, breaking down those silos, and determining how prevention efforts can be integrated so that we are not only changing one outcome but potentially changing many outcomes or reducing many types of violence. She also encouraged examining the intersection with other health outcomes and other health areas—for example, HIV infection or maternal and child health—to tap into existing prevention structures and expertise, acting accordingly, and possibly reducing multiple health problems. Her closing remark identified the challenge of really bridging science and practice. It is insufficient, she argued, just to identify effective programs. Determining how to disseminate those programs and policies and get them adopted in different settings and with different populations is critical—in other words, finding ways to accelerate what we do know that works. This is important not only for those who do this kind of work, but also for governments and the development community—everyone is a partner in making sure this is a reality.

David Hawkins, Rodrigo Guerrero, Elizabeth Ward, and Charlotte Watts gave presentations to summarize what is known about the effectiveness of different interventions, the importance of data collection in guiding prevention efforts, the types of interventions and their outcomes, the

characteristics or components that support effectiveness, and challenges for
effective programming and research.

## ADVANCES IN THE IDENTIFICATION OF
## EFFECTIVE POLICIES AND INTERVENTIONS

David Hawkins' presentation focused mainly on what is known about
youth violence prevention in the United States, the evidence base that
supports it, and what elements of effective interventions might be export-
able to developing countries for implementation in their epidemiological
contexts. The advances in youth violence prevention in the United States
and other developed countries have occurred only during the last 27 years;
prior to that, there had been only nine true experimental studies for delinquency prevention—and none of them were shown to be effective. The
basic premise of the science-based, public health approach to violence
prevention is that if you want to prevent a problem before it happens, you
need to identify the predictors of that problem. Longitudinal studies that
have followed children forward from birth or a bit older have identified
factors that, when present in earlier childhood development, predict negative outcomes. Some of these individual, family, and community risk factors include early and persistent antisocial behavior, friends who engage in
problem behaviors, alcohol and substance use, and constitutional factors
which are individual characteristics carried forward over time and can be
induced by the environment (ingestion of lead paint often leads to increased
violent behavior) or be genetically determined; family conflict or management problems (failure to monitor children or set clear behavioral expecta-
tions; caregivers' engaging in child maltreatment) and extreme economic
deprivation; availability of drugs and firearms, community norms that are
permissive of violence, and media portrayal of violence, respectively. Risk
factors were also identified in schools, such as academic failure. These
studies have identified not only risk factors, but also protective or promo-
tive factors that appear to promote healthy, crime- and violence-free child
development. These protective factors include high intelligence, resilient
temperament, and competencies and skills in individuals. In the social
domains of family, school, peer groups, and neighborhoods, they include
prosocial opportunities; reinforcement for prosocial involvement; social
bonding in family, schools, or neighborhoods; and healthy beliefs and clear
standards of behavior. Hawkins stressed that even though there is consistency across samples from developed nations for these risk factors, none
of them is a single cause of the adverse outcomes they can often predict in
youth—such as substance abuse, teen pregnancy and paternity, dropping
out of school, depression and anxiety, delinquency, and violence. They do,
however, provide a convenient catalogue of risk factors that are potential

targets for prevention intervention. Multiple risk factors may appear in a number of environments, as well as in the individual, and these factors are also predictive of violence—the more factors that are present, the greater is the likelihood of violence instead of successful or healthier outcomes. He stated that this reinforces the need for multidisciplinary efforts to address the same risk factors if the goal is to prevent youth violence.

## EVIDENCE FOR EFFECTIVE AND INEFFECTIVE PREVENTION INTERVENTIONS

Hawkins reviewed data from a number of controlled studies that have identified both effective and ineffective youth development policies and approaches. Some examples of ineffective approaches, also mentioned earlier by Irvin Waller, are Scared Straight, waivers to adult criminal courts, and gun buyback programs, which were associated with increased violent behavior after the supposed preventive or rehabilitative intervention. Hawkins asserted that we should not replicate these programs in developing countries if we are trying to profit from what has been learned in developed countries.

However, in the United States and other developed nations, there have been well-controlled, randomized trials that have shown policies or intervention strategies in 12 different areas (e.g., parental and infancy programs, early childhood education, see Box 5-1) to be effective in reducing youth

---

**BOX 5-1**
**Effective Policies and Programs Identified for**
**Youth Violence Prevention**

1. Prenatal and Infancy Programs
2. Early Childhood Education
3. Parent Training
4. After-School Recreation
5. Mentoring with Contingent Reinforcement
6. Youth Employment with Education
7. Organizational Change in Schools
8. Community Mobilization
9. School Behavior Management Strategies
10. Community and School Policies
11. Curricula for Social Competence Promotion
12. Classroom Organization, Management, and Instructional Strategies

SOURCE: Hawkins (2007).

violence or known risk or protective factors for youth violence. The Center for the Study and Prevention on Violence of the Institute of Behavioral Science at the University of Colorado at Boulder designed, launched and maintains the *Blueprints for Violence Prevention Initiative,* which identifies available programs that have been developed, tested, and shown to be effective. Their list of programs is available at http://www.colorado.edu/cspv/blueprints/. The *Communities That Care® Prevention Strategies Guide* produced by the U.S. Substance Abuse and Mental Health Services Administration (SAMHSA), also lists programs that have been tested and shown to be effective in well-controlled trials; it is available at http://preventionplatform.samhsa.gov/.

For effective strategies, the nurse-family partnership intervention has shown real evidence of long-lasting effects from a public health nurse visit during the second and third trimesters of pregnancy and the first two years of infancy, including reductions in prenatal health problems; maternal and child arrests and convictions; child abuse, neglect, and injuries; and welfare and food stamp use. Promoting Alternative Thinking Strategies (PATHS) is a school curriculum that is really involved in cognitive restructuring and in behavioral rehearsal—two potential pathways of intervention discussed by Dr. Garbarino—and can be implemented in the elementary grades for a cost of $82 per student in the first year, and half of that in the second year. Evidence for the effect of this program included improved self-control, improved understanding and recognition of emotions, improved conflict resolution strategies, and decreased conduct problems such as aggression. A minimal-cost program to prevent bullying in elementary and middle schools had the effects of reducing bullying by half, improving the school climate, and reducing antisocial behavior. Additional information on the costs and benefits of prevention programs is available at www.wa.gov/wsipp.

One of Hawkins' longitudinal studies in public schools of the Pacific Northwest has shown that creating opportunities for active involvement of children and reinforcing this involvement (from feeding classroom pets to working on team projects in schools or beautification projects in neighborhoods) reinforces social bonding, which subsequently reinforces positive norms and standards of behavior by which the child is likely to live. He stated that in America, the focus is on the standards that prohibit undesirable behavior but less on the process of promoting social bonding. By training everyday teachers and offering parenting workshops on emotional and skills development, they were able to see in six years, broad-ranging effects not only on lifetime violence, but also on alcohol use and sexual behaviors. Data from following the children to age 21 continued to show significant effects on those broad-ranging outcomes with the promotion of protective factors in high-risk environments.

In conclusion, Hawkins stated that investment in early childhood education, especially for low-income children, produces more benefits over the life of a child than it costs—with similar cost-benefit ratios seen in the nurse-family partnership interventions. Data collection to create epidemiological profiles of risk and protective factors to plan effective, multidisciplinary interventions, as well as data to document effective and ineffective programs, and dissemination at the community level to facilitate effective prevention planning, prioritization, and ownership are critically important. He also stated that efforts need to be made to reverse the trend, especially in the United States, of implementing programs that have been shown to be ineffective. Programs and policies that have been tested and shown to be effective can be used in developing countries, but they need to be adapted to the appropriate cultural context, and they have to be monitored and rigorously evaluated.

## INTERVENTION WITH MICROFINANCE FOR
## AIDS AND GENDER EQUITY (IMAGE) STUDY

Charlotte Watts discussed the Intervention with Microfinance for AIDS and Gender Equity study—a community, randomized controlled trial in eight villages in South Africa—designed in two phases and intended to address two social risk factors for women's vulnerability to violence and HIV: poverty and gender inequity. It was a collaborative effort between the London School of Tropical Medicine and Hygiene and the University of Witswatersrand's School of Public Health in South Africa. The study targeted community mobilization, as well changes in economic sufficiency for individuals that could reduce their risk of exposure to HIV and violence. Their community partnerships were with a local microfinance group that made small business loans to women in the poorest rural areas, as well as a local women's organization that addressed social and health issues facing women in the area. Participant selection was based on the usual selection processes of microfinance groups, which try to identify the poorest women in a community—more than half of whom had had to beg for their food the previous year. A total of 860 women were enrolled in the study. Their evaluation assessed the impact of this combination of microfinance and participatory activities around gender and violence on the women's economic and social empowerment as this related to the outcome of a woman's past-year exposure to physical or sexual partner violence. They also assessed any benefits to their households and other community members, especially adolescents in the household, by way of effect on knowledge, communication, voluntary counseling and testing, social mobilization, and sexual behavior as it related to the outcome of HIV infection. She stated that at the end of their study, the control groups also received the intervention.

She reported that in the first phase, they used their linkage with the microfinance program by adding a total of 10 educational sessions to their compulsory loan meetings, which prevented the participants from "opting out." The topics included gender issues, domestic violence, sexuality and HIV, and skill building for communication, conflict resolution, solidarity, and leadership. The second phase focused on helping participants take their concerns to the broader community using what is known as a natural opinion leader model. By offering additional training to a woman selected as a natural leader for her group after the initial 10-week session, they facilitated her ability to work with her loan group to identify and prioritize the concerns they would take to the community with the goals of developing an action plan and engaging men and youth. The investigators' use of a community participatory model disclosed that their preconceived ideas about prioritizing HIV and violence as the primary concerns for these women were altered when the women identified potable water, alcohol abuse, and a number of other issues for action.

Although Watts acknowledged the limited statistical power of their study, she did note that they were really attempting a proof of concept and trying to assess what effect size they could achieve around some of their indicators, given their limited statistical power. She also stated that the supplemental use of qualitative data helped them understand and explain some of the effect that could not be measured quantitatively. Their findings showed a significant impact on several of the different economic indicators of well-being, with improvement in household assets that may be suggestive of improvement in savings and expenditures. They did not see an effect on food security and school enrollments, but she explained that this may have been due to the broader contextual changes that were occurring in South Africa at the time and may have affected both their intervention and the control communities.

For broader measures of empowerment, they found positive trends in all of the indicators including self-confidence, challenging gender roles, communication with household members and partners, progressive attitudes toward violence, and autonomy in household decision making. The impact on women's past-year experience of physical and sexual violence was a reduction in levels of violence (pushing, hitting, forced sex, and fear to refuse) by 55 percent, a significant result, she stated, due to such an effect size. Qualitative data collection and analysis helped explain the reductions in violence by identifying changes in the women's relationships, a shift in women's attitudes toward violence, and an increased self-confidence attributed to their ability to earn income, as well as an elevated household status that may have facilitated their ability to challenge their experience of violence, including confidence in the option of leaving their abusive partners because of their newfound financial freedom. They also found fewer conflicts over finances, greater confidence to resolve conflict by improved communication with their partners, and evidence of group solidarity and influence that resulted from their participation in activities linked to their loan groups that enabled them to challenge what was happening in their individual lives, households, and communities in terms of violence.

For community mobilization, they were able to measure an increase in the number of marches including one to a local police station to protest the way cases of rape were being handled, meetings with local leaders, village workshops, new village committees targeting and monitoring rape and crime, and new partnerships among local organizations—all to raise community awareness, engage young men, provide assistance and advice to women in the community, and intervene individually when witnessing abuse. All are examples of diffusion that could not really be captured by their impact measures but were captured by their qualitative data collection and analysis.

The cost-effectiveness of interventions is a concern for everyone involved in the research on violence prevention and its translation. The IMAGE study was evaluated for cost-effectiveness by examining the costs of the research, the intervention, the trial, and the scaling-up of the intervention. Since the microfinance component was self-sustaining, the analysis really determined the incremental cost of adding the women's empowerment component with the local women's organization. In the trial, the cost (U.S. 2004 dollars) was found to be $24 per client, with a decrease to a final cost of $7 per person when scaled up to implementation, which exemplifies the economies of scale that can be obtained when increasing the coverage of this type of intervention.

An important finding of this study was that interventions can address the issue of gender-based violence, with all of its associated cultural issues, over relatively short time frames if the intervention is designed properly. Traditionally, Watts stated, it is assumed that interventions targeting cultural norms can bring about change over generations. She noted that other participatory interventions in South Africa and Brazil targeting issues around gender are showing evidence of impact by reducing male perpetration of intimate partner violence and other behaviors that are associated with norms that support gender inequities.

Watts echoed the need for long-term funding. For the IMAGE study, she explained that because violence did not fall clearly into the health objectives of many funders, they ended up "piecing together" funding from nine different donors. If funders want evidence on which to base their decisions, she implored them to prioritize funding rigorous research and evaluations. While she did not believe that randomized controlled trials could be conducted for all interventions, she said that there is no shortage of promising and innovative violence prevention interventions in developing countries that should be considered seriously for strategic evaluation to help build the evidence base. She gave two examples—Raising Voices, initiated in Tanzania and later replicated in Uganda and several other East African communities, and the Safer Schools intervention implemented in several countries and funded by the U.S. Agency for International Development. Her final observation was that not only rigorous evaluation, but also methodological work is needed to help conceptualize what these interventions are trying to achieve, to identify the process of change that will be promoted, and to define and measure key impacts and outcomes that are being assessed as part of the evaluation initiative.

## THE IMPORTANCE OF EPIDEMIOLOGICAL DATA
## FOR GUIDING PREVENTION

Rodrigo Guerrero and Elizabeth Ward discussed the use of epidemiological data in violence prevention planning in Colombia and the Caribbean. In Colombia, Guerrero stated that the public health approach to violence prevention has proven to be of crucial importance in interpersonal violence prevention efforts in the country, and also in the dissemination of their efforts in Cali, Colombia. Sharing data and their meaning was shown to be a very powerful tool for communities in bringing pressure to bear on policy makers and elected officials to engender continued support for the intervention. While serving as mayor of Cali, he stated that all crime 15 years ago was attributable solely to drugs and drug barons, but as they began data collection, they learned that 80 percent was due to firearms—with two-thirds occurring during the weekend. Data also indicated that alcohol intoxication played a role in the occurrence of crime. They instituted restrictions on carrying guns on weekends and actually banned gun carrying for local and national celebrations that permitted alcohol use to address these two risk factors, as well as restricting the sale of alcohol after 1:00 AM in public places. His policies were not without political risk because the gun restriction put his administration at odds with the Colombian army, which manufactures and sells guns in the country. Evaluation of the intervention showed that on the weekends for which the gun ban was in place, there was a 14 percent decrease in homicides compared to weekends that permitted gun possession. The gun ban combined with the restrictions on alcohol sales yielded a 35 percent reduction in homicides, which represented a reduction of nearly 700 homicides. Anecdotally, the mayor of Bogotá decided to implement the same ban on firearms in 1996 and, based on evaluation, saw similar reductions in firearm homicides in the city. From April to November of that same year, a legal battle ensued that questioned the authority of the mayors to institute such bans. The ban was not implemented in Bogotá during this time. As a result, an increase in firearms deaths occurred. Winning a ruling in the Colombian Supreme Court, the mayors were permitted the authority to institute such bans, and when they were reinstituted, the firearm and homicide rates once again declined.

According to Guerrero, this type of policy making and implementation requires reliable and opportune information, addressing multiple risk factors, political will and leadership, continuity, multisectoral efforts, and monitoring to make necessary corrections along the way.

## THE CARIBBEAN

Elizabeth Ward focused her comments on violence prevention efforts in Jamaica. She stated that Jamaica's rate of 54 homicides per 100,000 people surpassed that of the rest of the Caribbean as described by Bernice Bronkhorst. In addition, she acknowledged that the rate is affected by high rates of migration—both legal and illegal, including deportees—with people moving between the United States and the Caribbean, moving between the islands, and moving from South America. She spoke of the collaboration between the Jamaican Ministry of Health and the Centers for Disease Control and Prevention (CDC) to improve their surveillance and data collection and how the Ministry was eventually able to incorporate its computer-based system into nine of the largest hospitals, which cover 70 percent of hospital admissions. By collecting data such as the date of the violence-related injury, the place of occurrence and circumstances, method of injury, victim-perpetrator relationship, and geographic location, they have been able to prepare street-level "hot-spot" maps of Kingston and use this information to target their interventions. Their collaboration with a World Bank project enabled them to engage in a mapping of community assets that can be layered with violence mapping data and homicide data. Again, this mapping ability gave them valuable information for intervention planning, including where interventions were likely to have the greatest impact. Ward stated that by using these tools in a public health approach, they have successfully engaged communities to participate in their research and have validated the conclusions drawn from the data for multisectoral, community interventions. She noted that the Ministry of Health is an active participant in the Violence Prevention Alliance-Jamaica, which is modeled after that of the Violence Prevention Alliance spearheaded by the World Health Organisation (WHO).

## Examples of Interventions

The Peace Initiative is a community-based initiative housed in the Jamaican Ministry of National Security and is a collaboration between social workers and law enforcement. Another example is a U.S.-supported initiative that placed community workers in a specific community to address violence prevention and saw a significant reduction in the homicide rate from 11 percent to zero. Other community-based programs that Ward mentioned focus on violence prevention, including community policing, gang interventions, environmental improvements for safety, mediation and counseling, small-arms control, and domestic violence (including United Nations Development Fund for Women-supported activities). Some youth-focused programs that showed promise include programs at the YMCA, computer-based literacy projects (which she identified as a surprising protective factor against violence), and skills development linked with job opportunities. Some of these programs also utilize the entertainment media, photography, and sports programs as vehicles for effective and efficient communication and implementation. School-based programs in the region are utilizing some innovative cross-cultural activities, as well as some of the social-bonding techniques described by David Hawkins using interschool peer circles. A collaboration with the United Kingdom addressed drug trafficking between the two countries. This UK-Jamaica collaboration also targeted providing economic assistance to the families of offenders and has yielded an 80 percent reduction in the number of "drug mules" who are carrying drugs to the United Kingdom.

The private sector is also supporting some innovative strategies with matching donation campaigns, where employers make 2:1 donations for every employee-donated dollar to prevention programs, coupled with community-based interventions that include homework and scholarship programs. Wards stated that randomized, controlled trials of parenting programs that targeted home visits with toy play have even shown unintended positive effects such as improvements in self-esteem, fewer attention problems, and lower incidence of depression in both the intervention and the control groups. Other population-level interventions have shown promise, but they need to be properly evaluated.

## CHARACTERISTICS OF EFFECTIVE INTERVENTIONS

For Jamaica, Ward identified several characteristics of their successful and promising programs for sustainability including good organization, a holistic and comprehensive approach, good leadership, and community-based participation and assistance. Watts made similar observations about the importance of dissemination and community participation and mobilization in her discussion about the IMAGE project in South Africa, including the importance of linkages with other activities and organizations addressing economic development with an emphasis on choosing good partners and maximizing their comparative advantages. The synergy of linking participatory activities focused on gender with the microfinance program enabled them to take advantage of poverty alleviation strategies and processes that were already successful in the communities. She stressed the importance of taking the time to address the concerns of collaborators and other issues that might affect the study design. The microfinance organizations were concerned that collaborating with the researchers not only would affect their financial stability, but also might discourage the women from seeking loans if they were going to address sensitive issues such as intimate partner violence. This led to the linkage with local women's organizations to facilitate support and empowerment. They found that the collaboration did not jeopardize microfinance, but rather was enhancing, with improvements in various indicators of vulnerability of loan groups that microfinance organizations use for monitoring compared to interventions that offered microfinance only. The study also found a loan repayment rate of nearly 100 percent among the women enrolled as participants.

The rigorous evaluation of the IMAGE study and wide dissemination of its findings showed the potential influence of their findings because the South African National AIDS Plan now explicitly incorporates elements about addressing women's vulnerability to violence as part of the national AIDS strategy. Watts suggested that the participatory nature of the IMAGE study in challenging issues of gender and relationship took time and could not be done superficially and that researchers needed to think critically about intervention modalities that allow them to spend time with participants and really engage them in the issues of interest. The community mobilization component was also identified as important, but she cautioned it can be difficult because it could impact monitoring the effects of the study if the community chooses to mobilize around something that cannot be captured or measured.

## CHALLENGES FOR EFFECTIVE PROGRAMMING AND RESEARCH

In Jamaica, Ward identified the need for increased overall training, as well as community policing, health education for the importance of literacy and healthier lifestyles, strengthening information and monitoring systems, and some forms of income generation such as small business loans. Additional challenges identified include the need for sustained funding for long-term interventions, the need to translate small but effective programs to population-level interventions that are supported by community-based workers, the need to address social factors that affect families and communities, the need for widespread literacy and job skills training, the need to address political issues, and ensuring that efforts are multisectoral and geographically target areas with the highest incidence and prevalence of violence. Lastly, she stated the need for programmatic requirements to fund rigorous impact evaluation to help understand what interventions are making a difference.

Replicability and scaling up to a larger program are also of great concern to researchers, policy makers, funders, and implementers. The IMAGE study was a small intervention, but when it received additional funding, it was able to scale up to 1,800 clients—nearly double the original enrollment. Watts identified several issues for consideration when scaling up from a small research intervention to a much larger implementation including operational and organizational issues, whether there is programmatic compromise when scaling up occurs, whether any revisions have to be made, and whether there are health, social, and economic development mechanisms or vehicles for synergistic linkages and integration other than microfinance—such as literacy, HIV/AIDS, or malaria.

## QUESTIONS AND ANSWERS

The highlights of the discussion with participants focused on examples of the participatory approach in research coupled with epidemiological data from a specific program in El Salvador. The intervention was implemented by a former guerrilla, and while it targeted the entire community, it also targeted those at highest risk (18-25 years) for violence by focusing on job skill development, employment, and other structured activities that address alcohol and drug use to reduce the risk for this population. The community used data from the hospital injury surveillance system to monitor the violence-related injuries that occurred in the city.

# 6

# Words of Wisdom:
# Working with the Media and
# Nongovernmental Organizations

## RELATIONSHIPS WITH THE MEDIA

One of the participants raised the issue of engaging the public and the media, not only to help raise awareness about the prevalence of violence, but also to participate in interventions in their respective communities. Mr. John Donnelly's presentation addressed the issue of engaging the media. As reporter for the *Boston Globe* who focuses on global health, Mr. Donnelly stated that building relationships and having regular dialogue with reporters is critical to attracting the attention of journalists and obtaining "a good media outcome." He made five suggestions for improving relationships with the media. The first was to have a thorough understanding of their materials to make a strong presentation to the journalist, providing "good and bad" examples to illustrate trends and what is currently being done to address the problem. He remarked on the amazing evidentiary content of the World Health Organisation (WHO, 2002a) *World Report on Violence and Health* and that it was a fresh perspective for him to learn that so many types of violence could be addressed with the same public health approach for prevention, but that "it was all over the place." Cultivating a relationship with a reporter using new research findings that have not yet been published is also a possibility.

Secondly, he suggested that the example provided should be grounded in "real life" and that advocates should take the time to show the reporter why the focal issue is compelling. As an example, he recounted an experience when he traveled to India, at the recommendation of a WHO researcher, to learn about road traffic safety. In his conversation with a hospital adminis-

66

trator in Delhi, Donnelley still did not see the issue as compelling until the hospital administrator led him by the hand to a street near the hospital, where he saw tractor-trailer trucks, rickshaws, people running across the street, ox-drawn carts, motorcycles, passenger cars, and Metrorail above the street. In that chaotic activity, the hospital administrator was able to point to a spot on the road where one of his nurses was killed two weeks prior as she tried to cross. The available pedestrian crossings were each a half mile away, in opposite directions, from the hospital. This became a compelling example of the problem of road traffic safety.

His third suggestion was for participants to keep in mind that the media landscape is undergoing incredible transformation, especially in the United States. Economic survival has required many budgets to be reduced, which results in fewer domestic and international staff. These reductions have caused the traditional outlets that people are courting for media coverage to look internally and, as a result, to cover local issues more intensely. The fourth important suggestion is to develop relationships with various reporters. He readily admitted that this is not an easy task and it takes a long time—perhaps years of talking—and will not always result in a story. It's a conversation about national and international issues that permits you not only to become better acquainted with that journalist, but also to build trust. He even suggested that people could learn from each other by approaching colleagues to ask them about both positive and negative experiences with journalists.

His last suggestion might help increase the likelihood of getting an article in the press that one would actually be happy about in terms of accuracy in data and context. Here, the trusting relationship is very important, but other things that facilitate this include checking with the reporter for the accuracy of quotes while the article is being written, making oneself available to the reporter for clarification, helping him or her obtain additional information for the story or fact checking, and answering questions. This also extends to reporters working in countries where you are trying to change policies or invoke leadership to address issues—partnerships with reporters in those countries are essential. Donnelly cautiously ventured that people can also be a part of the media via "blogs" or publishing photographs or videos online. This attracts attention not only on the Internet, but also of reporters in the area since there is local interest in covering what is happening locally.

## Questions from the Audience

Donnelly addressed a few questions from the audience with an emphasis on specific opportunities for advocates and researchers to capture the media's attention and engage them to discuss or explore the root causes of violence and not the action that may be overshadowing the headlines. Timing, he suggested, is critical, along with the recognition that you may be contacted by a reporter or need to contact a reporter with whom a relationship has been developed with only a few hours' notice. He suggested that political reporters may also be interested, especially during presidential campaigns, not only in exploring the candidates' track records on violence prevention, but also in learning what they might do about the issue if they are elected. When asked why the media was reluctant to cover suicide, given that it accounts for more than 50 percent of violence-related deaths, Donnelley remarked that the media provides little coverage because of the shame and stigma often attached to suicide for families and communities. He added that journalists do not want to be accused of privacy violations. New research in suicide prevention may help increase coverage of the issue, and personal experiences of journalists with the topic may also encourage increased willingness to cover it. He also noted that training sessions for reporters on various health-related topics can be a useful tool in improving the way the media reports an issue.

## RELATIONSHIPS WITH NONGOVERNMENTAL ORGANIZATIONS

During the course of the workshop presentations and question-and-answer periods, there were multiple references to collaborating with other organizations that are engaged in research, programming, and advocacy for health issues that might intersect with violence or be impacted by violence. David Gartner spoke about the work of the Global AIDS Alliance and shared lessons learned from its advocacy for policies, resources, and programming to address the HIV/AIDS pandemic. In the course of his organization's work, it, along with other implementers, has come to realize that violence prevention must be an integral part of the global response to HIV/AIDS. His four-point recommendation for moving violence prevention forward was preceded by a brief overview of U.S.-based advocacy that has contributed to the success of the global response to HIV/AIDS, which includes a tenfold increase in the provision of antiretroviral treatment in Africa. Gartner noted that new multilateral institutions such as the Global Fund to Fight AIDS, Malaria, and Tuberculosis (Global Fund) and its operational structure that include equity in developing country membership and civil society as a full governance partner has also contributed to the rapidity of the response and successful resource mobilization. U.S. policy changes have enabled the use of low-priced generic drugs around the world. Gartner agreed with Donnelley's earlier call for marshaling evidence to make the case for policy development and resource mobilization for a cause, but also stated that accurate costing data grounded in what is actually needed for programmatic success are critical to helping multisectoral organizations coalesce around a common message and vision to work toward resource mobilization. The broad HIV/AIDS coalition was also able to generate bipartisan congressional support. He quoted Tip O'Neill as saying that "all politics is local," which Gartner thinks is particularly true for funding issues. All of these activities, combined with a political commitment from the Group of 8 (G8) to work toward universal treatment and access to AIDS services, has facilitated some progress toward this goal. He mentioned that at the same 2005 G8 Summit in Gleneagles, Scotland, summit where this commitment to universal access and treatment was announced, President Bush announced a new Women's Justice and Empowerment in Africa initiative to combat sexual violence and abuse against women. By Gartner's query to the audience, few had heard of the initiative—which, in his opinion, should have been a watershed moment for the violence prevention community—and his organization has had difficulty finding out the results of this initiative.

Mr. Gartner's first point for developing a strategy to put violence prevention on the U.S. policy agenda and mobilizing real resources is to ask for what is really needed, not what is "reasonable," which in Washington, D.C., is defined as "lacking ambition." Asking for what is needed and what a unified coalition of researchers, advocates, and organizations truly wants increases the likelihood that it will become a reality. Earlier, he mentioned the costing estimates from the Joint United Nations Programme on HIV/AIDS (UNAIDS) that helped create the unified voice that asked for multiple billions in funding. In the next several weeks after this workshop, and for the first time, these estimates will include costing for what is needed to internationally address violence prevention in the context of HIV/AIDS—which is only a first step to begin to address the global problem of violence. Mr. Gartner suggested that the entire community working on violence prevention would be able to rally around those costing estimates and build on the momentum for future funding and resource requests. To advocate for the domestic availability of these funds while expanding international funding for other initiatives, he contended that enormous pressure should be put on the congressional appropriators. With that said, billion-dollar initiatives do not come from Congress; so ideally, if the violence prevention community wants a new presidential initiative or linkage to an existing one, explicit language for major funding is needed that will go toward violence prevention and a structure for accountability. He echoed Donnelley's suggestion that the community should devote a lot of attention to this issue with the presidential candidates.

The second point acknowledged the importance of establishing linkages with other issues and movements, which has been responsible for the success for advocates working on other health issues. Even linkages outside of the health sector, with education for example, may be helpful to educate people and political candidates on the impact of violence. If they understand the dangers of exposure to HIV and sexual assault for many girls in schools without latrines or in walking to school, this could be an entry point for violence prevention dialogue. He stated that it will be nearly impossible for groups to obtain long-term funding in the hundreds of millions or more without these linkages. He offered concrete examples of funding for tuberculosis and services for orphans and other vulnerable children that effectively and synergistically linked to HIV/AIDS policy in recent years.

With the relationship between HIV transmission and violence, there may be opportunities for leveraging real AIDS funding for violence prevention. To date, the U.S. Congress has only asked for reports on AIDS and violence and issued a generic request for funds to train police and military to address gender violence where appropriate. This type of request and any similar to it, he cautioned, will not yield the results that are needed to scale up the kinds of programs that will work in violence prevention. It is an important part of the response to violence, but a more significant way to address gender-based violence and equity would be to implement broader empowerment interventions. These could include providing access to a safe education for all girls, which may come from abolishing school fees, as well as linkages to economic empowerment strategies that contain violence prevention messages, such as microcredit financing programs illustrated by the Intervention with Microfinance for AIDS and Gender Equity (IMAGE) study. Education and economic empowerment are clearly linked to decreasing the vulnerability of women and young girls and may play a role in addressing risk factors for young girls especially—because they often marry older men for economic security but are subsequently exposed to HIV and intimate partner violence.

In Gartner's messages about linkages, he stated he was not suggesting that violence prevention would become subsumed by other issues but rather that concurrent activities could take place. He clarified that his suggestion was to advocate for a presidential initiative and congressional legislation for violence prevention *while* linking with existing programs of key implementers for public violence prevention education and intervention integration. He noted that these collaborations might even educate many foundations and increase the funding they make available for violence prevention initiatives.

Accountability for funds requested and appropriated was his third point. Any violence prevention initiative should have clear and measurable performance targets that become a part of the reporting process, as well as an entity with oversight for the initiative and the power to deliver programmatic management to reach the performance targets. This would be similar to the Office of the Global AIDS Coordinator, which has real authority and reports directly to the Secretary of State and the White House.

His final point was that multilateral organizations are essential to real success. While most of his comments have focused on the U.S. response to HIV/AIDS, it is important to recognize that every U.S. dollar contributed to the Global Fund leverages an additional $2 for most other European donors. In addition, multilateral aid is not subject to what he termed "the beltway tax" or the high overhead rates that prevent important money from reaching the ground where it is most needed. He identified a small multilateral vehicle that has been addressing the prevention of violence against women for the last decade—the United Nations Development Fund for Women (UNIFEM). The United States has increased its contributions to $1.8 million of the $1 billion UNIFEM budget. He did articulate support for the recommendation to create an agency for women as part of the United Nations, which Stephen Lewis mentioned as a possibility for an appropriate multilateral mechanism. If this recommended agency does not evolve, he suggested that people should support the UNIFEM to become a major multilateral mechanism that can leverage money from the rest of the world.

## Questions from the Audience

In response to questions from the audience, Gartner pointed out that addressing violence, like other issues in global health, is not only an issue of compassion, but also clearly one of national security. India, Russia, and China—all countries with rising HIV rates and climbing rates of violence—are nuclear powers. He stated that we are risking state failure in many countries of sub-Saharan Africa, with the possibilities of future civil conflicts and the alarming and escalating numbers of children who will be orphaned in many southern African nations. Recent events have shown that drug-resistant tuberculosis can cross borders quickly. All of these examples and many others point to the health dimensions that link violence to issues directly related to the security of the United States.

When asked about the usefulness and impact of reports from the Institute of Medicine (IOM) for influencing Congress and the administration, he identified the IOM's recently released report *PEPFAR Implementation: Progress and Promise* (IOM, 2007; available at http://www.nap.edu/) as being enormously helpful in the HIV/AIDS community's efforts to remove budgetary allocations from the U.S. Global AIDS Initiative's legislation that are affecting the effectiveness of U.S. prevention policy in the program. He also stated that he thought an IOM report (a consensus study) would be helpful in catalyzing the operational and policy definitions for what could constitute scientifically sound violence prevention interventions, as well as linking together the issues that need to be addressed.

# 7

# Scaling Up International Support for Violence Prevention

As a precursor of, but relevant to, this session, Mark Rosenberg provided a context for the focus of the second day's presentations—the critical step of resource mobilization. He provided an overview of the workshop's three main messages: violence is preventable, but questions remain about the application of what is known to be effective in developing countries; demonstrating effectiveness in developing countries is the first step in widespread implementation of this important approach; and the mobilization of resources to lay the groundwork for this demonstration capacity in developing countries is necessary for its eventual widespread dissemination and implementation. He referenced the papers of Zaro et al. (2007) and Mercy et al. (2007) (see Appendix C) as complementary conceptual frameworks that can be used to think about implementing violence prevention in developing countries. He also noted that they can also be useful for addressing many other public health problems. Mercy et al. (see Appendix C) identified five key elements for building strong, national foundations for violence prevention: (1) developing a national action plan and identifying a lead agency; (2) enhancing the capacity for data collection; (3) increasing collaboration and exchange of information; (4) implementing and evaluating specific actions to prevent violence; and (5) strengthening care and support systems for victims. They further identified strategies for primary, secondary, and tertiary prevention and suggested types of interventions for these strategies that might be appropriate to implement in developing countries. Zaro et al. (see Appendix C) attempted to put all of the ideas together in the action plan and identified five different domains in which activities are necessary (leadership, research and data collection, capacity building

72

and dissemination, intervention development, and victim services), as well as the inputs for desired impacts and outcomes, with the ultimate goal of preventing violence to promote health and well-being in developing countries. In his concluding remarks before introducing the moderator of the panel that would address resource mobilization, Rosenberg stressed the need for strong and effective collaborations and partnerships. Discussions at the networking dinner following the first day's presentations revealed that it took 24 months to build the partnerships in the Intervention with Microfinance for AIDS and Gender Equity (IMAGE) study and even longer, sometimes years, for other partnerships to be built for long-term interventions. Rosenberg also noted that these collaborations often need strategies, management, structure, and investments to get things accomplished.

Rodney Hammond moderated this session and explained that the speakers were asked to organize their presentations around the themes of identifying the groundwork they are laying to internationally expand and scale up the public health approach, identifying what more needs to be done to support effective efforts, and providing examples of the investments and activities that suggest a strategy for widespread adoption of effective methods to prevent violence.

## INTERNATIONAL DEVELOPMENT ASSISTANCE AND VIOLENCE PREVENTION

Collective, interpersonal, or self-directed violence has extensive and pervasive long-term implications for development and health. Moreover, these effects are themselves multi-layered and can undermine development at individual, communal, and national levels. Although the different paths by which violence exerts such economic strains remain unclear, the Millennium Development Plan is a useful framework for examining the wide-ranging impacts of violence on different sectors and systems. Violence and underdevelopment may be linked in a vicious circle where each perpetuates the other. There is also a vicious cycle between poverty and violence. On the one hand it is well established that poverty, particularly in the context of economic inequality and especially when geographically concentrated, contributes to high levels of violence by weakening intergenerational family and community ties, control of peer groups, and participation in community organizations. In turn, evidence from the World Bank indicates that high rates of violence in a community reduce property values and undermine the growth and development of business, thus contributing to the very inequalities and concentrations of poverty that play a role in causing violence (see Appendix C, Matzopoulos et al., 2007).

Alexander Butchart acknowledged various bilateral efforts of the United States in South Africa and Jamaica, the United Kingdom in South Africa, and the German Technical Cooperation Department in various Central American countries that have been instrumental in supporting violence prevention in these countries. He focused his remarks on the Violence Prevention Alliance, starting with a brief background of the organization, which is a loose network formed in 2004 of countries that share a similar vision about using science to prevent violence in developing countries. Its secretariat is housed at the World Health Organisation (WHO) and includes development agencies, governments, foundations, and nongovernmental organizations. Its objectives are to strengthen the support for science-based violence prevention, to increase collaboration and exchange of information on violence prevention, and to facilitate implementation of the recommendations of the *World Report on Violence and Health*. The government of Belgium hosted a Violence Prevention Alliance strategy meeting in 2006, where it was agreed to form a working group that would advocate with official development aid agencies for their increased support of science-based violence prevention programming. The working group included government representatives, development agencies, national agencies, centers, and councils—for example, the Centers for Disease Control and Prevention (CDC), the South African Medical Research Council, and nongovernmental organizations, one of which was in Denmark. The group decided to use a practical approach within the official development agencies agenda, which is driven by the Millennium Development Goals, and human rights- and human security-based approaches. The working group developed a discussion document (forthcoming, with the working title of *Reducing the Impact of Violence on Health, Security, and Growth: How Development Agencies Can Help*) representing a coherent Violence Prevention Alliance viewpoint to make the case for increased attention to violence prevention, to assess the gaps in programming and the way the discourse of official development agencies is engaging the problem, to suggest an agenda of action, and to stimulate ongoing dialogue among official development agencies on violence prevention.

To determine what is needed for further action, the Violence Prevention Alliance conducted a content analysis of 22 official development agency websites to discern the visibility and level of priority given to the seven types of violence defined in the workshop's materials. Data showed that collective violence, intimate partner and sexual violence, and violence against children received considerable but insufficient attention. Youth violence (especially male-on-male violence, which is a leading contributor to homicide death and to severe physical injuries) received little attention, as did elder abuse and self-directed violence. With a few exceptions, they generally found policy and program guidance to be very weak, with little focus on upstream or primary prevention—as if there were no existing evidence base for violence prevention. Guidance for fundamental processes and systems—information systems, leadership, and national plans—was found to be lacking in many of the sites. Crosscutting strategies for prevention and care were largely absent, with people looking at different types of violence in isolation from one another.

As for what needs strengthening or increased attention, Butchart identified an inadequate focus on high-risk groups that are not defined in terms of human rights and Millennium Development Goals. In addition to the lack of support for fundamental processes, there is also a great need to address piecemeal prevention approaches and to present better arguments for approaches that deal with different types of violence and shared underlying risk factors. The Violence Prevention Alliance made a number of international and national recommendations for strengthening the official development agencies' agenda on violence prevention, some of which were similar to the frameworks mentioned by Rosenberg. These include foundation building, specific violence prevention activities, and an approach to using the science and evidence base in their efforts. The international recommendations include developing common criteria between different agencies and different United Nations groups for upstream violence prevention programming, recognizing and using the evidence base in developing an official development agencies' agenda which includes violence prevention and expanding the sectoral entry points for violence prevention, so that health, education, employment, and welfare can be included as important partners. They also recommended the inclusion of violence prevention indicators in routine poverty and development surveys. The national recommendations were similar to the international and will be partially informed by the preparations for and proceedings of this workshop. Lastly, the Violence Prevention Alliance has proposed an array of violence prevention interventions according to what is known about their effectiveness; comments about the difficulties, challenges, and opportunities of implementing them; and descriptions of crosscutting interventions that are likely to deal with multiple types of violence simultaneously.

## LESSONS LEARNED FROM
## LONG-TERM FUNDING COMMITMENTS

Gary Yates provided some considerations for lessons learned from a $70 million, 10-year, public health-based initiative to prevent gun violence, injury, and death of youth, funded by the California Wellness Foundation. The initiative was prompted in response to epidemiological data that showed handgun violence as the leading cause of death for young people in California in the early 1990s. Yates stated that the initiative, which was really aimed at reducing the lethality of violence, was thought to be a comprehensive approach combining research, policy advocacy, media advocacy, community programs, and leadership development and recognition programs—wrapped in a multimillion-dollar public education campaign. He identified a few outcomes from the initiative. In a state that had never been able to even get a bill out of committee to regulate handguns, by 2003 California had the toughest gun control legislation in the country. The foundation's investment of $7 million a year was actually larger than the state's investment of $5 million a year for youth violence prevention, but by 2003, the state was investing nearly $400 million a year in youth violence prevention. Most importantly, by 2003, the number of young people dying from gun violence in California had been reduced nearly by half. He was quick to acknowledge that the foundation certainly was not the only contributing factor to all of those things, but it was a contributing factor to what happened in California over that decade.

As for the lessons learned, Yates identified eight from the initiative. The first, *convening stakeholders,* was an extremely important part of promoting the partnerships and networking that Dr. Rosenberg mentioned earlier. He identified this as one of the reasons the foundation funds the World Health Organisation and continues to help fund its annual conference on global violence prevention. The annual conference model is now applied to all of the Wellness Foundation's health initiatives, but it began with the violence prevention initiative's annual conferences. Next, *persistence and patience are extremely important.* He noted that this is true for legislation and policy efforts, as well as for the provision of funding and leveraging of resources. After seven years of that grant making program, not a single bill had been signed into law to regulate firearms in California. By the eighth year however, five legislative bills had been signed into law, including banning the sale and manufacture of Saturday night specials. Every year since, additional gun control measures have been passed in California. The eighth or ninth year reflected substantial, annual, state-budgeted financial investments made to the level described previously. Third lesson, *research and advocacy are both necessary.* Yates stated, "data is important, but data in and of itself will not move policy. Passion is important, but passion in and of itself will not move policy." When the two are combined, there is much greater potential to have an effect not only on policy makers, but on opinion leaders, who tend to have an effect on policy makers, as was mentioned by David Gartner. The fourth lesson is *consistency of message matters* over time. When the foundation first launched the Violence Prevention Initiative in 1993, the concept of violence being a public health issue was not well understood, even in public health circles in California, and only one health department had a public health program in violence prevention. When the foundation was preparing to send out requests for proposal for research or for community work, very few programs were self-identified as focusing on violence prevention. So the fact that violence might be able to be prevented was an important message over time. The other important message was that handguns were the number-one killer of young people in California, and a conservative state attorney general incorporated that message in a public speech during the fifth year of the initiative. Next, *a multidisciplinary approach* that includes law enforcement and community residents in local community programming is critical for effectiveness. For at least one-third of the 18 community sites funded that were above the bar in terms of effect, in every case, community residents were very much involved. Other disciplines, including law enforcement, public health, academia, and social work, were also involved. The sixth lesson focused on *leadership programs*, which can have a very powerful long-term effect. The Wellness Foundation's leadership programs were two-year academic fellowships and two-year community fellowships, as well as a leader recognition program. Over the decade that the initiative was in place, approximately 300 individuals went through one or more of those programs. Today, Yates noted, many of the people who participated in these leadership programs are still active in violence prevention, some as national and California state policymakers. He viewed this as a ripple effect for more than just the development program in and of itself. Seventh, is that *human behavior doesn't take place in a laboratory*, especially in society. He suggested that "researchers can't control all the variables they would like to control to prove to a $p$-value" that the intervention being used had an effect. However, he noted that there is value in common sense and an ability to observe. "If the numbers go down the way they went down in California, you don't really have to worry about the $p$-value. There are thousands of lives saved over that period of time." The final lesson: *it is really important for organized philanthropy and government to continue funding and to continue implementing the programs when true positive effects are seen.* He explained that there is a tendency for money to go elsewhere and programs to go away when things get better. He suggested that this is the worst thing to do, especially when the effort is beginning to have an effect on something. The Wellness Foundation continues to invest in violence prevention with $5 million a year, and the State of California, even during really serious budget deficits, kept that violence prevention amount at the $400 million level. Additionally, Yates stated that "the real credit goes to the advocates that put together a very powerful movement and network in California. They didn't back off once the numbers got better—they kept pushing. That is extremely important." Additional information about the evaluation of the Wellness Foundation's violence initiative and lessons learned is available at www.tcwf.org.

## THE UNITED KINGDOM'S EFFORTS IN
## ARMED VIOLENCE PREVENTION

Kate Joseph's presentation focused on discussing the rationale for the involvement of the Department for International Development (DFID), which has a budget of nearly $12 billion, in violence prevention. She also addressed strategies for elevating the issue onto the agenda of the international donor community. She reminded the group that many donors, perhaps most donors, base their interventions or their programs around the Millennium Development Goals, which cover a range of different things—eradicating extreme poverty, achieving universal primary education, maternal health, child mortality, HIV/AIDS, tuberculosis, malaria, and others. She pointed out that the framework from which her department has to operate does not make a single reference to violence, conflict, or even governance. This reinforced her rationale that careful thought and attention should be paid to how the work that DFID does impacts those indicators because they drive the donor community.

She observed that DFID has a history of working on conflict prevention, post-conflict recovery, security, and justice. Due to the multifaceted nature of the work, her department often collaborates with the UK's Foreign Office and the Ministry of Defense. She stated that the UK experience in Iraq and Afghanistan has very much "colored our engagement in conflict prevention and post-conflict recovery." Mistakes in the post-conflict period, she further explained, should facilitate careful thinking about how this kind of work is done in the future and the order in which things are done to prevent a relapse into conflict and, perhaps more importantly and more seriously, to prevent the post-conflict environment from turning into an environment of lawlessness, chaos, disorder, and violent crime. However, she acknowledged that the United Kingdom does have more positive experiences in conflict resolution and social reconstruction in Sierra Leone. The efforts on security and justice essentially started as a set of projects about building the capacity of the military to ensure state security. It quickly realized that state security wasn't particularly important for development; rather, individual and personal security was important so that people could feel safe to go about their daily lives and therefore engage in economic activity that would drive development. Providing that security was only one-half of the coin, the other half being access to fair and speedy justice. Joseph stated that this work on security and justice was just as much about involving the community in deciding what it needed for its own security. Lastly, DFID has been doing a lot of work on small arms or gun control.

Originally, the small arms control efforts were very much about controlling the supply of weapons—controls on exports and imports, controls on arms brokers. DFID realized that these types of control don't really have much impact or benefit unless they are accompanied by a whole set of measures that address the context in which weapons are used—why people feel the need to acquire weapons and why they feel the need to use them. This is now essentially the focus of DFID's work and the dialogue in which it is trying to engage others. Also, while it has legal requirements to spend 90 percent of the money in low-income countries, a lot of the countries that have very high rates of gun violence—Brazil, for example—are middle-income countries. There is a close relationship between high levels of violence and extreme poverty in those countries, and her department is struggling to resolve this dilemma.

She explained that the primary purpose of all this aid is poverty reduction, not violence prevention or conflict reduction. Her department's skepticism about diverting its resources into this area mirrors that of the donor community and national governments in what they perceive to be the "securitization" of aid—spending aid on security objectives with the extreme end of that spectrum being spending on counterterrorism. In 2005, DFID attempted to recast a lot its work on security in terms that would resonate with the development community, which she stated may also facilitate its ability to meet the target of putting 0.7 percent of the gross domestic product (GDP) into development. Ms. Joseph explained that violence was reclassified to be consistent with DFID's particular focus on service delivery by stating that security is a basic service to which everybody, especially the poor, has a right—just the same as a right to health, education, and food.

### Evidentiary Needs for the Development Agenda

Joseph observed that many donor agencies or development actors treat violence as a "kind of external shock" with which they have to deal or cope, likely by working around it, but not actually addressing it. It is necessary to help donors and development agencies understand that there is something that can and should be done and—if it is done—will actually make a huge difference in the success of development interventions. She emphasized the need for evidence that violence impedes development and that violence prevention is effective in order to elevate it to the development agenda, and she hailed public health, and criminal justice to a lesser degree, for providing some of the best evidence to date.

Improved monitoring and evaluation of this area with the inclusion of economic indicators are essential to be able to explain this issue in economic terms. Joseph stated that it is not enough to say that intervention X is actually reducing the level of violence; rather, go the extra mile to say that a reduced level of violence is creating economic opportunities and that economic indicators are going up. Consistent with Butchart, Mercy et al., and Zaro et al., she also identified the need to build a capacity for systematic data collection in developing countries, including having governments build the kinds of datasets that underlie the United Nations Development Programme's Human Development Index or the World Bank's World Development Index. These data help donors assess whether countries are meeting the Millennium Development Goals. She said that many successes in this area are community-based or local and queried how they can be scaled up to the national level. She also cautioned that donors have a lot of pressure to obligate and allocate money quickly, and that it can most easily and preferably be done through governments, usually central government. The seemingly counterintuitive challenge, she stated, is to figure out how donors can fund larger, longer-term programs—spend more money, not less. Joseph identified analytical tools, models, programming ideas, and good practice as areas that need strengthening. Although she recognized that there is no one-size-fits-all approach or a true model, she identified the need to facilitate better understanding of the types of interventions that are being talking about.

Ms. Joseph acknowledged a trade-off between integrating violence prevention into existing work and developing stand-alone initiatives by querying whether it is really a matter of putting a violence prevention lens on the development work that is already being done or whether it is something else. Almost all donors have committed to the principle of country-level development defined in the Paris Declaration on Aid Effectiveness—this means letting a country decide its own priorities for action. So, donor action is rightly and increasingly led by a country's priorities, with donor support for the budget as a whole or for a particular sector. Simply stated, violence prevention also has to be a priority for developing country governments who will then request funding for it. If countries don't prioritize violence and continue instead to concentrate on universal primary education or other issues, it is difficult for donors to suggest elevating the issue on the country-identified agenda. She observed that decision making for countries to prioritize violence prevention may be affected by political influences, which can contribute to differences in "outsider" and "insider" perspectives. To outsiders, the violence may seem chaotic, but to insiders, not only may there be vested interests in perpetuating violence, but also it may be quite organized. Lastly, to address many of the necessary, but missing, elements to elevate violence prevention on the development agenda, DFID is working within the Organisation for Economic Cooperation and Development's Development Assistance Committee to develop guidance for donors on programming for prevention of armed violence. As a result of the workshop, she also identified a potential collaboration with the WHO-led Violence Prevention Alliance in this regard.

## UNICEF AND PREVENTION OF VIOLENCE AGAINST CHILDREN

Alan Court described the United Nations Children's Fund (UNICEF) programs for children up to the age of 18 years and stressed that while violence prevention is a multisectoral issue, child protection also involves health, nutrition, education about HIV/AIDS, and employment opportunity. He explained that violence against children is neither a minor nor a small-scale issue. It is diverse and covers harmful traditional practices such as genital mutilation and cutting of 100 million to 140 million women and girls worldwide; armed conflict and armed violence, which are responsible for 200,000 deaths and 53,000 homicides annually; physical punishment in schools and other institutions; and sexual exploitation and trafficking of an estimated 1.2 million children annually—but as Ms. Joseph mentioned, it is something that can actually be described to enable an agency to mobilize the resources to be able to address it.

In UNICEF, they talk about the protective environment for children and are dealing with a whole range of issues from government commitment to life skills development of children themselves, how parents get involved, and community awareness. He identified community awareness as really important since the political and legal environments in countries can influence the age of criminality. For example, the pressure from the public in Central America is to lower the age of criminal responsibility—in contrast to Amnesty International, which advocates a change in 100-year-old Iranian law to raise the age of criminality to 18 years, no longer permitting children (girls at age 8 and boys at age 12 years) to be executed for crimes.

UNICEF proposed a range of solutions to address violence against children, including dealing with legislative frameworks and justice systems; expanding the knowledge base to understand what is going on, as several speakers have spoken about data collection at national, regional, and global levels; supporting national assessments and national plans of action to address issues; strengthening social welfare and service delivery systems, which are chronically weak in both low- and middle-income countries; emphasizing coordination and partnerships; and leveraging the resources needed for children.

He discussed the *World Report on Violence Against Children,*[1] independently commissioned by the UN Secretary-General, that has received the widespread endorsement of countries around the world—developing countries, industrialized countries, middle-income countries—and will guide some of the future work of the organization. In the United States, he mentioned Washington was very much involved in discussions, prior to its launch, about the content of the report, which provided the first

---

[1]Available at http://www.violencestudy.org or http://www.unicef.org.

comprehensive global picture of violence in five different settings—home and family; schools and educational settings; care and justice institutions; places of work; and the community. The study concluded that violence against children occurs everywhere—in every single country, in one way or another—and suggested that violence in the home and family, especially here in the United States, could be more problematic to address than the others. However, for appropriate interventions, in his view it is important to differentiate not only the type of violence, but also where it occurs. The report also stated, "No violence against children is justifiable, and all violence is preventable." So the questions he posed were whether we recognize it, whether we are willing to address it, and whether we are willing to make it a societal concern rather than an individual concern. For female genital mutilation, for example, UNICEF found that this is an issue that can only be addressed by society as a whole, not by individuals or individual families, and the most effective thing is to provide data and information to communities who are much more likely to make their own decisions to drop the practice as evidenced in Senegal. He also noted that the World Economic Forum in Amman actually concluded that issues of high unemployment are linked to violence among youth and the tendency toward greater violence among young people because of the inability of the educational systems throughout the Middle East to provide the necessary education to produce the labor force that is necessary throughout the country.

Court mentioned that upcoming UNICEF programs on the prevention of violence and responding to violence against children will be based on the findings of the *World Report on Violence Against Children*. A finding of particular importance is the need to systematically collect and synthesize information. Although there are data and evidence, he stated that they are by no means sufficient or of sufficient quality to actually build up programs. One major UNICEF activity under way is a review of the Graça Machel study of children in armed conflict that was started in 1996. The goals of the review are to understand the changing nature of conflict in the past decade, to review systemic-level developments, to assess policy frameworks of the United Nations and others, and to develop recommendations to define a platform for next decade. This review will be presented in October 2007 by the Secretary-General's special envoy for children in armed conflict. Additionally, UNICEF is undertaking research on the direct and indirect impacts of small weapons and light arms on children. Related to human security, he noted that Japan, along with other countries, is examining how post-conflict, social reconstruction might be something different in terms of a way for people to get back together that will sow the seeds of peace. Often something as simple as reintegrating refugees can, in fact, cause future conflict between them and those who never left.

Another area he emphasized for minimizing violence against children is legislation and advocacy, with UNICEF work already under way. In 2006, various international standards, laws, and amendments on violence against women and children that do exist were adopted by 15 countries. UNICEF and the French government cosponsored a February 2007 meeting in which the Paris Commitment (different from the one on aid effectiveness) was codified and adopted by 59 countries. This declaration is a commitment on freeing children from armed conflict as victims of and participants in conflict. He stated that Lebanon's and Israel's recent use of cluster munitions has increased the international impetus to reduce or ban the use of this type of munitions, while noting that many countries including the United States and the United Kingdom have still not banned the use of cluster munitions.

Mr. Court identified other UNICEF efforts including strengthening institutional capacity, especially where there are weak social assistance or social welfare programs, in 64 countries around the world. Included in this capacity-building effort is the examination of tracing systems, reintegration programs in emergency settings, and what is set up in post-conflict countries. UNICEF's collaborative partnerships have produced and disseminated handbooks on child protection, child trafficking, violence in general, and reducing gun violence. UNICEF has a multisectoral child survival strategy, which examines and considers indirect and direct causes of childhood death, including communicable disease and malnutrition. UNICEF is also examining recent evidence from the University of the West Indies and others on the problems relating to young child development and preschool, as well as research that examines the effect of events and activities during pregnancy and postpregnancy that may have a direct influence on the development of children.

When asked about organizational resources that would be needed to address the many components he described, Court stated UNICEF estimates, based on a five-year follow-up to the UN study on violence against children, would total $25 million annually. Fiscal resources for follow-up of the steps needed to address female genital mutilation and cutting were estimated through the year 2015 and totaled $240 million. He stated that he thought these estimates to be eminently reachable. He noted, however, that improved collaboration, not a continuation of "individual work on individual strands of the problem," would move violence prevention forward as a collective action on multiple agendas.

## GENDER-BASED VIOLENCE IN THE CARIBBEAN

Elsie LeFranc reiterated that violence is a major health problem in the Caribbean, being one of the top three contributors to years of life lost, with the heaviest toll among young people. She stated that it is now clear that the health and economic burden of violence and injury should no longer be measured only in terms of the effects of death and injury on the immediate victims. Of great importance also, she stated, are the likely short- and longer-term consequences—including the hindrance that these kinds of problems are likely to be to the economic development of these countries. She hypothesized that these factors likely persuaded the Wellcome Trust of the importance of investing in basic research to examine and better understand the socioeconomic determinants of the problem to assist in development of the kinds of preventive efforts that need pursuit.

In her research, she described use of the Conflict Tactics Scale to measure levels of interpersonal violence by examining a number of social variables that include migration, social networks, family structures, psychosocial factors, demographics, and the usual socioeconomic variables. She highlighted a few findings from the study. First, she and her colleagues were struck by the fact that there were roughly equivalent levels of physical violence on men and on women. Secondly, men were more at risk of physical abuse by strangers, while women were more at risk of abuse from persons known to them. Thirdly, there was more reported sexual abuse of women than of men, but it should be noted that sexual abuse of men by women can be high. Of the things that stood out, she pointed to the lack of any serious gender differential in the levels of exposure and the magnitude of the problem, especially between partners. When looking at some of the data on the perpetration of violence within partnerships, she stated that while there is probably some female overreporting or male underreporting, it is nonetheless interesting to see that fewer men were perpetrators of physical violence. She also noted that there were no statistical gender differences in sexual coercion. These findings queried the attitudes of violence that would be found in this kind of environment. LeFranc and colleagues also utilized qualitative data in their study suggesting that violent attitudes and the preference for violent conflict resolution tactics may not only be widespread, but also begin at very early ages.

She also discussed the findings from a UNICEF-supported study on violence against children in Dominica. LeFranc and her colleagues were surprised by the preponderance of violence-oriented responses perpetrated by children for seemingly mundane, nonviolent offenses such as being pushed in the schoolyard or peers ruining homework papers—which garnered responses such as cutting, stabbing, choking, hitting, beating, and sexual assault in retaliation. The data also indicated that the punishment strategies at home and at school could be harsh and violent. Certainly, where an average of only 14 percent of the children in the discussions had never been hit by a teacher and only 15 percent had never been hit at home, violent corporal punishment is widespread, possibly indiscriminate, and probably encouraging the high tolerance levels they found. The data also identified the type of instruments used for punishment including scissors, stones, screwdrivers, needles, blades, cutlasses, brooms, bottles, forks, galvanizing, or being burned at least once by a candle, hot iron, or cigarette. A study in Jamaica reinforced high rates of verbal aggression or physical violence in the home (97 percent) and schools (87 percent), while another UNICEF review of the region conducted within the last year yielded similar findings.

From these findings, LeFranc hypothesized that many of the traditional explanations of interpersonal violence and their associated interventions may not be as helpful as previously hoped. Most of the explanations, she stated, assume that a social pathology perpetrated by a small percentage of the population needed to be addressed. Within that conceptual framework, many studies look for social problems and dysfunction that could help explain those deviant behaviors and also search for linkages with other deviant, delinquent, and criminal behaviors. However, she explained that the data showing the commonality of the phenomenon among peers and between parents, children, and teachers really suggests a culture of violence and adversarial relationships—a culture in which violent and even aggressive behaviors appear to be a fairly normal and even valued means of social intercourse and negotiation. It may then be, as suggested by one study they did in Barbados and another done by other researchers in the United States, that violence is deemed necessary to maintain a workable relationship and even a "normal and deserved response to a spot of bother." In terms of the debate about whether people are inherently violent or pacific, this conclusion would support the view that violence may be inherently inevitable and is only held in abeyance.

If this assumption were true, it would imply that preventive approaches at the most scaled-up levels possible are certainly critical. LeFranc cautioned, however, that very careful thought must be given to the types and variety of entry points utilized. She advocated for interventions to target early childhood development when children begin to appreciate another person's point of view, as well as behavior and value modification with emphasis on finding necessary structural and institutional supports for sustainability. Early analysis of their data has so far indicated the importance of focusing on social capital types of variables. However, the picture is not at all straightforward. She stated there is also some evidence from other studies indicating that those involved in intimate partner violence are not necessarily involved in violence outside the domestic context. From her study, the data indicated that more attention needs to be given to the types of social institutional structures and arrangements that seem to encourage violent forms of social dialogue, as well as to parenting practices, punishment strategies, the dynamics and tactics of relationship management, and dispute resolution strategies.

In terms of what more is needed, Dr. LeFranc stated that a great deal more work is necessary to sort out the precise pathways for action in different countries. Male battery, she noted, needs to be recognized and understood for inclusion in violence prevention efforts since its predictors may differ from those for female battery. Lastly, in accordance with the remarks of Dr. Garbarino, she advocated for increased differentiation in measures according to social contexts for a better understanding of the different types or arenas of violence and therefore the different risk factors in those social contexts in which the violence and aggression are being perpetrated.

## NATIONAL AND INTERNATIONAL PERSPECTIVES OF SCALING UP PREVENTION PROGRAMS

Carl Bell explored lessons learned about suicide prevention from the Institute of Medicine (IOM, 2002) report *Reducing Suicide: A National Imperative*,[2] as well as his research on HIV prevention in Africa. He reviewed a variety of risk and protective factors (biological, psychological, social, and environmental) and urged that an integrated understanding of both is needed, emphasizing that risk factors are not always predictive because of the moderating effect of protective factors. The extensive literature on protective factors, which he described as "being all over the place," does identify some universal concepts (social fabric, social skills, monitoring children, and minimizing trauma) that could benefit from synergistic, science-based approaches to maximize resources and outcomes.

His current violence and HIV prevention work is based on a previous collaboration with Brian Flay and Flay's triadic theory of influence, which includes all of the theories that focus on health behavior change used in the last two decades. In his simplified version of this complex biopsychosocial model, Dr. Bell identified several things needed for intervention—a social fabric that connects people together, access to modern technology to monitor behavior in the population and to create an "adult protective field" for children, self-esteem, social skills, and strategies to minimize the effects of trauma. Prior collaboration with former U.S. Surgeon General David Satcher and Bell's current work have identified necessary elements for successful interventions and for constructing social fabric, many of which were reiterated in the lessons presented by Gary Yates—bringing all of the stakeholders together, the need to collect data and evidence to create synergistic and integrated systems, the importance of leadership to develop a common language and vision, and sustaining funding and programs after positive effects are noted.

---

[2] Available at http://books.nap.edu/catalog.php?record_id=10398.

His violence prevention work informed his HIV prevention work domestically and in Durban, South Africa. By working at the individual, family, and community levels, this work has had positive effects with multiple family and group interventions in terms of neighborhood social control and organization, increased primary and secondary social networking, and improved communication between youth and their parents. In South Africa, Bell focuses on social skills, teaching parents how to parent children—how to bond, how to attach, how to supervise, and how to monitor children's behavior. He noted that creating self-esteem, a sense of power, a sense of uniqueness, a sense of model, a sense of being connected—all of these things seemed to decrease the need to engage in risky behaviors. The adult protective shield in terms of monitoring children is very important. He noted that when you have neighbors monitoring other neighbors in terms of domestic violence, people modify their behavior and there are improvements in terms of punitive parenting. Bell's HIV prevention work was also found to be effective in reducing the stigma of HIV for both children and adults.

From research in the Chicago Public Schools it has been shown that when children, teachers, and parents are connected and attached; the findings indicate less violence, less suicide, delayed sexual debut, and fewer other disruptive behaviors among children, which appears to be consistent with Hawkins' findings with social bonding. Bell's research on bonding and attachment dynamics in the same school system, using Aban-Aya's Afrocentric risk behavior prevention curriculum, focused on teaching refusal skills for social or peer pressures and skills for assertiveness, negotiation, and conflict resolution. The study provides youth the opportunity to practice these skills to aid in their ability to avoid high-risk health behaviors. These social skills are taught in the context of also teaching decision making (Stop, Think and Act) and problem solving skills. Bell's work also promoted opportunities for children to become attached to their schools by creating an environmental structure during the school year and summer months, with academic and recreational activities and serving meals.

Dr. Bell's research to address child abuse and neglect domestically reduced significantly the numbers of African American children who were being removed from their homes in McLean County, Illinois. At the start of the study, 35 children per 1,000 were being removed and at the end of their initiative, the number was reduced to 14 per 1,000 children, higher than children of other races and ethnicity. He reiterated that exposure to child abuse and neglect, along with other adverse experiences such as witnessing violence against one's mother, living with household members who are substance abusers, living with household members who are mentally ill or suicidal, or living with ex-offender household members are major drivers of adult mental and physical health problems. Bell also stated that various studies have shown a range of people who experience trauma, from

52 to 78 percent—evidence of its ubiquitous nature. His research in South Africa has indicated that minimizing the effect of trauma as part of violence prevention efforts can reduce physical illness in the country's population, and he suggested that we need more research to understand how protective factors may promote resilience to posttraumatic stress disorder and other stress-related disorders.

In summation, Bell reiterated the need for more research to build the knowledge and evidence base and the need for public will to address violence prevention. He also advocated for the discontinuation of programs that have been shown to be ineffective. For youth violence prevention, he strongly encouraged participants to read Surgeon General Satcher's report[3] for guidance in moving forward.

## QUESTIONS AND ANSWERS

A number of issues were raised during this period, but the one that prompted the most discussion was how to bring all of the perspectives that have been discussed, including public health, human rights, and developmental issues together to support violence prevention in low- and middle-income countries. The panelists' responses addressed the importance of evidence gathering and dissemination of findings on the determinants, magnitude, and consequences of violence as critical to this synthesis; providing data on the costs and benefits of violence prevention; and building and strengthening capacity for design, implementation, and research. Other important elements identified included repetition of the message; convening and engaging key stakeholders; persistence in engagement; identifying provisional or proximal indicators that can be measured as part of a review or assessment of long-term initiatives for midcourse corrections if necessary; advocacy with the national governments in countries to get them to prioritize violence prevention in health and development investment; and greater dissemination of the success of long-term violence prevention initiatives such as that of the California Wellness Foundation, which does not treat its investment like a pilot project. Further remarks suggested examining the promising and innovative work that is already being conducted in low- and middle-income countries such as Brazil and others for strategic decision making for evaluation efforts; acknowledging and using the positive effects of advocacy for international conventions, especially for children's issues; examining issues that affect the credibility of governments and donors to advocate with a human rights-based approach; and being inclusive when creating coalitions and multisectoral collaborations.

---

[3] Available at http://www.surgeongeneral.gov/library/youthviolence/youvioreport.htm.

# 8

# Opportunities and Challenges for U.S. Agencies and Organizations to Focus on Violence Prevention in Developing Countries

Fran Henry moderated this session and began by explaining the different format of the session, as well as its objectives to hear about opportunities and obstacles to advancing violence prevention from people who administer U.S. federal agency programs and from representatives of a multilateral bank and an international nongovernmental organization. This is the last opportunity in context of this Institute of Medicine (IOM) workshop to interact with the people who can influence policy, programming, and funding on all kinds of issues that can relate to violence prevention. Unlike the previous sessions, the representatives from these agencies and organizations presented a brief overview of their organizational activity related to domestic and international violence prevention, followed by a dialogue around questions posed by the moderator. This section first presents the overview of each organization, followed by a summary for each question posed.

## ORGANIZATIONAL PROFILES OF VIOLENCE PREVENTION ACTIVITIES

Tom Insel of the National Institute of Mental Health (NIMH), one of the 27 institutes and centers of the National Institutes of Health, explained that its mission is to reduce the burden of mental disorders through research on the mind, brain, and behavior. Much of the focus is on curing disease with an interest in autism, schizophrenia, and mood and anxiety disorders. NIMH is not a service delivery agency, but it does conduct studies of what the evidence base will be for specific services that could be delivered. The

NIMH has an annual budget of nearly $1.5 billion, much of which comes from Congress, to conduct research within the United States for cures that will make a difference to the American people. This being said, about 220 grants each year—as of 2006—were international grants and many of them were concerned with HIV. These grants were made partially because the principal investigators were domestic, but working in an international or global context. Perhaps 10 percent of those grants were actually to principal investigators outside the United States. For the most part, that 10 percent was funded outside the United States because there was some special expertise or some special value to the United States in supporting someone in Iceland, South Africa, or China to do the research.

In the context of this meeting, much of NIMH research really looks not so much at violence per se, but at the consequences of violence, which he stated is also true for its international portfolio. NIMH studies posttraumatic stress disorder in Israel, mothers and children following Chernobyl, the effect of HIV infection on mothers and children in South Africa, the influence of torture in Nepal, and the victims of war in Kuwait. He described a second component relevant to how they engage in violence prevention with long-term NIMH funding for projects such as the nurse visitation studies of David Olds for nearly 30 years. He stated that there are now several replications of this nurse visitation intervention in pregnancy and postdelivery that show the efficacy and the cost-effectiveness of reducing violence both of children and to children. The greatest impact of the past and current NIMH work is a focus on self-directed violence. He reiterated the statistic of 54 percent of violent deaths globally being related to suicide. This remains a problem of great and often understated importance in the United States with 30,000 suicides each year, relative to about 18,000 homicides, and of global importance with 800,000 deaths annually. NIMH has projects in Russia, China, and Scandinavia—three of the countries with the highest rates of suicide—examining how suicide can be reduced and how to improve monitoring. In conclusion, he stated that a great deal of the suicide rate in both the United States and the rest of the world is related to mental illness and there is abundant evidence that treating depression, substance abuse, and mental illness reduces the rate of suicide. He also stated that reducing access to weapons is equally important to this goal.

Kent Hill, of the U.S. Agency for International Development (USAID), stated that the agency considers violence to be a pervasive public health and human rights problem and that, programmatically, USAID has been making efforts to respond to victims' needs, as well as to prevent violence, since the early 1990s. He identified three important areas of its work: (1) conducting demographic and health surveys, particularly for the issues of female genital cutting and domestic violence to support accurate data collection; (2) providing grants for building global capacity to address violence prevention and for working with service providers, program managers, and policy makers in various countries; and (3) programmatically addressing the connection of HIV to violence because of the gender issues involved in human rights violations and gender-based violence. He stated that it is not possible to address gender-based violence unless the right to abstinence and the double standards that are often involved in male behavior, let alone coercive male behavior, are addressed and that USAID hopes to make an impact on HIV prevention. It also attempts to address victims' needs in dealing with the tragic consequences of gender-based violence. He mentioned that in 2002, the President's Emergency Plan for AIDS Relief (PEPFAR) spent $104 million for 240 activities to address gender-based violence. While he thinks this amount was too low, it was at least movement in the right direction. Programs in Rwanda, South Africa, and Uganda—costing $1.8 million—were offered as examples to address gender-based violence and to assist survivors in accessing comprehensive treatment. Hill stated that more work could be done to address male behaviors. Finally, Dr. Hill mentioned that USAID tries to work within the interagency cooperative process and the PEPFAR Gender-Based Violence Working Group that deals with this, so that agency programs do not overlap unnecessarily. He encouraged participants to refer to USAID's publication *Addressing Gender-Based Violence Through USAID's Health Programs* for more information about its programs, as well as to PEPFAR's report on gender-based violence and HIV/AIDS. These documents are available from PEPFAR and USAID websites.[1]

Stephen Blount from the U.S. Centers for Disease Control and Prevention (CDC) said CDC recognizes that violence in developing countries has an important impact on U.S. citizens and therefore our national interests. CDC attempts to be a resource to the World Health Organisation (WHO), the international community, and developing countries. In the area of insecurity, Blount stated that it is clear to CDC that violence breeds chaos and chaos breeds violence. Additionally, it recognizes the impact of violence on economic growth in developing countries and therefore the impact on commerce and trade for the global community, including the U.S. economy. CDC also recognizes the safety risks to U.S. citizens who travel and work abroad. Blount acknowledged the link between violence and other health problems in developing countries, and because of this, CDC works very closely with USAID in PEPFAR activities. Through CDC's programmatic activities abroad and its extensive history and experience of working in developing countries, it addresses the unfortunate link of violence with broader reproductive health issues, issues of refugee health, substance abuse, and many other problems. Dr. Blount also acknowledged that some

---

[1]Available at http:// www.pepfar.gov and http://www.usaid.gov/.

of the lessons learned in the United States can help inform the research agenda and programmatic work in developing countries.

For all of CDC's recognition and programmatic efforts, he acknowledged that with an agency budget of $9 billion, it invests about $1 billion in international activities. However, less than $1 million of that amount is invested in activities related to violence prevention (compared to zero dollars five years ago). Blount explained that this investment supports partnerships with the Inter-American Coalition for the Prevention of Violence, WHO, the Pan-American Health Organization (PAHO), and the Violence Prevention Alliance. CDC attempts to make contributions to the four steps of the public health approach described by Mark Rosenberg. To define the problem, it works closely with WHO and, in 2004, collaboratively published guidelines for conducting community surveys on injuries and violence. In 2007, the first expert meeting on improving collection and analysis of data on violence and injuries would be held. CDC has recently completed a report on sexual violence against female children in Swaziland based on the first national survey to be conducted on this topic in that country. This report documents the magnitude of the problem and subsequent analyses will address risk and protective factors. In 2004, it supported another WHO publication *The Economic Dimensions of Interpersonal Violence*, which it hopes will be a key step to speaking the language of decision makers, particularly ministers of finance, who will be making the important investments in violence prevention at a national level. To develop and test prevention strategies, proven and promising prevention practices in the WHO handbook are currently being piloted in a number of countries. CDC also supported the 2003 PAHO publication *Violence Against Women: The Health Sector Responds* and is now working with the its Chinese counterpart on a national plan for suicide prevention. To ensure widespread adoption of proven policies, CDC is working with the partnerships mentioned above to advance and make available these best practices.

Marco Ferroni of the Inter-American Development Bank (IDB) described the operational institution that finances projects and investments, provides technical expertise and assistance in the design and implementation of policies and programs, and offers platforms for learning in many different sectors, including this particular sector of citizen security and crime and violence. The Inter-American Development Bank is a regional development bank that works around the world, and his focus is in Latin America and the Caribbean—a region where crime and violence are endemic and growing and where the problem of crime and violence is increasingly recognized as a development problem. IDB recognizes violence as both a public health and a law enforcement problem and even concedes that, sectorally speaking, it may be many other things; but its perspective is that violence is a development problem that affects the business climate, and therefore the growth potential, of the countries in the region. Like Bell, Ferroni explained that violence also affects the scope for human development aid by infringing on the factors that determine social cohesion, affecting how societies operate. The learning platforms that he mentioned have shown that there are thousands and thousands of municipalities and small towns in the region where the authorities and the population in general do not know what they can do or what has already been achieved in the very region—for example, in Colombia. Therefore, he explained that these communities often address the problem of crime and violence by means of populist measures that have little chance of getting at the multiple, often subtle, and usually very complex roots of the problem. He proposed that more outreach and more platforms for learning are needed.

The IDB is currently engaged in 12 countries, with projects that have been requested by the countries' governments. Dr. Ferroni noted that government demand for these projects is increasing. He described its approach as holistic, since this is a multidimensional and multicausal challenge and said it seeks to address causes rather than symptoms. The approach is intended to be epidemiological in nature in the sense that different risk factors are assessed and factored into an integrated risk management approach that relies on contributions from many departments and many sectors—health, education, family welfare, urban infrastructure, law enforcement, justice sector reform, police reform, and the role of the media. The IDB approach recognizes that data and information systems are needed to inform policy and communication strategies and that programs have to be monitored and evaluated in order to create a basis for learning and do better next time around. The approach, which he also described as being about building citizenship, substantive democracy, and democratization, also calls for an engagement of the community and all stakeholders—that is, civil society, neighborhoods, the business sector, opinion leaders, government at all levels, the media, police, and law enforcement. Ferroni also stated that this approach rests on the belief that violence is often a learned behavior, thereby positioning domestic violence as a precursor of violent behavior in the street. IDB projects, therefore, in many cases address issues or aspects of domestic violence, youth violence, and violence in schools, which can condition young people for violent behavior.

Holly Burkhalter of the International Justice Mission (IJM), a faith-based nongovernmental organization based in the United States, described its function as a law firm for poor people by providing free legal assistance to victims of violent abuse and injustice. It has 14 overseas offices, largely staffed by nationals who are members of the bar associations in their own countries and employs an unusual casework model. The types of crimes addressed in their 14 offices in Latin America, Africa, South Asia, and Southeast Asia are forced labor, police abuse, seizure of widows' land, child rape, and child prostitution. IJM lawyers represent the victims and help them access services, take their cases to the authorities, and help investigate those cases—basically "walking alongside the authorities"—to attempt national court prosecution of "crimes that would never have seen the light of day."

She described the IJM work in Guatemala with a staff of about six people, including lawyers, investigators, and social workers, as a concrete example of its operational model. This small staff undertook the exclusive prosecution of cases of child sexual abuse and child rape (some of them involving foreign pedophiles). Since October 2006, of the 11 cases IJM investigated, brought to the authorities, and helped to prosecute, there have been convictions and jail time in all 11 cases, which she described as an "unheard-of record in a country that can barely prosecute anything." She said that there was will and conviction on the part of the authorities to prosecute, but they just didn't have the resources or the knowledge to accomplish this. In all cases, Burkhalter stated, the idea was to bring immediate relief to the victim, followed by securing perpetrator accountability, and finally, attending to the aftercare needs of the victim, which in the particular case of child rape and child prostitution could go on for many, many years.

Through its efforts, IJM hopes to create a social demand for seeing the system work for the poorest and, eventually, to assist the government's response by developing the skills it needs to do the job of governance. IJM also hopes to scale up and replicate its work when a working model has been proven. IJM has received a $5 million grant from the Bill and Melinda Gates Foundation for a study in a new location, which will include an evaluation component to measure the impact on the incidence of the crime itself in a high child-trafficking incident area, and also to measure the impact on the local police and justice system. The larger implications of successful prosecution of many child prostitution cases, which are basically economic crimes since sex trafficking is a "money maker" accompanied by debt bondage and enforced labor, may force adjustments in the brothel community and among traffickers. In the area of child prostitution in Cambodia where IJM has been involved the longest, it has helped bring 85 cases to conviction with serious jail time.

IJM is also now engaged in trying to study the implications on the crime itself—researching whether deterrence can occur in real time (not waiting until poverty has been eradicated and a functioning justice system created) in countries, even given their flawed justice systems, many of which are corrupt, all of which are poor. Anecdotally, Ms. Burkhalter stated that IJM believes this to be the case in Thailand and Cambodia where it has done work.

Thomas Feucht of the National Institute of Justice (NIJ) of the U.S. Department of Justice described the sole function of the institute as the independent research, development, and evaluation arm of the Department of Justice. NIJ is housed in a family of agencies that are focused principally on state and local issues, including the Office of Justice Programs, the Bureau of Justice Statistics, and the Office of Juvenile Justice and Delinquency Prevention. It has an annual budget for social and behavioral science, which is Feucht's area of responsibility, of approximately $14 million. To this workshop audience, one of the most important contributions of NIJ is its violence against women research portfolio, which over the last 12 years he thinks has made huge strides in understanding and solving problems of victims of violence against women in the United States.

NIJ also conducts basic research that is focused on the operation of justice—how police operate and issues of corrections and sentencing. Sometimes, Feucht stated, this puts NIJ on the side of more law, less order. He identified this research as perhaps one of the most important contributions that NIJ can make and an important commodity that can be of great value as this effort goes forward—NIJ's familiarity with and investments in the way in which police operate, understanding how police have changed in this country, for instance. During the workshop breaks, Feucht's discussions reaffirmed the important transition that police have made in this country from crime control to crime prevention. In some important ways, he stated, police have embraced their principal responsibility not as catching criminals, but as preventing people from engaging in criminal behavior. Feucht observed that the notion of community policing, which is not more than 15-20 years old, has reshaped policing.

In conclusion, Dr. Feucht also noted that the National Institute of Justice has an extremely slender window through which it is able to conduct international activities and international research since it cannot make grants to non-U.S. taxpaying entities. It does, however, have an international center and a very slender statutory mission, but he stated that the federal government was built principally of inward-looking domestic agencies and all agencies within it act accordingly. He encouraged participants to think about what kinds of resources, expertise, knowledge, research, and evidence these inward-looking, domestically oriented agencies might be able to bring to bear on international issues if the agencies were statutorily licensed and directed—not just encouraged, but ordered or expected—to think and act globally.

## ROUND-ROBIN QUESTIONS WITH THE PANELISTS

The panelists were engaged in dialogue with questions posed by the moderator, based on the assumption that agencies would need larger budgets but that this issue would not be the premise of the questions. Rather, Ms. Henry first asked whether the organizations had the authority to "go upstream" to focus on violence prevention, if this were something they would indeed be interested in doing, and whether they needed advocacy from civil society groups to obtain the authority if they did not currently have it. In response, Dr. Insel stated that NIMH has authorization to engage in violence prevention research and has been doing so for 40 years. He believes that there is sufficient evidence from studies conducted in the United States to know how to prevent violence, especially in the family setting, but the question is how to disseminate and implement what is known. Insel also stated his belief that many of the interventions are cost-effective and not high-tech interventions; he would expect cultural variations in the programs but thinks they would look basically the same everywhere and that it's worth the investment to begin to try.

Dr. Ferroni agreed with Insel in that we have enough evidence, but that the issue is about how to bring together a community of practice that involves many different types of actors—from government officials to civil society in its many expressions of the private sector, the business sector, and so on. This coalition would need to rally around a concept that might work in a particular society, a particular culture—coming up with action and an evaluation framework that would enable those who are participating to know whether progress is being made during the process of implementation. Ferroni stated that talking about how to create the authorizing environment is essentially how the problem seems to be presenting itself to his institution. He also mentioned that latent demand needs to be developed into explicit needs and explicit designs of projects and operations; depending on who is being engaged for participation, you may run into a whole range of opinions that are not compatible with each other, at least not in the short run, and a lot of discussion will be needed. For example, when talking about police reform for response and prevention, multiple issues must be addressed including improving police effectiveness and capacity for response, the need for civilian and social control, and accountability.

Ms. Burkhalter responded that for the types of crimes and violence the International Justice Mission addressed, she is unsure whether there is a way to focus on prevention without deterrence. She also stated that the human rights community has not looked to national governments and local public justice systems and judiciaries as a form of deterrence and protection. Rather, her lifelong experience in the human rights field, until now, has been that the authorities are the source of human rights abuses, and in some of the countries where IJM works, this is indeed the case. Even if the authorities are often the source of abuse, they are also the only recourse, which means there is not a "workaround for the poorest." By showing that the system can work, IJM eventually hopes it will be possible for people to actually think of going to the police when they need the help, instead of running from the police. She argued that this will not happen without some form of carrot-and-stick and pressure on international donors to make resources available, as well as a sense of communal expectation that the police will do the job they are supposed to do. As a nongovernmental organization, IJM can help with this but cannot be a substitute for it. Burkhalter does not believe that prevention is achievable through public education, and this makes the success of IJM's work even more essential; but she firmly stated that the major donors and other nongovernmental organizations cannot "hang back forever waiting to prove that a local justice system should be expected to protect the poorest. . . . We have to test that system, make demands on that system, and help that system do that job."

Dr. Hill agreed with Burkhalter's assessment of "not putting teeth to the rhetoric and working on a prosecution system" as a recipe for failure. He stated that USAID certainly has the authority to move ahead and in his opinion—with its decades-long expertise in social marketing, whether condoms, water sanitation tablets, or insecticide-treated nets—ought to use that expertise to work on behavior change in other areas, such as male norms. Hill predicted that to successfully engage lawyers and police to do what they should or lawmakers to put the right laws in place, need to aggressively attack the issue of changing male norms—which is an example of pushing ahead on several fronts simultaneously.

In response to the query of authorization to work in the area of violence prevention, Dr. Blount stated it is very clear that over the last 10 years, CDC's role as a technical agency has evolved, first and foremost in the area of HIV. AIDS has been defined as a national security issue for the United States, as well as a development issue, which has helped shape CDC's collaboration with USAID on PEPFAR and the President's Malaria Initiative. He stated that CDC "feels fully authorized, but . . . not appropriated very much," which means it makes contributions to the global effort in the settings in which it works collaboratively.

Dr. Feucht replied that the idea of moving upstream has a couple of connotations, in terms of moving from response and treatment to prevention. Over the last couple of days of the workshop, he has noticed a theme emerge—maybe not a sense of despair, but a sense of willingness to move ahead without justice agents—without police, without courts, without prosecutors—because they are just not making the move; they are the drag effect; they are the source of the problem, which he agreed is true in a lot of places. However, he offered the story of domestic violence in the United States over the past 30-40 years, and the police response to domestic violence in this country, as a hopeful story to tell. Feucht characterized it as a story of the professionalism of the police in agencies across this country, where communities that would never have taken their problems to the police now go directly to them. The success includes community oversight boards and methods of accountability. Dr. Feucht stated that "the bad news is that it has not been so long that policing and justice agencies in the United States have begun to emerge from the dark ages, but the good news is that it can be done."

Before turning the panel over to questions from the participants, Ms. Henry asked if there were some way we could form better partnerships between the federal agencies and the experts here in this room or among the recipients of the workshop report. She asked how the panel would best like to work with people who are interested in the report. She also queried about the kind of interaction that has been lacking to date and how to facilitate what is needed.

Dr. Ferroni replied that this is linked to how he thinks about going upstream. IDB is an intergovernmental institution that works with government, but it consults with many others, including civil society. Many on the staff are development economists that are used to analyzing developmental issues. Traditionally the problem of crime and violence was not considered a developmental issue, but rather more the quintessential issue of infrastructure. Ferroni stated that the work of nongovernmental groups, such as what Ms. Burkhalter has been talking about, can over time widen the range of topics that those in the agencies can discuss officially with other governments.

Dr. Blount reiterated CDC's more circumscribed role of helping to build a case, testing interventions, monitoring and evaluating those interventions, and sharing that information with the public health community. He stated that using the Institute of Medicine's workshop report to garner support and interest, both internationally and domestically, will be very important. Blount suggested that it is time to take what we already know, what we have reviewed together here over the last couple of days, and move toward both an international strategy, perhaps developed via the convening of WHO and others, and a domestic U.S. strategy, so that those in the United States can contribute to meeting the goals of an international strategy. He stated that the broad strategy would have to address the interests of the business community, the faith community, foundations, and nongovernmental organizations. These are the people, in his estimate, who will make things happen, including at the level of the federal government. Blount stated that "the case has been made, but it needs to be made better."

Dr. Hill proposed the adoption of more inclusive strategies to address gender-based violence in both male and female behaviors and norms in several contexts. These contexts include health, human rights, educational needs of women and children, and participatory civil society. For example, the evidence suggests that women and girls who are abused don't go to school. If interventions that focused on addressing the factors that promotes the violence against girls (i.e. sexual assault at or on the way to school), were integrated with programs that address the needs of women and girls, the likelihood of girls attending school may increase. Hill acknowledged that large, well-funded interventions already exist for many activities that address the needs of women and girls. He suggested that the group develop proposals in those areas that have a gender-based violence component, explaining how an intervention here will help them reach the objectives of those other interventions.

Dr. Insel reminded the group about the tragic April 2007 shooting on a university campus by a young, psychotic student who killed 32 people, then himself. While many in the audience may be familiar with this story, Insel stated that what is probably not known is that in the same week, the same number of people died, at the same age—that is, college-age people—from suicide. Dr. Insel stressed that the same number of students die from suicide every week throughout the year but that these facts are not in anyone's headline or on anyone's newscast. He emphasized that there is a need to make sure that people understand what the data tell us, which is that when talking about violent death, whether in the United States or globally, it's more likely to be self-directed than other-directed, and continued ignorance of this fact is at our own peril. Addressing this does not require a criminal solution, and 90 percent of these suicides are a reflection of having an illness of the brain that is treatable. He identified this issue as a potential point of influence for the group where it could have a major impact by renewing the focus on thinking about this part of the problem, which is correctable, not so much through criminal deterrence as through simple medical intervention. For the most part, Insel noted that these interventions do not exist in the United States and aren't even on the agenda in much of the developing world.

Ms. Burkhalter replied that she would like to see the kind of rigor that was developed in the HIV/AIDS treatment movement and response applied to the kind of human rights interventions and infrastructure development that is required in judiciaries in poor countries. She stated that while many may be critical of the president's global AIDS program, it has totally changed the landscape in terms of the rights of poor people to antiretrovirals and health. If donors could make that same kind of rigorous demand on justice systems that they want to help, then the question of human rights won't disappear and an infrastructure can be built as we are doing for HIV/AIDS interventions. She identified the protection of orphans and vulnerable children as the area in which this can be done most quickly. Hundreds of thousands of children are grieving and they are uniquely vulnerable to abuse. From its work in the AIDS-burdened countries in sub-Saharan Africa—Rwanda, Uganda, Zambia, and Kenya—IJM sees governments with some willingness to comply, good laws, and some infrastructure, but they lack a child protection system. Weekly, IJM receives multiple cases of children in foster care and institutional settings who are victims of sexual abuse. She noted that Kenya, a case in point, has authoritative will, but no resources, no database, no capacity for follow-up, and no training or ability to recognize child sexual abuse. The WHO *World Report on Violence and Health* didn't have much to say about deterrence and justice systems, but it did talk about the need for national planning. Burkhalter reiterated that lessons from the AIDS prevention and treatment movement showed that national planning, accountability, metrics, baselines, and money are necessary to build the infrastructure and capacity.

## QUESTIONS FROM PARTICIPANTS

This section highlights the questions and the discussions around them. One question addressed the need for integrating efforts and developing a common agenda for violence prevention. While there seemed to be agreement on this notion, it was emphasized that a common agenda and strategy for violence prevention does not have to obliterate the differences between dealing with self-directed violence and other-directed violence: that is, between treating suicide as an illness of the brain, and requiring a criminal justice response and prevention work for issues of sexual violence and partner violence. It was suggested that this is one of the challenges of this workshop and figuring out how to use the subsequent summary to build this common agenda, while still respecting the individual differences that each of our agencies and perspectives brings. The issue of how much evidence is needed for action sparked further discussion since many of the presenters identified the need for more rigorous data collection and evaluation and pleaded for greater collaboration and funding from CDC, NIMH, and other government agencies to do this. The clarification provided by some panelists was that there is enough evidence, especially for prevention, to implement and test interventions in the United States and in developing countries without having to wait for all of the research related to these issues to be conducted. The evidence, it was pointed out, also makes a case for cost-effectiveness, as well as an ability to reduce family violence and improve outcomes even for the next generation, but this simply is not done—which is a tragedy—knowing something can be done and not applying it. It was also suggested that if translation from research to practice cannot be pushed forward, then examining why it can't could also be a research question that should attempt to resolve the conundrum.

The next question that garnered a good deal of discussion dealt with the issue of agency and organizational flexibility in providing funding to civil society, nongovernmental organizations, and small communities and municipalities that have great initiatives and are trying to find solutions on their own, but need funding for implementation and evaluation. Some of the panelists indicated that they do have flexibility, but underscored the importance of working through central governments and ministries of finance to try to build capacity and sustainability, despite the bureaucracy and corruption that sometimes exist.

In response to a query from the audience about collaboration, it was acknowledged among the panelists that their participation in this workshop session was the first time they have been "in the same room at the same time." Multiple comments made it apparent that many in the room, including participants, were captivated by the potential of what could be accomplished with a concerted amalgamation of the panelists' programming and research portfolios, budgets, and expertise. The last question addressed the issue of ignoring the data about self-directed violence by asking about the potential impact of the Wellstone bill for mental health parity and the president's New Freedom Commission report on the need to transform the mental health system of the United States. The response indicated that there are a great number of people in the mental health workforce, but the majority of them are not trained to do anything that has an evidence base to it. Addressing this workforce issue will not be easy and will require bringing on a new cohort of people who are actually trained to do what needs to be done. The importance of integrating mental health into the umbrella of primary health care, in a way that has not previously occurred, was also identified. In one panelist's opinion, the irony of this workshop meeting did not go unnoticed because this integration happens much better in some countries than it does in the United States, which he likened to a Third World country in terms of the quality of care that is developed and the access to care that people have. This workshop meeting was one place where, interestingly, we could actually learn from other opportunities in global health, and he mentioned that an awful lot can be learned from the rest of the world about how to do this better. Lastly, it was commented that the human rights-based work that is being done should not be overlooked as part of the common agenda in terms of the opportunities it creates for recovery from trauma, healing, justice, and accountability for victims of violence.

# 9

# Taking Global Violence Prevention
# to the Next Step:
# Questions for the Workshop Participants

Specific actions, tasks, and considerations were suggested by the panelists, but this chapter summarizes the suggestions from participants for moving violence prevention forward. Although the Institute of Medicine (IOM) does not make recommendations in workshop summaries, the participants were asked to provide feedback and suggestions for facilitating global dialogue about violence prevention dialogue and movement on the global public health agenda. The suggestions that follow should not be construed as recommendations of or endorsement by the IOM and are the opinions of the workshop participants. The suggestions for action were obtained during group sessions in which participants were asked to respond to the following specific questions: (1) How do we make a strong case that the United States has an interest in preventing violence in the rest of the world in general and in developing countries in particular? (2) How do we get sustained commitment and support from funders, especially the U.S. government agencies and foundations that fund global health work, and expand the purview of key U.S. agencies that now focus solely on violence prevention within the United States? (3) What are the important research and programmatic priorities that should be undertaken to create a solid foundation for successful violence prevention? (4) How do we encourage collaborative efforts among nations, U.S. agencies, international agencies, and private enterprise to engage in the work of violence prevention? (5) What steps should be taken by U.S. agencies to truly implement the public health approach to violence prevention in developing countries? The sections that follow are summaries of the groups' responses to those questions.

## MAKING THE CASE FOR THE U.S. INTEREST IN
## PREVENTING GLOBAL VIOLENCE

To address global violence generally and particularly in developing countries, participants suggested that economics, health, and security must be added to the moral imperative. These elements mirrored the presentations of several of the panels. Several workshop presentations showed that violence affects trade and tourism, and diminishes economic viability and market stability. Participants made the economic argument that the U.S. is part of the global economy which depends on stability. Since violence hinders investment, especially foreign investments that are more likely to be made in stable, nonviolent states, which would be seen as "better investment climates," violence prevention could be a compelling reason for greater U.S. economic interests. The groups felt it important to strengthen the "business" argument with more concrete figures for a country's investment in violence prevention (similar to World Bank and World Health Organisation [WHO] data). The health arguments were to portray violence as a risk factor and burden for other health issues (e.g., the huge impact on the spread of HIV/AIDS and its prevention, almost everyone acknowledged, cannot be accomplished without violence prevention). It was also suggested that violence prevention be incorporated into the public health agenda for maternal and child health. Popular messaging in the past around infectious disease management has stated that "viruses know no borders." A tag line that includes violence was suggested: "Bacteria do not have passports, nor does violence."

In terms of human security, the participant groups focused on the role of violence as a destabilizing force for nations and how a cycle of violence—interpersonal violence, collective violence, and terrorism—is created among unstable countries. Participants suggested that dialogue to confront the failed state argument for lack of intervention (e.g., Somalia) could be heightened and Rwanda could be seen or used as an example for success in acknowledgment of what transpired during the genocide, the provision of trauma counseling, and other activities. The groups noted that high-violence regions may cultivate individuals who reject U.S. or other outside interventions, which necessitates collaborating with local leadership to avoid negative impressions and fear of what the U.S. motives are in supporting violence prevention measures. Migration was also added as an issue to be addressed in making the case since violence cannot be expected to remain localized and isolated, which underscores the vital interest in preventing violence in the United States. Additionally, the participants suggested that violence serves as a stimulus for illegal and legal immigration, and while greater countrywide stability discourages some citizens from leaving, the "brain drain" created by those who do leave paralyzes countries that most need citizens in their technical and professional capacities. Finally, the participant groups stated that it can be important to address migration as part of the business argument because the U.S. workforce overseas incurs high costs on behalf of global violence.

Communication strategies were also identified as part of the case-building argument and included things such as adding global violence as a focus to the upcoming Institute of Medicine (IOM) study on global health, a sequel to its previous report *America's Vital Interest in Global Health* (IOM, 1997).[1] Convention of an IOM consensus committee to study the issue of violence prevention in developing countries was suggested even though it takes time to organize, fund, and conduct such a study. This committee would be able to make recommendations that oftentimes carry more weight than a workshop of this nature. Other strategies suggested included establishing definitions that build on those of the *World Report on Violence and Health* (WHO, 2002a) to foster unity and facilitate multilateral-interorganizational dialogue and promote coalition building. In making a unified and consistent argument for violence prevention, it was emphasized that the argument must be tailored to those to whom the case is being made, with precise definitions of key issues and terms.

## GARNERING SUSTAINED COMMITMENT AND SUPPORT FROM U.S. AGENCIES AND ORGANIZATIONS

This question asked participants to explore how to expand the purview of key U.S. agencies and organizations in the public and private sectors that may or may not focus solely on violence prevention within the United States or abroad, and how to secure sustained commitment and funding for global violence prevention. The groups' suggestions for securing sustained funding commitments are targeted to three actors—the U.S. government, corporate and private philanthropy, and the advocacy community.

For government, suggestions included taking advantage of the government's propensity to follow public opinion and establish a five-year advocacy strategy for major congressional commitment, advocacy for tax structures (federal and state) to have specific revenue attached to violence prevention (i.e., tourism tax), latching onto current initiatives already on the drawing board for government that can become the focused attention of grassroots advocacy, resurrecting the work done by government organizations to prevent gender violence, and considering the possibility of modifying the statutory authority with regard to federal agencies' abilities to act globally.

For corporate and private philanthropy, they suggested developing critical collaborations for capacity building and dissemination of tools

---

[1]Available at www.nap.edu.

and skills for *long-term sustainability*, identifying key stakeholders and sources of funds that can develop a viable business plan and measures to illustrate the value of violence prevention to their own corporate interests, and illustrating how sustained commitment can be conceptualized and made more manageable "in pieces" that make it attractive to potential funders. Other suggestions included broadening the focus of potential and emerging funders (i.e., women's and human rights groups who might consider violence prevention as an area in which to "make their mark") and recognizing good will, innovation, and effective interventions and efforts with global awards.

For advocacy, the ideas included strategic use of alliances and interest groups by pairing professional associations with grassroots organizations, putting a human face on violence prevention when making the case and using the media to gain more widespread support, building a broader constituency, supporting Fran Henry and Global Violence Prevention Advocacy by formalizing relationships with an advisory board, and broadening the coalition (i.e., Carnegie Endowment). Other examples included support for the International Violence Against Women Act, which will be introduced in Congress, as well advocacy for the creation of a cabinet-level Department for Peace in the U.S. government, which is a current focus of the U.S. Institute for Peace.

Finally, the groups suggested creating a national, government organization or agency dedicated to violence prevention that would serve as a unifying force and interact on an international level (i.e., partner with WHO), speak to national security issues internally and externally, address all types of violence, and have the seed money with which to start. They acknowledged that this entity would not necessarily have to be a government agency and queried whether it could be a business in the corporate sector with an appropriate plan similar to business plans for other ventures.

## IDENTIFYING RESEARCH AND PROGRAMMATIC PRIORITIES

To create a solid foundation for successful violence prevention, the participant groups prioritized evaluating the cost-effectiveness and success of outcomes, meta-analyses of current data, archiving current international violence prevention data to serve as basis for future efforts, and listening to people on the ground—learning from what has been successful in developing countries and what has been successful in the United States *with symbiotic translations from* "practice to research and research to practice." Additional ideas included developing true partnerships, increasing investment in training for research and programs, assessing root causes of violence and the benefits of prevention, and compiling country-level data so that countries can make evidence-based decisions with the ethical framework and capacity-building aspects for studies on suicide and child maltreatment using WHO (2005) *Multi-Country Study on Women's Health and Domestic Violence Against Women* as a template. Other suggestions included an overall effort to create an infrastructure for a violence prevention movement by building a field or discipline, pursuing research infrastructure grants and funding streams, archiving or warehousing best practices from around the globe, creating a pipeline for instituting relationships and collaborations between researchers and community members, and fostering a research infrastructure of those who are interested in interdisciplinary violence prevention. Finally, the groups queried whether there is a need for a specialty—which they termed "vioelentology"—to provide interagency details to promote knowledge and dialogue that would include conferences to assess the impact of violence across the life span, including its economic burden and implications as a part of the specialty.

## ENCOURAGING COLLABORATIVE EFFORTS

Participant suggestions included appealing to specific interests in varied sectors for violence prevention including faith-based organizations, civil society organizations, corporations, and government agencies; advocating for interagency details to promote knowledge and dialogue; and advocating for a 10-year formal and funded cooperative agreement from the U.S. Agency for International Development to the Centers for Disease Control and Prevention (CDC), similar to the funding for the reproductive health agreement that would give CDC more funds and more of a mandate to provide aid and tactical assistance to developing countries. The United Nations Special Representative on Violence Prevention was identified as a potentially important voice and platform to utilize. The participants' most comprehensive suggestion seemed to be to develop a *plan of action* that identifies countries that have supported violence prevention work to date and ensures that advocates and effective populations are "at the table" with businesses, nongovernmental organizations, governments, and others. The plan would also call together a representative sample of groups (not solely of academics) under the "violence umbrella" and ensure that research is participatory and would recognize the need for findings to be communicated in the vernacular back to the target community so that they are usable in real time.

## NEXT STEPS FOR U.S. AGENCIES TO IMPLEMENT
## THE PUBLIC HEALTH APPROACH

The participants concluded their group work by making suggestions for specific next steps for U.S. agencies to implement the public health approach in violence prevention. To top the list, they suggested that congressional, executive, or administrative authority and appropriations be given to U.S. agencies that engage in violence prevention work domestically to expand to an international focus. Next, conduct in-country analysis and use it as a guide for capacity building, inventory current efforts to document progress, identify gaps, and bring in other groups and other countries to develop more encompassing definitions and program efforts. This would ensure that there would be one place in which all of this information could be found, including the research and findings presented during this workshop. Next, they suggested coordinated meetings between key agencies and serious consideration of establishing an interagency task force to focus on violence prevention. Lastly, they suggested targeting PEPFAR (President's Emergency Plan for AIDS Relief) countries for violence prevention effort "add-ons" to current AIDS work.

## CONCLUDING OBSERVATIONS

Pat Kelley, Mark Rosenberg, and Etienne Krug offered some thoughts about the workshop and the next steps. Dr. Kelley stated that the IOM report of this workshop's proceedings would capture many of the ideas presented that might serve the larger scientific and implementing communities in their efforts to move the agenda on violence prevention forward. He mentioned that the report might also serve the upcoming dialogue around the reauthorization of PEPFAR, as well as the IOM's Board on Global Health for consideration in its future study portfolio. Dr Krug, on behalf of the World Health Organisation, stated this was a very important meeting because the latest evidence on what is known in the United States about violence prevention and the study of violence is of great interest to him and his colleagues. He also suggested that the way in which this workshop meeting was organized and done could become a model for repetition in other countries, because, he noted, the lack of involvement of the U.S. government can also be said for the governments of the United Kingdom, France, and many other donor governments. Dr. Krug stated that the follow-up to this meeting would be critically important and expressed his hope that the momentum and networking created during the workshop would spur Congress to empower U.S. agencies to do more in this field. He stated that the suggestions that the participants generated were considered valuable, but the most important to WHO would be for the United States Agency for International Development, the National Institutes of Health, the Centers for Disease Control and Prevention, and many other U.S. government agencies be empowered to technically, politically, and financially support international violence prevention efforts.

Dr. Rosenberg talked about John Seely Brown's four stages of knowledge development, through which he generated a scorecard to rate the current violence prevention movement's efforts. The first stage is generating knowledge—it involves research, discovery, and finding new things. In this stage, he gave a rating of "A–" because of the impressive findings of the last two decades to move this field forward. The second stage of dissemination is the spread of what we know—communications. This received a rating of "B–." The *World Report on Violence and Health* was published and a lot of copies were disseminated, but he stated that most policy makers in the United States and around the world don't really understand violence prevention; he acknowledged that adding the knowledge from the Institute of Medicine might help. Integration is the third stage, where existing knowledge on the same issue is brought together from different studies and fields. It involves bringing together different types of violence and the knowledge from violence prevention in different countries—the global south together with the global north, and the low- and middle-income countries with the wealthy countries. Finally, it involves integrating what we know about violence prevention with what others have learned about other diseases. He gave this a "C" rating because of the great deal of work that remains, in his estimate, for knowledge integration. Rosenberg stated that this workshop meeting was good in bringing people together from different fields, but that integration of the National Institute of Justice, the people who work in policing and law enforcement, those who prosecute people after violence has been done, the people who build justice systems, those who work in health and public health, the people who work in sociology, and the anthropologists and psychologists is still needed to break down programmatic and institutional silos. Finally, Brown talked about application—using this knowledge to improve the world. Rosenberg rated this area a "D" because he stated that there is much to be done to counter both the madness that engenders so much violence and our lack of action as we professionally, personally, and societally witness its consequences when we know what can be done to prevent it.

# References

Bell, C. 2007. *Risk factors are not predictive factors due to protective factors.* Presented to the Workshop on Violence Prevention in Low- and Middle-Income Countries: Finding a Place on the Global Agenda, Board on Global Health, Institute of Medicine, June 26-27, Washington, DC.

Blount, S. 2007. *A review of activities of the Centers for Disease Control and Prevention for violence prevention.* Presented to the Workshop on Violence Prevention in Low- and Middle-Income Countries: Finding a Place on the Global Agenda, Board on Global Health, Institute of Medicine, June 26-27, Washington, DC.

Bronkhorst, B. 2007. *Why the world should be more invested in violence prevention: The socioeconomic costs of violence in the Caribbean.* Presented to the Workshop on Violence Prevention in Low- and Middle-Income Countries: Finding a Place on the Global Agenda, Board on Global Health, Institute of Medicine, June 26-27, Washington, DC.

Burkhalter, H. 2007. *A review of activities of the International Justice Mission for violence prevention.* Presented to the Workshop on Violence Prevention in Low- and Middle-Income Countries: Finding a Place on the Global Agenda, Board on Global Health, Institute of Medicine, June 26-27, Washington, DC.

Butchart, A. 2007. *Violence prevention and official development assistance (ODA) agencies.* Presented to the Workshop on Violence Prevention in Low- and Middle-Income Countries: Finding a Place on the Global Agenda, Board on Global Health, Institute of Medicine, June 26-27, Washington, DC.

Caine, E. 2007. *Frameworks for suicide prevention.* Presented to the Workshop on Violence Prevention in Low- and Middle-Income Countries: Finding a Place on the Global Agenda, Board on Global Health, Institute of Medicine, June 26-27, Washington, DC.

Campbell, J. 2007. *Global perpective on violence against women and women's health.* Presented to the Workshop on Violence Prevention in Low- and Middle-Income Countries: Finding a Place on the Global Agenda, Board on Global Health, Institute of Medicine, June 26-27, Washington, DC.

Campbell, J., M. Baty, R. Gandhour, J. Stockman, L. Francisco, and J. Wagman. 2007. The intersection of violence against women and HIV/AIDS. In *Workshop on Violence Prevention in Low- and Middle-Income Countries*, Board on Global Health, Institute of Medicine. Washington, DC: The National Academies Press.

CDC (Centers for Disease Control and Prevention). 2002. *Sexual violence surveillance: Uniform definitions and recommended data elements*. Atlanta, GA: CDC.

CDC. 2007. *Report on child maltreatment surveillance: Uniform definitions and recommended data elements*. Atlanta, GA: CDC (forthcoming).

Court, A. 2007. *Violence prevention in low- and middle-income countries: Finding a place on the global agenda*. Presented to the Workshop on Violence Prevention in Low- and Middle-Income Countries: Finding a Place on the Global Agenda, Board on Global Health, Institute of Medicine, June 26-27, Washington, DC.

DHHS (U.S. Department of Health and Human Services). 2001. *Youth violence: A report of the Surgeon Genera*. Washington, DC: U.S. DHHS.

Donnelley, J. 2007. *Establishing successful relationships with the media*. Presented to the Workshop on Violence Prevention in Low- and Middle-Income Countries: Finding a Place on the Global Agenda, Board on Global Health, Institute of Medicine, June 26-27, Washington, DC.

Ferroni, M. 2007. *A review of the activities of the Inter-American Development Bank for violence prevention*. Presented to the Workshop on Violence Prevention in Low- and Middle-Income Countries: Finding a Place on the Global Agenda, Board on Global Health, Institute of Medicine, June 26-27, Washington, DC.

Feucht, T. 2007. *A review of the activities of the National Institute of Justice of the U.S. Department of Justice for violence prevention*. Presented to the Workshop on Violence Prevention in Low- and Middle-Income Countries: Finding a Place on the Global Agenda, Board on Global Health, Institute of Medicine, June 26-27, Washington, DC.

Garfield, R. 2007. *Collective violence and conflict*. Presented to the Workshop on Violence Prevention in Low- and Middle-Income Countries: Finding a Place on the Global Agenda, Board on Global Health, Institute of Medicine, June 26-27, Washington, DC.

Gartner, D. 2007. *Lessons learned from nongovernmental organizations for elevating violence prevention on the global health agenda*. Presented to the Workshop on Violence Prevention in Low- and Middle-Income Countries: Finding a Place on the Global Agenda, Board on Global Health, Institute of Medicine, June 26-27, Washington, DC.

Gordis, L. 2000. *Epidemiology* (Second Edition). Philadelphia, PA: W.B. Saunders Company.

Guerrero, R. 2007. *Importance of information for designing violence prevention strategies*. Presented to the Workshop on Violence Prevention in Low- and Middle-Income Countries: Finding a Place on the Global Agenda, Board on Global Health, Institute of Medicine, June 26-27, Washington, DC.

Hawkins, J.D. 2007. *Preventing youth violence in the U.S.: Implications for developing countries*. Presented to the Workshop on Violence Prevention in Low- and Middle-Income Countries: Finding a Place on the Global Agenda, Board on Global Health, Institute of Medicine, June 26-27, Washington, DC.

Hill, K. 2007. *A review of the activities of the United States Agency for International Development for violence prevention*. Presented to the Workshop on Violence Prevention in Low- and Middle-Income Countries: Finding a Place on the Global Agenda, Board on Global Health, Institute of Medicine, June 26-27, Washington, DC.

Insel, T. 2007. *A review of the activities of the National Institute for Mental Health of the National Institutes of Health for violence prevention*. Presented to the Workshop on Violence Prevention in Low- and Middle-Income Countries: Finding a Place on the Global Agenda, Board on Global Health, Institute of Medicine, June 26-27, Washington, DC.

IOM (Institute of Medicine). 1997. *America's vital interest in global health: Protecting our people, enhancing our economy, and advancing our international interests.* Washington, DC: National Academy Press.

IOM. 2002. *Reducing suicide: A national imperative.* Washington, DC: The National Academies Press.

IOM. 2006. *Posttraumatic stress disorder: Diagnosis and assessment.* Washington, DC: The National Academies Press.

IOM. 2007. *PEPFAR Implementation: Progress and Promise.* Washington, DC: The National Academies Press.

IOM-NRC (National Research Council). 2007. *PTSD compensation and military service.* Washington, DC: The National Academies Press.

Joseph, K. 2007. *The United Kingdom's efforts in armed violence prevention.* Presented to the Workshop on Violence Prevention in Low- and Middle-Income Countries: Finding a Place on the Global Agenda, Board on Global Health, Institute of Medicine, June 26-27, Washington, DC.

Krug, E. 2007. *Violence prevention: A global public health challenge.* Presented to the Workshop on Violence Prevention in Low- and Middle-Income Countries: Finding a Place on the Global Agenda, Board on Global Health, Institute of Medicine, June 26-27, Washington, DC.

LeFranc, E. 2007. *Interpersonal violence in the Caribbean.* Presented to the Workshop on Violence Prevention in Low- and Middle-Income Countries: Finding a Place on the Global Agenda, Board on Global Health, Institute of Medicine, June 26-27, Washington, DC.

Matzopoulos, R., B. Bowman, and A. Butchart. 2007. Violence, health, and development. In *Workshop on Violence Prevention in Low- and Middle-Income Countries,* Board on Global Health, Institute of Medicine. Washington, DC: The National Academies Press.

Mercy, J. 2007. *The impact of child maltreatment on health in developing countries.* Presented to the Workshop on Violence Prevention in Low- and Middle-Income Countries: Finding a Place on the Global Agenda, Board on Global Health, Institute of Medicine, June 26-27, Washington, DC.

Mercy, J.A., A. Butchart, M.L. Rosenberg, L. Dahlberg, and A. Harvey. 2007. Preventing violence in developing countries: A framework for action. In *Workshop on Violence Prevention in Low- and Middle-Income Countries,* Board on Global Health, Institute of Medicine. Washington, DC: The National Academies Press.

Muenning, P. 2002. *Designing and conducting cost-effectiveness analyses in medicine and health care.* San Francisco: Jossey-Bass.

NIJ (National Institute of Justice) and CDC (Centers for Disease Control and Prevention). 2006. *Extent, nature, and consequences of rape victimization: Findings from the National Violence Against Women Survey.* Washington, DC: U.S. Department of State.

NRC (National Research Council). 2002. *Elder mistreatment: Abuse, neglect, and exploitation in an aging America.* Washington, DC: The National Academies Press.

NRC and IOM (National Research Council and Institute of Medicine). 2000. *From neighborhoods to neurons: The science of early childhood development.* Washington, DC: National Academy Press.

PAHO (Pan American Health Organization). 2003. *Violence against women: The health sector responds.* Washington, DC: PAHO.

Rosenberg, M.L. 2007. *Global violence prevention: The storyline.* Presented to the Workshop on Violence Prevention in Low- and Middle-Income Countries: Finding a Place on the Global Agenda, Board on Global Health, Institute of Medicine, June 26-27, Washington, DC.

Rosenberg, M.L., J.A. Mercy, J. Campbell, A. Butchart, D. Hawkins, and G. Alleyne. 2007. *Taking global violence prevention to the next step: Workshop suggestions.* IOM Planning Committee. Presented to the Workshop on Violence Prevention in Low- and Middle-Income Countries: Finding a Place on the Global Agenda, Board on Global Health, Institute of Medicine, June 26-27, Washington, DC.

Sidel, V., and B. Levy. 2007. Collective violence: Health impact and prevention. In *Workshop on Violence Prevention in Low- and Middle-Income Countries,* Board on Global Health, Institute of Medicine. Washington, DC: The National Academies Press.

UNDOC–WB (United Nations Office on Drugs and Crime–The Latin America and Caribbean Region of The World Bank). 2007. *Crime, violence, and development: Trends, costs, and policy options in the Caribbean.* Washington, DC: The World Bank.

Waller, I. 2007. *Ounce of (smart) prevention (delivered) worth a pound of (reactive) enforcement.* Presented to the Workshop on Violence Prevention in Low- and Middle-Income Countries: Finding a Place on the Global Agenda, Board on Global Health, Institute of Medicine, June 26-27, Washington, DC.

Ward, E. 2007. *Violence prevention work in the Caribbean: Successes, promises, and challenges.* Presented to the Workshop on Violence Prevention in Low- and Middle-Income Countries: Finding a Place on the Global Agenda, Board on Global Health, Institute of Medicine, June 26-27, Washington, DC.

Watts, C. 2007. *The IMAGE study.* Presented to the Workshop on Violence Prevention in Low- and Middle-Income Countries: Finding a Place on the Global Agenda, Board on Global Health, Institute of Medicine, June 26-27, Washington, DC.

WHO (World Health Organisation). 1999. *Report of the consultation on child abuse prevention, 29-31 March 1999.* Document No. WHO/HSC/PVI/99.1. Geneva, Switzerland: WHO.

WHO. 2002a. *World report on violence and health.* Geneva, Switzerland: WHO.

WHO. 2002b. *Revised global burden of disease (GBD) 2002 estimates.* http://www.who.int/healthinfo/statistics/gbdwhoregionmortality2002.xls (accessed July 30, 2007).

WHO. 2004. *The Economic dimensions of interpersonal violence.* Geneva, Switzerland: WHO.

WHO. 2005. *WHO multi-country study on women's health and domestic violence against women.* Geneva, Switzerland: WHO.

Yates, G. 2007. *Long-term commitment and funding of violence prevention: Lessons learned from the California Wellness Foundation.* Presented to the Workshop on Violence Prevention in Low- and Middle-Income Countries: Finding a Place on the Global Agenda, Board on Global Health, Institute of Medicine, June 26-27, Washington, DC.

Zaro, S., M.L. Rosenberg, and J.A. Mercy. 2007. A logical framework for preventing interpersonal and self-directed violence in low- and middle-income countries. In *Workshop on Violence Prevention in Low- and Middle-Income Countries,* Board on Global Health, Institute of Medicine. Washington, DC: The National Academies Press.

# Appendix A

# Workshop Agenda

**WORKSHOP ON VIOLENCE PREVENTION IN
LOW- AND MIDDLE-INCOME COUNTRIES:
FINDING A PLACE ON THE GLOBAL AGENDA**

June 26-27, 2007
Keck Center of the National Academies, Room 100
500 Fifth Street NW, Washington, D.C.

*Tuesday, June 26, 2007*

8:30-9:00 a.m.        *Registration (Continental Breakfast Provided)*

9:00-9:15 a.m.        *Welcoming Remarks*

Patrick Kelley, M.D., Dr.P.H.
Director, Board on Global Health
Institute of Medicine (IOM)

9:15-9:30 a.m.        *Welcoming Remarks*

Mark L. Rosenberg, M.D., M.P.P.
Chair, IOM Violence Prevention Workshop
    Planning Committee
Executive Director, The Task Force for Child
    Survival and Development

9:30-10:15 a.m.            *Keynote Speaker*

                          Stephen Lewis
                          Former United Nations Special Envoy for HIV/
                             AIDS in Africa
                          Chairman of the Board, Stephen Lewis
                             Foundation

10:15-10:30 a.m.          *Break*

10:30 a.m.-12:30 p.m.     *Why the World Should Be More Invested in
                          Violence Prevention: Violence as a Health,
                          Criminal Justice, Human Development, and
                          Economic Problem*

                          Sir George Alleyne, M.D. (**panel moderator**)
                          Director Emeritus, Pan American Health
                             Organization
                          Member, IOM Violence Prevention Workshop
                             Planning Committee

                          Etienne Krug, M.D., M.P.H.
                          Director, Department of Injuries and Violence
                             Prevention
                          World Health Organization

                          Irvin Waller, Ph.D.
                          Director, Institute for the Prevention of Crime
                          Professor, University of Ottawa

                          James Garbarino, Ph.D.
                          Maude C. Clarke Chair in Humanistic
                             Psychology,
                          Director, Center for the Human Rights of
                             Children
                          Loyola University Chicago

                          Bernice van Bronkhorst, M.Sc.
                          Urban Specialist, Sustainable Development Group
                             in the Latin America and Caribbean Region
                          The World Bank

12:30-1:00 p.m.           *Lunch (provided)*

1:00-1:30 p.m.          *Lunch Speaker (Keck 100)*

                        John Donnelly
                        2007 Kaiser Media Fellow
                        Reporter, Washington Bureau
                        *The Boston Globe*

1:30-3:30 p.m.          *The Intersection of Violence and Health: The*
                        *Impact of Violence on Health Conditions*
                        *Including Beyond Immediate Physical Injury*
                        *and as a Consequence of Other Forms of*
                        *Violence*

                        Jacquelyn Campbell, Ph.D., R.N. (**panel
                            moderator**)
                        Anna D. Wolf Chair, Johns Hopkins University
                            School of Nursing
                        Johns Hopkins University
                        Member, IOM Violence Prevention Workshop
                            Planning Committee

                        Richard Garfield, Dr.P.H.
                        Clinical Professor of International Nursing
                        Coordinator of World Health Organization/
                            Pan American Health Organization Nursing
                            Collaborating Center
                        Columbia University

                        Eric Caine, M.D.
                        Chair, Department of Psychiatry,
                        John Romano Professor of Psychiatry,
                        Professor of Psychiatry and Neurology
                        University of Rochester Medical Center

                        James Mercy, Ph.D.
                        Special Advisor for Strategic Directions
                        Division of Violence Prevention, National Center
                            for Injury Prevention and Control
                        U.S. Centers for Disease Control and Prevention
                        Co-Chair, IOM Violence Prevention Workshop
                            Planning Committee

3:30-3:40 p.m.          *Break*

| 3:40-5:30 p.m. | *What Is Working Around the World in Violence Prevention? Potentially Effective Interventions for Developing Countries* |
|---|---|

Linda Dahlberg, Ph.D. (**panel moderator**)
Associate Director for Science,
Division of Violence Prevention, National Center
    for Injury Prevention and Control
U.S. Centers for Disease Control and Prevention

David Hawkins, Ph.D.
Endowed Professor of Prevention, School of
    Social Work
Founding Director, Social Development Research
    Group
University of Washington at Seattle

Rodrigo Guerrero, M.D., Dr.P.H.
President of the Board, Vallenpaz
Cali, Colombia

Elizabeth Ward, M.D.
Director, Disease Prevention and Control
Division of Health Promotion and Protection
Ministry of Health, Jamaica

Charlotte Watts, Ph.D.
Sigrid Rausing Chair in Gender Violence and
    Health
Director, Health Policy Unit
London School of Hygiene and Tropical Medicine
University of London

| 5:30-6:30 p.m. | *Networking Reception Sponsored by Global Violence Prevention Advocacy* |
|---|---|

| 6:30-8:00 p.m. | *Networking Dinner Sponsored by Global Violence Prevention Advocacy with a Program on Violence Prevention Advocacy (Keck Atrium, 3rd Floor)* |
|---|---|

Fran Henry, M.B.A.
Project Coordinator
Global Violence Prevention Advocacy

*Wednesday, June 27, 2007*

8:30-9:00 a.m.          *Registration (Continental Breakfast Provided)*

9:00-9:30 a.m.          *Plenary Session: Presentation of Frameworks*
                        *for Violence Prevention in Developing Countries*
                        *Developed and/or Commissioned by the*
                        *Workshop Planning Committee*

                        Mark L. Rosenberg, M.D., M.P.P.
                        Chair, IOM Violence Prevention Planning
                            Committee

9:30-11:30 a.m.         *Scaling Up International Support for Violence*
                        *Prevention: The Groundwork for Violence*
                        *Prevention and Scaling Up of Interventions and*
                        *Research*

                        Rodney Hammond, Ph.D. (**panel moderator**)
                        Director, Division of Violence Prevention,
                            National Center for Injury Prevention and
                            Control
                        U.S. Centers for Disease Control and Prevention

                        Alexander Butchart, Ph.D.
                        Coordinator, Prevention of Violence in the
                            Department of Injuries and Violence Prevention
                        World Health Organization
                        Member, IOM Violence Prevention Planning
                            Committee

                        Kate Joseph, M.A.
                        Security Policy Advisor
                        Department for International Development
                        United Kingdom

                        Gary L. Yates
                        President and Chief Executive Officer
                        The California Wellness Foundation

                        Alan Court, M.A.
                        Director of Programme Division
                        United Nations Children's Fund

Elsie Le Franc, Ph.D.
Professor Emeritus and Adjunct Professor,
Sir Arthur Lewis Institute of Social and
    Economic Studies
University of West Indies

Carl Bell, M.D.
President and Chief Executive Officer,
    Community Mental Health Council
Director of Public and Community Psychiatry,
Professor of Psychiatry and Public Health
University of Illinois at Chicago

11:30 a.m.-12:00 p.m.   *Lunch (provided)*

12:00-12:45 p.m.        *Lunch Speaker (Keck 100)*

David Gartner, J.D.
Policy Director
Global AIDS Alliance

12:45-1:00 p.m.         *Break*

1:00-2:45 p.m.          *Participant Breakout Groups*

Discussion locations:
Group A: Keck 101
Group B: Keck 105
Group C: Keck 109
Group D: Keck 700
Group E: Keck 800
Group F: Keck 1024
Groups G and H: Keck 100

2:45-3:15 p.m.          *Break*

(Facilitators of groups meet in Keck 109 and
summarize for the report back)

| 3:15-3:30 p.m. | *Group Report* |
| | |

Jacquelyn Campbell, Ph.D., R.N.
Member, IOM Violence Prevention Workshop
   Planning Committee

| 3:30-5:00 p.m. | *Opportunities and Challenges for U.S. Agencies and Organizations to Focus on Violence Prevention in Developing Countries* |

Fran Henry, M.B.A. (**panel moderator**)
Program Coordinator
Global Violence Prevention Advocacy

Holly Burkhalter
Vice-President, Government Relations
International Justice Mission

Marco Ferroni, Ph.D.
Deputy Manager, Sustainable Development
   Department
Inter-American Development Bank

Thomas Feucht, Ph.D.
Deputy Director for Research and Evaluation
National Institute of Justice

Stephen Blount, M.D., Ph.D.
Director, Coordinating Office for Global Health
U.S. Centers for Disease Control and Prevention

Kent Hill, Ph.D.
Assistant Administrator, Bureau for Global
   Health
U.S. Agency for International Development

Tom Insel, M.D.
Director
National Institute of Mental Health

5:00-5:30 p.m.          ***Concluding Remarks***

                        Patrick Kelly, M.D., Dr.P.H.
                        Etienne Krug, M.D., M.P.H.
                        Mark Rosenberg, M.D., M.P.P.

# Appendix B

# Participant List

Tanya Abramsky
Erik Alda
George Alleyne
Andrew Alonge
Roseanna Ander
Mark Anderson
Bernard Auchter
Susan Aziz
Karen Babich
Karen Bachar
Marlene Beckman
Carl Bell
Jocelyn Bell
Lanny Berman
Stephen Blount
Linda Bowen
Laurence Branch
David Brown
Nelle Temple Brown
Alexander Butchart
Eric Caine
Jacqueline Campbell
Madeline Carter
Shannan Catalano
Carme Clavel Arcas

Larry Cohen
Karen Colvard
Alberto Concha-Eastman
Marie-Therese Connolly
Linda Dahlberg
Renae Diegel
John Donnelly
Deborah Donovan Rice
Howard Dubowitz
Alan Eccleston
Joshua Edward
Mary Ellsberg
Jamie Ferrell
Marco Ferroni
Martin Finkle
Leilani Francisco
Meg Gage
James Garbarino
Claudia Garcia-Moreno
Richard Garfield
Nicole Gaskin-Laniyan
Jill Gay
Amanda Geppert
Michael Gerber
Jess Gersky

Andrea Gielen
James Gilligan
Nancy Glass
Karen Goraleski
Stuart Grudgings
Rodrigo Guerrero
Rodney Hammond
Stephen Hargarten
Pat Harner
Barbara Hatcher
Frances Henry
Irene Hoskins
Adnan Hyder
Robin Ikeda
Christine Johnson
Wanda Jones
Kate Joseph
Manisha Joshi
Naomi Karp
Meredith Kerley
Kathy Kidd
Johann Koehler
Walter Korzec
Mary Koss
Etienne Krug
Jorge Lamas
Bandy Lee
Elsie LeFranc
Jennifer Levy
Gail Lippert
Catalina Lopez
Virginia Lynch
Elizabeth Maag
Bob Mazer
James Mercy
Maurice Middleberg
Carrie Mulford

Elena Nightingale
William Omondi Odongo
Anne Outwater
Pamela Pine
Aron Primack
Frank Putnam
Paul Quinnett
Jerry Reed
Winnie Reed
Lainie Reisman
Avid Reza
Mark Rosenberg
Jaime Rothbard
Charles Russell
Prachi Sanghavi
Lisa Schechtman
Joan Serra Hoffman
Vic Sidel
Susannah Sirkin
Susan B. Somers
Susan Sorenson
Sidney Stahl
Richard Stanley
Maxine Stein
Kiersten Stewart
Rachel Sturke
Aimee Thompson
Meredith Tuller
Andres Villaveces
Katherine Vittes
Irvin Waller
Rita Webb
Stephanie Whittier
Marcia Wolf
Gary Yates
Diego Zavala

# Appendix C

# Background Papers for
# June 2007 Workshop

# PREVENTING VIOLENCE IN DEVELOPING COUNTRIES:
## A FRAMEWORK FOR ACTION

*James A. Mercy*[1, 4]
*Alex Butchart*[2]
*Mark L. Rosenberg*[3]
*Linda Dahlberg*[1, 4]
*Alison Harvey*[2]

## Introduction

In the year 2002, there were an estimated 1.6 million deaths due to violence throughout the world. This was around half the number of deaths due to HIV/AIDS, roughly equal to deaths due to tuberculosis, somewhat greater than the number of road traffic deaths, and 1.5 times the number of deaths due to malaria.[1] The largest number of violent deaths was due to suicide: 870,000 cases or 54 percent. Homicide accounted for 560,000 deaths or 35 percent. There were 170,000 deaths directly due to war.[1] Less than 10 percent of all violence-related deaths occur in high-income countries.[2] For every death, nonfatal injuries due to violence lead to dozens of people hospitalized, hundreds of emergency department visits, and thousands of doctor appointments. Over and above these deaths and injuries, some highly prevalent forms of violence (such as child maltreatment and intimate

[1]James A. Mercy and Linda Dahlberg are with the Division of Violence Prevention National Center for Injury Prevention and Control (NCIPC), Centers for Disease Control and Prevention (CDC), Atlanta, Georgia, USA.

[2]Alex Butchart and Allison Harvey are with the Department of Injuries and Violence Prevention of the World Health Organization, Geneva, Switzerland.

[3]Mark L. Rosenberg is Executive Director of the Task Force for Child Survival and Development, Decatur, Georgia, USA.

[4]The findings and conclusions of this paper are those of the authors and do not necessarily represent the views of the CDC.

NOTE: The papers in this appendix contain the views and opinions of the author(s) and do not necessarily reflect those of the Institute of Medicine.

partner violence) have been shown to have numerous noninjury health consequences, including high-risk behaviors such as alcohol and substance misuse, smoking, unsafe sex, eating disorders, and the perpetration of violence, and via these risk behaviors contribute to such leading causes of death as cardiovascular disorders, cancers, depression, diabetes, and HIV/AIDS.[3] Although the negative effects of violence are felt by all, violence also disproportionately affects the development of low- and middle-income countries. In poorer countries the economic and social impacts of violence can be very severe in terms of slowing economic growth, undermining personal and collective security, and impeding social development. Development agencies, therefore, have a major stake in preventing violence so as to ensure that their investments are not undermined by the economic and social costs of violence.

There are no simple solutions for preventing violence. Violence is, however, a public health problem that can be understood and changed. We have learned a great deal about violence prevention in recent decades, but it has become clear that violence prevention will not be achieved through a vaccination or a single piece of legislation. Rather, preventing violence will require a sustained commitment to the application of good science and the implementation of effective programs in a rapidly changing world.

We define violence as the intentional use of physical force or power, threatened or actual, against oneself, another person, or a group or community that either results in or has a high likelihood of resulting in injury, death, psychological harm, maldevelopment, or deprivation.[2] Three general types of violence are encompassed by this definition: interpersonal, self-directed, and collective. Interpersonal violence includes forms perpetrated by an individual or small group of individuals, such as child abuse and neglect by caregivers, youth violence, intimate partner violence, sexual violence, and elder abuse.[2] Self-directed violence includes suicidal behavior as well as acts of self-abuse, where the intent may not be to take one's own life.[4] Collective violence is the use of violence by groups or individuals who identify themselves as members of a group, against another group or set of individuals, to achieve political, social, or economic objectives. It includes war, terrorism, and state-sponsored violence toward its own citizens.[5]

This paper articulates a framework for violence prevention that is grounded in the wealth of knowledge we have gained in recent decades from research and programmatic efforts in both rich and poor countries of the world. The framework content draws on carefully considered recommendations that have been presented in major international reports on violence over the past decade. These include the *World Report on Violence and Health*, the *World Report on Violence Against Children*, the *Secretary General's In-depth Study of All Forms of Violence Against Women*, and the chapter on interpersonal violence in the second edition of *Disease Control*

*Priorities in Developing Countries.*[3, 6-8] This framework can be used by both developing countries and funding agencies as a guide for the types of processes and actions that are most likely to be successful in building strong foundations for ongoing violence prevention efforts, and for identifying those violence prevention strategies that are most likely to be effective. This framework is divided into two parts. The first part addresses the processes required to develop and support effective violence prevention interventions, programs, and policies. The second part identifies broad strategies for preventing violence. Strategies for preventing violence from occurring in the first place (primary prevention) are discussed as well as those for preventing violence from reoccurring and mitigating its consequences.

Ideally we would like to provide a short list of specific interventions or "best buys" that have been proven to be effective and are ready for application in developing countries now. Unfortunately, few violence prevention interventions have been implemented in developing countries with the capacity to evaluate the outcomes over a sustained period of time and collect the data needed to measure cost-effectiveness. We know that we need cost-effectiveness data to market this public health approach to violence prevention; we know that we are marketing to an increasingly sophisticated set of decision makers, and this is a good thing. Unfortunately, however, we are in a vicious circle. We have a good idea about the extensive toll that violence takes in developing countries and we have very good data to show that interventions to prevent interpersonal and self-directed violence are effective in developed countries. But we don't have the resources necessary to develop the capacity for implementing and evaluating these interventions in developing countries, where we believe they would do the most good. For this reason, we need to make the strongest case possible for investing in building the capacity to take interventions that are proven effective in developed countries and systematically implement and evaluate them in the developing world.

### Building the Foundation for Violence Prevention

To succeed in preventing violence requires building a foundation that supports the development, implementation, maintenance, and monitoring of interventions, programs, and policies. This foundation draws on many of the same skills and capacities that are needed and, in some cases, have been developed for other public health problems. Therefore, wherever possible and reasonable, efforts should be made to build upon the infrastructure that has been developed to address other public health problems to also address violence prevention. The following elements are critical for building this solid foundation (see Box C-1).

---

**BOX C-1**
**Key Elements in Building a Strong Foundation for Violence Prevention**

- Develop a national action plan and identify a lead agency
- Enhance the capacity for collecting data
- Increase collaboration and the exchange of information
- Implement and evaluate specific actions to prevent violence
- Strengthen care and support systems for victims

---

*Develop a National Action Plan and Identify a Lead Agency*

Developing a national plan is a key step toward effective violence prevention. A national plan should include objectives, priorities, strategies, and assigned responsibilities, as well as a timetable and mechanism for evaluation.[3, 9] It should be based on input from a wide range of governmental and nongovernmental actors.[10] It should also be coordinated by an agency with the capacity to involve multiple sectors in a broad-based implementation strategy.[10]

*Enhance the Capacity for Collecting Data*

Data are necessary to set priorities, guide the development of interventions, programs, and policies, and monitor progress.[3, 6-8] A basic goal of enhancing data collection should be to create a system that routinely obtains descriptive information on a number of key indicators that can be accurately and reliably measured.[9] The contributions of violence to other public health problems (e.g., HIV, mental health) should be documented and the baseline measurements for violence and its consequences should be routinely measured along with other health problems.

*Increase Collaboration and the Exchange of Information*

The work of violence prevention engages many different societal sectors. In particular, health, criminal justice, and social service institutions play a critical role in addressing the needs of victims and formulating and implementing prevention strategies. The success of violence prevention efforts depends to a substantial degree on the ability of these sectors to work together and, in many cases, integrate their efforts. Violence prevention efforts in developing countries should give dedicated attention to ways to enhance effective collaboration between these sectors.[3, 7]

Much has been learned about violence prevention in both rich and poor countries over the past several decades. Working relations and communications between international agencies, governmental and nongovernmental agencies, researchers, and practitioners engaged in violence prevention should be improved so that valuable lessons can be shared.[3] Systems and processes for collaboration and exchange of information are critical both inter- and intranationally.

*Implement and Evaluate Specific Actions to Prevent Violence*

The development of information that assesses and evaluates what programs and policies are most effective is critical.[3, 6-8] While there are no simple solutions to the problem of violence, there are a number of effective and promising strategies that can be adapted and implemented in developing countries.[3, 6-8] It is critical that such efforts be carefully evaluated in order to ensure that they are working and to build the prevention knowledge base.

*Strengthen Care and Support Systems for Victims*

Health, social, and legal support systems for victims of violence are critical for treating and mitigating the psychological, medical, and social consequences of violence.[3, 6-8] These systems can help to prevent future acts of violence, reduce short- and long-term disabilities, and help victims cope with the impact of violence on their lives.[9] Violence prevention efforts should be integrated into the health systems that are developed for the diagnosis, treatment, and evaluation of interventions and treatments for other health problems. Strengthening integrated health systems should include strengthening the capacity to do violence prevention.

## Key Strategies for Violence Prevention

Based on the scientific literature on the epidemiology, etiology, and prevention of violence, several strategic foci for violence prevention have emerged that are important for developing countries and funding agencies to consider as they decide where to invest limited resources.

## Strategic Foci for Primary Prevention

Ultimately the goal of public health is to prevent violence from occurring in the first place. While moving toward that end it is important to remember that interpersonal, self-directed, and collective violence are related to one another in several ways.[11] These types of violence share common risk factors, often occur together, and one may cause the other (e.g., child maltreatment is a risk factor for suicide). Common underlying risk factors for these different forms of violence include, for example, certain cultural norms, social isolation, substance abuse, income inequality, and access to lethal methods.[2] Prevention efforts addressing common underlying risk factors have the potential to simultaneously decrease different forms of violence. The following primary prevention strategies are scientifically credible, can potentially impact multiple forms of violence, and represent areas where developing countries and funding agencies can make reasonable investments (see Box C-2).

*Increase Safe, Stable, and Nurturing Relationships Between Children and Their Parents and Caretakers*

Decades of research in the neurobiological, behavioral, and social sciences clearly indicate that exposure to maltreatment and other forms of violence during childhood negatively impacts brain development and increases subsequent vulnerability to a broad range of mental and physical health problems, ranging from anxiety disorders and depression to cardiovascular

---

**BOX C-2**
**Key Strategies for Violence Prevention**

*Primary Prevention Strategies:*
- Change cultural norms that support violence
- Promote gender equality and empower women
- Reduce economic inequality and concentrated poverty
- Increase safe, stable, and nurturing relationships between children and their parents and caretakers
- Reduce access to lethal means
- Reduce availability and misuse of alcohol
- Improve the criminal justice and social welfare systems
- Reduce social distance between conflicting groups

*Secondary and Tertiary Strategies:*
- Engage the health sector in violence prevention
- Provide mental health and social service services for victims of violence
- Improve emergency response to injuries from violence
- Reduce recidivism among perpetrators

disease and diabetes.[12-15] Young children experience their world through their relationships with parents and other caregivers.[16, 17] These relationships are fundamental to healthy brain development and consequently our physical, emotional, social, behavioral, and intellectual capacities.[16] From a public health perspective the promotion of safe, stable, and nurturing relationships is therefore strategic in that, if done successfully, it can benefit a broad range of health problems and contribute to the development of skills that will enhance the acquisition of healthy habits and lifestyles. Moreover, evidence for the effectiveness of targeting violence prevention programs toward children or people who influence children in the early stages of the developmental cycle is greater than for interventions targeting adults. Early interventions have the potential to shape the attitudes, knowledge, and behavior of children while they are more open to positive influences and also to affect their behavior over the course of their lifetimes.[18]

Three general approaches to increasing safe, stable, and nurturing relationships are parenting training, provision of social support for parents and families, and the creation of social environments that support and protect children (e.g., policies that protect children from victimization at school). The most basic approach to facilitating safe, stable, and nurturing relationships is through the education of parents in child-rearing and management strategies. There is good evidence that these types of programs are effective at influencing the child-rearing practices of families as well as, in the cases of early child home visitation and hospital-based shaken baby prevention programs, reducing maltreatment.[12, 19-22] Early child home visitation programs include, to varying degrees, training of parents on child care, development, and discipline.[22] They may also provide support by facilitating parent group meetings or in the form of daycare, transportation, and family planning services. These programs are typically targeted at low-income families, but not exclusively. These programs, however, are relatively expensive and have not yet been rigorously evaluated in developing countries. Hospital-based shaken baby prevention programs disseminate information about the detrimental impact of violent infant shaking to both parents before an infant is discharged following birth.[21] These programs are relatively inexpensive to implement; however, there is only limited evidence for their effectiveness.

An important dimension of safe, stable, and nurturing relationships is parental monitoring and supervision. Inadequate monitoring and supervision and lack of parental involvement in the activities of children and adolescents are well-established risk factors for youth violence.[22] There is also evidence that a warm, supportive relationship with parents or other adults is protective against antisocial behavior.[22] Given these factors an increase in youth violence would be expected where families have been disintegrated through wars or epidemics, or because of rapid social change.[23] Mentoring programs that match high-risk children and youth with a positive adult role model are a potentially effective antidote to family disintegration. Although not widely evaluated, there is limited evidence that they can be effective in reducing youth violence.[24, 25] In general efforts to increase positive adult involvement in the lives of children and youth appears to be an important element in the primary prevention of violence.

## Reduce Availability and Misuse of Alcohol

Although levels of alcohol consumption, patterns of drinking, and rates of interpersonal violence vary widely between countries, across all cultures there are strong links between the two. Each exacerbates the effects of the other with a strong association between alcohol consumption and an individual's risk of being either a perpetrator or a victim of violence. Harmful alcohol use directly affects physical and cognitive function.[26] Reduced self-control and ability to process incoming information makes drinkers more likely to resort to violence in confrontations,[27] while reduced ability to recognize warning signs in potentially violent situations makes them appear easy targets for perpetrators.[28, 29] Individual and societal beliefs that alcohol causes aggressive behavior can lead to the use of alcohol as preparation for involvement in violence, or as a way of excusing violent acts.[30, 31] Dependence on alcohol can mean individuals fail to fulfill care responsibilities or coerce relatives into giving them money to purchase alcohol or cover associated costs.[32, 33] Experiencing or witnessing violence can lead to the harmful use of alcohol as a way of coping or self-medicating.[34, 35] Uncomfortable, crowded, and poorly managed drinking settings contribute to increased violence among drinkers.[36, 37] Alcohol and violence may be related through common risk factors (e.g., antisocial personality disorder) that contribute to the risk of both heavy drinking and violent behavior.[38] Prenatal alcohol exposure resulting in fetal alcohol syndrome or fetal alcohol effects are associated in infants with increased risk of their maltreatment, and with delinquent and sometimes violent behavior in later life, including delinquent behavior, sexual violence, and suicide.[39]

Central to preventing alcohol-related violence is to create societies and environments that discourage risky drinking behaviors and do not allow alcohol to be used as an excuse for violence. The evidence base for the effective prevention of alcohol-related violence is mainly from high-income countries. Much less is known about the effectiveness of interventions elsewhere with differences in drinking cultures, societal attitudes toward violence, and laws surrounding the sale and consumption of alcohol being important considerations. Increased alcohol prices through higher taxation can reduce levels of violence.[40] In the United States, it has been estimated that a 1 percent increase in the price of alcohol will decrease the probability of wife abuse by about 5 percent, while a 10 percent increase in the excise tax on beer will reduce the likelihood of severe child abuse by around 2 percent.[41, 42] Locally, minimum price policies can reduce access to cheap alcohol in licensed premises if adhered to by all vendors.[43] Reducing the availability of alcohol can reduce consumption levels and related violence. In Diadema, Brazil, prohibiting the sale of alcohol after 23:00 helped prevent an estimated 273 murders over 24 months;[44] conversely, removal of the government control of off-license beer sales in Finland led to a 46 percent increase in consumption and increased alcohol problems.[45] Drinking venues that are poorly managed are associated with higher levels of violence.[46] Interventions to improve management practice include training programs for managers and staff, use of licensing legislation to enforce change (e.g., door supervisor training), and implementation of codes of practice.[47] In Australia, a community-based initiative to improve management practice of drinking venues in North Queensland led to a reduction in arguments (by 28 percent), verbal abuse (by 60 percent), and challenges or threats (by 41 percent) within those premises.[48]

## Reduce Access to Lethal Means

The lethality of interpersonal, self-directed, and collective violence is affected by the means people use to carry out this violence. Reducing access to these lethal means may help to minimize the health consequences of violence. For example, a primary means of attempting and completing suicide in many developing countries is self-poisoning by use of pesticides. In Samoa, the introduction of paraquat was associated with a 367 percent increase in suicide rates between 1972 and 1981.[49] Efforts to control access to paraquat began in 1981 and the suicide rate dropped by more than two-thirds by 1988. Similarly, controlling access to lethal doses of sedatives such as barbiturates has also been found to help reduce suicide.[50]

Firearms are another common means for committing homicide and suicide. A wide variety of strategies have been employed to restrict access to firearms, such as mandating waiting periods before purchase, promoting safe storage, and limiting where firearms can and cannot be carried. In the mid 1990s, Colombian officials in Bogotá and Cali, noting that homicide rates increased during weekends following paydays and national holidays and near elections, implemented a ban on carrying handguns during these times, resulting in an almost 14 percent reduction in homicide rates.[51] In the Australian state of Victoria, firearm-related suicides, assaults, and unintentional deaths decreased following two periods of legislative reform: the 1988 implementation of legislation requiring the registration of all firearms and the 1996 strengthening of licensing regulations and addition of a mandatory waiting period.[52] However, the evidence to determine whether or not such strategies are effective in reducing firearm-related homicides is currently insufficient,[53] although several policies hold promise.[54, 55]

There is some evidence that homicide rates tend to increase after wars.[56] One factor contributing to this may be that weapons remaining in war-stricken regions contribute to mortality and injuries even after wars are over.[57] Many of the weapons used during the wars in Mozambique, Angola, and Namibia, for example, are now in the hands of criminals.[58] The relationship between collective and interpersonal violence may help explain why in regions like sub-Saharan Africa rates of both homicide and war-related deaths are high.[11] Efforts to disarm former combatants may help to reduce the lethality of violence that often occurs in the aftermath of wars.

### Promote Gender Equality

Inequality with respect to gender is strongly associated with interpersonal and self-directed violence.[7, 59, 60] Gender inequality has many faces. For example, cultural traditions that favor male over female children, early marriage for girls, male sexual entitlement, and female "purity" place women and girls in a subordinate position relative to men and make them highly vulnerable to violent victimization.[61, 62] More subtle cultural attitudes and beliefs about female roles may also contribute to violence and exist, to varying degrees, in every part of the world.[63] An ethnographic study of wife-beating in 90 societies concluded that it occurs most often in societies where men hold the household economic and decision-making power, where divorce is difficult for women to obtain, and where violence is a common conflict resolution tactic.[64] Rape is also more common in societies where cultural traditions favoring male superiority are strong.[65]

Maintaining the sexual purity of girls is a powerful cultural value that is associated with violence in many parts of the world. Female genital mutilation, for example, is a practice usually performed on girls before puberty in many parts of Africa, some Middle Eastern countries, and immigrant communities around the world.[66] An estimated 80 to 135 million women and girls worldwide have undergone female genital mutilation.[66, 67] "Honor killings," another extreme outcome of cultural traditions found mainly in Middle Eastern and South Asian countries, occur when a female is killed by her own family after her virginity or faithfulness has been brought into question because of, for example, infidelity or rape.[64, 68] Data on this phenomenon are limited, but a study of homicides in Alexandria, Egypt, found that 47 percent of female victims were killed by a relative after they had been raped by another person.[69]

The cultural preference for male children is associated with high levels of female infanticide in China, Middle Eastern countries, and India.[11] In China, the preference for sons is particularly strong in rural areas, where traditional cultural beliefs have their strongest hold.[68] It has also been suggested that the "one couple, one child" policy in China may have exacerbated the problem of female infanticide.[68, 70]

Suicidal behavior can be both a direct and an indirect consequence of cultural traditions that support male dominance. As an indirect consequence, women exposed to intimate partner violence are at greater risk of suicidal behavior.[59] The subordination of women has also been more directly linked to high rates of suicidal behavior, particularly among women in their childbearing years.[59] In India and Nepal, for example, culturally related phenomena like dowry disputes and arranged marriages have been linked with suicidal behavior among young women.[64, 71] In China young rural women are at particularly high risk of suicide; their rates are 66 percent higher than rates among young rural men.[72] Low status, limited opportunities, and exposure to various forms of domestic violence may partially explain their elevated rates.[73]

Examples of effective programs to prevent violence against women by promoting gender equality are limited, but there are some promising approaches. For example, in South Africa, Stepping Stones is an HIV prevention program that aims to improve sexual health through building stronger, more gender-equitable relationships with better communication and less violence between partners.[74] A randomized controlled trial of the program found that, in addition to reducing HIV infection, the men in the program disclosed lower rates of perpetrating severe intimate partner violence at 12 and 24 months post-intervention.[75] In a 3-year randomized study involving women from the Sekhukhuneland District of South Africa's Limpopo Province, the Intervention with Microfinance for AIDS and Gender Equity Study examined whether the provision of a microfinance program combined with education on gender and HIV/AIDS could socially and economically empower women and reduce intimate partner violence and HIV infection.[76] The study was a joint initiative of the University of the Witwatersrand (Johannesburg), the London School of Hygiene and Tropical Medicine, and the Small Enterprise Foundation in South Africa with funding from South Africa's Ministry of Health and the United Kingdom's Department for International Development. The intervention consisted of providing small loans (500 to 1,000 Rand) to help women start up businesses (e.g., dressmaking, fruit and vegetable sales) and involving the women in training sessions at loan repayment meetings over 6 months that explored issues such as gender roles, culture, sexuality, communication, relationships, violence, and HIV/AIDS. Results showed that experiences of physical and sexual violence were reduced by half among women participating in the intervention compared to a control group of women.[76] Levels of economic well-being improved and social changes were observed with evidence of changes in women's empowerment.

*Change Cultural Norms That Support Violence*

The cultural context plays an important role in violent behavior. Social and cultural norms that promote or glorify violence toward others, including physical punishment; norms that diminish the status of the child in parent-child relationships; and norms that demand rigid gender roles for males and females can increase the incidence of violence.[12, 59, 77] Cultural norms can also be a source of protection against violence such as in the case of traditions that promote equality of women or respect for the elderly. While evidence for the effectiveness of modifying cultural norms and values as a violence prevention strategy is limited, this approach has been an important dimension of addressing other public health issues such as smoking and drunk driving in the United States and many other high- and middle-income countries. This approach has also been undertaken, with some success, in some low-income countries. For example, in the Kapchorwa district of Uganda, the Reproductive, Education, and Community Health Program enlists the support of elders in incorporating alternative practices to female genital mutilation that are consistent with their original cultural traditions.[78]

Public awareness campaigns are a common approach to changing the cultural norms that underlie violence. For instance, the 16 Days of Activism Against Gender Violence Campaign is a movement that has generated a variety of awareness-raising activities around the world. Approximately 1,700 organizations in 130 countries have participated in the annual campaign since 1991.[79] Activities include disseminating messages through mass media channels (television, radio, newspapers, magazines, posters, and billboards) and other awareness-raising mechanisms such as town meetings or community theatre. To date, however, the link between public awareness campaigns and intimate partner and sexual violence behavior change is not well established.[79]

In South Africa, the Institute for Health and Development Communication has won acclaim for using mass media to change attitudes and basic social norms around intimate partner violence through a broadcast series called Soul City.[3] A multilevel intervention was launched over 6 months consisting of the broadcast series itself, print materials, a helpline, partnership with a national coalition on intimate partner violence, and an advocacy campaign directed at the national government with the aim of achieving implementation of the Domestic Violence Act of 1998. The strategy aimed for impact at multiple levels: individual knowledge, attitudes, self-efficacy, and behavior; community dialogue; shifting social norms; and creating an enabling legal and social environment for change. An independent evaluation included a national survey pre- and post-intervention, and focus groups and in-depth interviews with target audience members and stakeholders at various levels. The evaluation showed that the program had a positive impact on implementation of the Domestic Violence Act of 1998, positive changes in social norms, and changes in individual knowledge of where to go for help and beliefs that intimate partner violence is a private matter. Attempts were made to measure impact on violent behavior but numbers were not sufficient to determine the impact.[80]

*Improve the Criminal Justice and Social Welfare Systems*

Cross-national studies show that the efficiency and reliability of a nation's criminal justice institutions and the existence of programs that provide economic safety nets are associated with lower rates of homicide.[81, 82] In Bahia, Brazil, one study concluded that dissatisfaction with the police, the justice system, and prisons increased the use of unofficial modes of justice.[83] From the perspective of the primary prevention of violence, maintaining a fair and efficient criminal justice system contributes to the general deterrence of violence. Similarly, social welfare institutions provide basic supports for individuals and families in dire economic circumstances and, therefore, may serve to mitigate the effects of income inequality. Improvements and reforms in these systems should be considered as potentially important dimensions of national violence prevention policies and programs.[84]

*Reduce Social Distance Between Conflicting Groups*

Hate-motivated violence appears to flourish in societies and communities where racially or ethnically distinct groups hold dearly to negative beliefs and stereotypes about each other. The occurrence of this type of violence may be associated with the social distance that separates such groups.[85, 86] The greater the social distance as reflected, for example, in the frequency of interaction, the level of functional independence, and degree of cultural disparity between two groups, the greater the frequency and severity of collective violence.[87, 88] One study attempting to explain the presence and absence of communal violence between Hindus and Muslims in India provides support for this theory.[89] The findings suggest that the presence of strong associational forms of civic engagement, such as integrated business organizations, trade unions, political parties, and professional associations, appear to protect against outbreaks of ethnic violence. In relatively peaceful communities, the existence of these forms of association created a context that essentially reduced the social distance between these ethnic groups. In those settings, violence came to be seen as a threat to business and political interests that were shared across ethnic groups, thereby increasing the motivation to nip rumors, small clashes, and tensions in the bud, rather then let them fester.[89] Consequently interventions and policies that support the creation and maintenance of formal mechanisms of association between social groups, otherwise at odds with one another, may be a useful tool in the prevention of collective violence, particularly where conflicting groups are in close geographic proximity.

### Reduce Economic Inequality and Concentrated Poverty

Poverty is consistently found to have a strong and positive correlation with interpersonal violence, especially homicide.[90] However, when other community factors distinct from, but related to, poverty are controlled, this association is substantially weakened, suggesting that the effect of poverty on interpersonal violence may be conditional on other factors. These factors include community change associated with high residential mobility, concentrations of poverty, family disruption, high population density, and community disorganization as reflected in weak intergenerational family and community ties, weak control of peer groups, and low participation in community organizations.[91, 92] The juxtaposition of extreme poverty with extreme wealth appears to be an important ingredient in the recipe for violence as well. Income inequality, for example, has been found to be strongly linked with homicide rates in both industrialized and developing countries.[93-95] Furthermore, the high geographic concentration and social isolation of poor people, typically associated with high levels of economic inequality, compounds many problems that contribute to interpersonal and collective violence.[50] Interventions and policies that seek to deconcentrate poverty by dispersing poor people within more economically and socially heterogeneous communities may help to reduce their isolation from jobs, positive role models, marriage partners, and good schools.[96] For example, one evaluation of a housing voucher program (i.e., where residents of public housing are given vouchers that can be used to rent housing in the private market in any location) in the United States found that enabling families to move from public housing complexes into neighborhoods with lower levels of poverty substantially reduced violence by adolescents.[97] A systematic review of evaluations of the effects of housing voucher programs found them to also be effective in reducing violent victimization and property crime.[98] Economic programs or policies to reduce the inequalities and extreme concentrations of poverty that exacerbate these inequalities may be among the most powerful strategies for preventing violence, although the evidence base for such interventions needs to be more firmly established.

## Strategic Foci for Secondary and Tertiary Prevention

While an emphasis on primary prevention is essential for reducing the health burden associated with violence in the long term, secondary and tertiary prevention programs and services are necessary for addressing some of its more immediate consequences. In addition to their value for treating and reducing the severity of the physical and psychological sequelae of interpersonal, self-directed, and collective violence, these types of interventions are important for intervening in the cycle of violence. Violence in families and other intimate relationships is often repetitive and can occur repeatedly over long periods of time. In many cases of youth violence and hate violence, retaliation for prior acts of violence is an important motive. Moreover, children may learn to engage in violent behavior as a result of observing the use of such behavior by other important persons in their lives. Several strategic foci for the secondary and tertiary prevention of violence have emerged from our existing knowledge base that are important considerations in violence prevention planning.

## Engage the Health Sector in Violence Prevention

Physicians and other health professionals are key gatekeepers in efforts to monitor, identify, treat, and intervene in cases of interpersonal and self-directed violence. In fact, some studies show that more cases of interpersonal violence come to the attention of health care providers than to police.[99] The potential role of health care providers in these efforts is not widely understood or embraced and there are many institutional and educational barriers limiting the effectiveness of even committed providers.[100] Programs to educate health care providers are an essential first step in this process and a variety of such efforts are under way around the world.[12, 49, 101] Screening programs to identify victims of intimate partner violence, child maltreatment, sexual violence, elder abuse, or suicidal behavior are also being used in many emergency departments, doctor's offices, and clinic settings around the world, although the effectiveness of these interventions in reducing subsequent violence is not well understood.[12, 49] Despite our limited understanding of the effectiveness of various strategies for engaging the health care sector in violence prevention, activities in this area should be carefully considered as potentially important components of comprehensive efforts to prevent interpersonal violence.

## Provide Mental Health and Social Service Services for Victims of Violence

The health and social consequences of violence are much broader than death and injury. They include very serious consequences for the physical and mental health and development of victims.[12, 49, 101, 102] Studies indicate that exposure to violence can lead to risk factors and risk-taking behaviors later in life (depression, smoking, obesity, high-risk sexual behaviors, unintended pregnancy, alcohol and drug use) as well as some of the leading causes of death, disease, and disability (heart disease, cancer, suicide, sexually transmitted diseases).[12, 49] Violence also begets violence. Suicidal behavior, for example, is a well-documented consequence of intimate partner violence, child maltreatment, and sexual violence.[4, 12, 49] Given the potential for violence to impact upon a broad range of costly health outcomes, mental health and social services to intervene and reduce these costs should be considered an important component of secondary and tertiary prevention efforts. Mental health services, for example, are provided to victims in many parts of the world; however, while there is research that suggests these types of interventions can improve the mental health of victims, there is less information available on their other benefits.[12, 103]

*Improve Emergency Response to Injuries from Violence*

Unless death occurs immediately, the outcome of an injury from interpersonal violence depends not only on its severity but also on the speed and appropriateness of treatment.[104] Acute treatment of the injured requires a special approach. The establishment of trauma systems designed to more efficiently and effectively treat and manage injured victims, including those injured in violence, is an important factor in reducing the health burden of violence that does occur. Research has suggested that reductions in the lethality of criminal assault in the United States, for example, is largely explained by the application of developments in medical technology and medical support services to the treatment of victims of interpersonal violence.[105]

*Reduce Recidivism Among Perpetrators*

Data from the United States have indicated that a minority of serious violent offenders are responsible for a majority of serious violent crime.[106] Whether this is also true in developing countries has yet to be determined, but it suggests that strategies that reduce the risk that an offender will repeat acts of violence are a potentially important part of addressing this problem. Meta-analyses of treatment programs designed to reduce recidivism, particularly among delinquent and violent youth, suggest that effective treatment programs can divert a significant proportion of violent youth from future violence.[107] Those programs that have been found to be most effective in developed countries include multimodal, behavioral, and skills-oriented interventions, family clinical interventions such as Family Functional Therapy and Multisystemic Therapy, therapeutic foster care, and wraparound services used by justice systems to intensively supervise and provide tailored services to delinquent youth.[106-108]

## Conclusion

As developing countries seek to improve the health of their citizens, the impact of violence on health can no longer be ignored. In 1996 the World Health Assembly adopted a resolution declaring violence as a major and growing public health problem across the world. A framework for approaching violence prevention was first put forth in the *World Report on Violence and Health* and has been further refined and expanded in subsequent reports including the *World Report on Violence Against Children*, the *Secretary General's Study of All Forms of Violence Against Women*, and the chapter on interpersonal violence in the *Second Edition of Disease Control Priorities in Developing Countries*. The 1996 World Health Assembly resolution was cosponsored by a developing country, South Africa, and a developed country, the United States; both recognized the importance of making violence prevention a global public health priority even before evidence of effectiveness could be collected. Eleven years after the resolution, both developing and developed countries have applauded and adopted many recommendations included in this series of reports, signaling the beginning of an exciting, new agenda for public health.

A great deal of progress has been made in violence prevention. There is strong reason to believe that the interventions under way and the capacity to implement violence prevention will make a difference.[8] The lessons learned to date during public health's short experience with violence prevention are consistent with the lessons from public health's much longer experience with the prevention of infectious and chronic diseases. Violence can be prevented in developing countries if their governments, their citizens, and the global community start now, act wisely, and work together.[8]

## References

1. WHO Global Burden of Disease (GBD) mortality database for 2002 (Version 5), Geneva, Switzerland.
2. Dahlberg LL, Krug EG. Violence—a global public health problem. In: Krug E, Dahlberg LL, Mercy JA, Zwi AB, Lozano R, eds. *World Report on Violence and Health*. Geneva, Switzerland: World Health Organization, 2002; 3-21.
3. Krug E, Dahlberg LL, Mercy JA, Zwi AB, Lozano R, eds. *World Report on Violence and Health*. Geneva, Switzerland: World Health Organization, 2002.
4. Deleo D, Bertolote J, Lester D. Self-directed violence. In: Krug E, Dahlberg LL, Mercy JA, Zwi AB, Lozano R, eds. *World Report on Violence and Health*. Geneva, Switzerland: World Health Organization, 2002; 185-212.
5. Zwi AB, Garfield R, Loretti A. Collective violence. In: Krug E, Dahlberg LL, Mercy JA, Zwi AB, Lozano R, eds. *World Report on Violence and Health*. Geneva, Switzerland: World Health Organization, 2002; 213-239.
6. Pinheiro PS. *World Report on Violence Against Children*. Geneva, Switzerland: United Nations, 2006.

7. United Nations. *Secretary General's In-Depth Study on All Forms of Violence Against Women*. Geneva, Switzerland: United Nations, 2006.
8. Rosenberg ML, Butchart A, Mercy J, Narasimhan V, Waters H, Marshall MS. Interpersonal violence. In: Jamison DT, Breman JG, Measham AR, Alleyne G, Claeson M, Evans DB, Prabhat J, Mills A, Musgrove P (eds.). *Disease Control Priorities in Developing Countries*, 2nd Edition. Washington, DC: Oxford University Press and The World Bank, 2006; 755-770.
9. Butchart A, Phinney A, Ckeck P, Villaveces A. *Preventing Violence: A Guide to Implementing theRrecommendations of the World Report on Violence and Health*. Geneva, Switzerland: Department of Injuries and Violence Prevention, World Health Organization, 2004.
10. World Health Organization. *Milestones of a Global Campaign for Violence Prevention*. Geneva, Switzerland: World Health Organization, 2004.
11. Reza A, Mercy JA, Krug E. Epidemiology of violent deaths in the world. *Injury Prevention* 2001;7:104-111.
12. Runyan D, Wattam C, Ikeda R, Hassan F, Ramiro L. Child abuse and neglect by parents and other caregivers. In: Krug E, Dahlberg LL, Mercy JA, Zwi AB, Lozano R, eds. *World Report on Violence and Health*. Geneva, Switzerland: World Health Organization, 2002; 59-86.
13. National Research Council and Institute of Medicine. *From Neurons to Neighborhoods: The Science of Early Childhood Development*. Committee on Integrating the Science of Early Childhood Development. Shonkoff JP, Phillips DA (eds.). Board on Children, Youth, and Families, Commission on Behavioral and Social Sciences and Education. Washington, DC: National Academy Press, 2000.
14. Felitti VJ, Anda RF, Nordenberg D, Williamson DF, Spitz AM, Edwards V, Koss MP, Marks JS. The relationship of adult health status to childhood abuse and household dysfunction. *American Journal of Preventive Medicine* 1998;14:245-258.
15. Kendall-Tackett KA. *Treating the Lifetime Health Effects of Childhood Victimization*. Kingston, NJ: Civic Research Institute, Inc., 2003.
16. Repetti RL, Taylor SE, Seeman TE. Risky families: family social environments and the mental and physical health of offspring. *Psychological Bulletin* 2002;128(2):330-366.
17. National Scientific Council on the Developing Child. *Young Children Develop in an Environment of Relationships*. Working paper no. 1. Accessed August 10, 2006, from http://www.developingchild.net/reports.shtml. 2004.
18. Mercy JA, Rosenberg ML, Powell KE, Broome CV, Roper WL. Public health policy for preventing violence. *Health Affairs* Winter 1993;12(4):7-29.
19. Taylor TK, Biglan A. Behavioral family interventions for improving child-rearing: a review of the literature for clinicians and policy-makers. *Clinical Child and Family Psychology Review* 1998;1(1):41-60.
20. Lundahl B, Risser HJ, Lovejoy MC. A meta-analysis of parent training: moderators and follow-up effects. *Clinical Psychology Review* 2006;26:86-104.
21. Dias MS, Smith K, deGuehery K, Mazur P, Li V, Shaffer ML. Preventing abusive head trauma among infants and young children: a hospital-based, parent education program. *Pediatrics* 2005;115(4):470-477.
22. U.S. Department of Health and Human Services. *Youth Violence: A Report of the Surgeon General*. Rockville, MD: U.S. Department of Health and Human Services, Centers for Disease Control and Prevention, National Center for Injury Prevention and Control; Substance Abuse and Mental Health Services Administration, Center for Mental Health Services; and National Institutes of Health, National Institute of Mental Health, 2001.

23. Mercy JA, Butchart A. Farrington D, Cerda M. Youth violence. In: Krug E, Dahlberg LL, Mercy JA, Zwi AB, Lozano R, eds. *World Report on Violence and Health*. Geneva, Switzerland: World Health Organization, 2002;23-56.

24. Grossman JB, Garry EM. *Mentoring: A Proven Delinquency Prevention Strategy*. Washington, DC: United States Department of Justice, Office of Justice Programs, 1997 (Juvenile Justice Bulletin, No. NCJ 164386).

25. Thornton TA, Craft CA, Dahlberg LL, Lynch BS, Baer K. *Best Practices of Youth Violence Prevention: A Sourcebook for Community Action*. Rev. ed. Atlanta, GA: Centers for Disease Control and Prevention, National Center for Injury Prevention and Control, 2002.

26. Peterson JB et al. Acute alcohol intoxication and neuropsychological functioning. *Journal of Studies on Alcohol* 1990;51:114-122.

27. Graham K. Social drinking and aggression. In: Mattson M, ed. *Neurobiology of Aggression: Understanding and Preventing Violence*, 1st ed. Totowa, NJ: Humana Press, 2003.

28. Abbey A et al. Alcohol and sexual assault. *Alcohol Research and Health* 2001;25:43-51.

29. Testa M, Livingston JA, Collins RL. The role of women's alcohol consumption in evaluation of vulnerability to sexual aggression. *Experimental and Clinical Psychopharmacology* 2000;8:185-191.

30. Hunt GP, Laidler KJ. Alcohol and violence in the lives of gang members. *Alcohol Research and Health* 2001;25:66-71.

31. Tryggvesson K. The ambiguous excuse: attributing violence to intoxication—young Swedes about the excuse value of alcohol. *Contemporary Drug Problems* 2004;31:231-261.

32. Department of Social Development. *Mothers and Fathers of the Nation: The Forgotten People—the Ministerial Report on Abuse, Neglect and Ill-Treatment of Older Persons*. South Africa, Department of Social Development, 2001.

33. Bradshaw D, Spencer C. The role of alcohol in elder abuse cases. In: Pritchard J, ed. *Elder Abuse work: Best Practice in Britain and Canada*, 1st ed. London, England:Jessica Kingsley Publishers, 1999;332-353.

34. Widom CS, Ireland T, Glynn PJ. Alcohol abuse in abuse and neglected children followed-up: are they at increased risk? *Journal of Studies on Alcohol* 1995;56: 207-217.

35. Wingood GM, DiClemente RJ, Raj A. Adverse consequences of intimate partner abuse among women in non-urban domestic violence shelters. *American Journal of Preventative Medicine* 2000;19:270-275.

36. Graham K et al. Aggression and barroom environments. *Journal of Studies on Alcohol* 1980;41:277-292.

37. Homel R, Clark J. The prediction and prevention of violence in pubs and clubs. *Crime Prevention Studies* 1994;3:1-46.

38. Moeller FG, Dougherty DM. Antisocial personality disorder, alcohol and aggression. *Alcohol Research and Health* 2001;25:5-11.

39. Kelly SJ, Day N, Streissguth AP. Effects of prenatal alcohol exposure on social behaviour in humans and other species. *Neurotoxiciology and Teratology* 2000;22:143-149.

40. Cook PJ, Moore MJ. Violence reduction through restrictions on alcohol availability. *Alcohol Health and Research World* 1993;17:151-156.

41. Markowitz S. The price of alcohol, wife abuse, and husband abuse. *Southern Economic Journal* 2000;67:279-304.

42. Markowitz S, Grossman M. Alcohol regulation and domestic violence towards children. *Contemporary Economic Policy* 1998;16:309-320.

43. Møller L. *Global Alcohol Policy Alliance*. The Globe; 1:2. http://www.ias.org.uk/publications/theglobe/04issue1,2/globe0412_p5.html. html (accessed October 10, 2005), 2000.

44. *The Prevention of Murders in Diadema, Brazil: The Influence of New Alcohol Policies.* Pacific Institute for Research and Evaluation, Maryland. http://resources.prev.org/resource_pub_brazil.pdf. html (accessed October 10, 2005), 2004.
45. Mäkelä P, Tryggvesson K, Rossow I. Who drinks more or less when policies change? The evidence from 50 years of Nordic studies. In: Room R, ed. *The Effects of Nordic Alcohol Policies: What Happens to Drinking and Harm When Control Systems Change?* (Publication 42). Helsinki, Finland: Nordic Council for Alcohol and Drug Research, 2002. Cited in Babor T et al. *Alcohol: No Ordinary Commodity. Research and Public Policy.* New York: Oxford University Press, 2003.
46. Graham K, Schmidt G, Gillis K. Circumstances when drinking leads to aggression: an overview of research findings. *Contemporary Drug Problems* 1996;23:493-557.
47. Graham K et al. The effect of the Safer Bars programme on physical aggression in bars: results of a randomized controlled trial. *Drug and Alcohol Review* 2004;23:31-41.
48. Homel R et al. Making licensed venues safer for patrons: what environmental factors should be the focus of interventions? *Drug and Alcohol Review* 2004;23:19-29.
49. Bowles JR. An example of a suicide prevention program in a developing country. In: Diekstra RFW, Gulbinat W, Kienhorst I, de Leo D (eds.). *Preventive Strategies in Suicide.* Geneva, Switzerland: World Health Organization, 1995.
50. Oliver RG. Rise and fall of suicide rates in Australia: relation to sedative availability. *Medical Journal of Australia* 1972;18;2(21):1208-1209.
51. Villaveces A, Cummings P, Espitia VE, Koepsell TD, McKnight B, Kellermann AL. Effect of a ban on carrying firearms on homicide rates in 2 Colombian cities. *JAMA* 2000;283(9):1205-1209.
52. Ozanne-Smith J, Ashby K, Newstead S, Stathakis VZ, Clapperton A. Firearm related deaths: the impact of regulatory reform. *Injury Prevention* 2004;10:280-286.
53. Hahn RA, Bilukha OO, Crosby A, Fullilove MT, Liberman A, Moscicki EK, et al. First reports evaluating the effectiveness of strategies for preventing violence: firearms laws. *Morbidity and Mortality Weekly Report* 2003;52(RR14):11-20.
54. Hemenway D. *Private Guns, Public Health.* Ann Arbor, MI: University of Michigan Press, 2004.
55. Ludwig J, Cook PJ (eds.). *Evaluating Gun Policy.* Washington, DC: The Brookings Institution, 2003.
56. Ember CR, Ember M. War, socialization, and interpersonal violence: a cross-cultural study. *Journal of Conflict Resolution* 1994; 38(4):620-646.
57. Meddings DR. Weapons injuries during and after periods of conflict: retrospective analyses. *British Medical Journal* 1997;315:1417-1419.
58. Smith C. The international trade in small arms. *Jane's Intelligence Review* 1995 September;7(9):427-430.
59. Heise L, Garcia-Moreno C. Violence by intimate partners. In: Krug E, Dahlberg LL, Mercy JA, Zwi AB, Lozano R, eds. *World Report on Violence and Health.* Geneva, Switzerland: World Health Organization, 2002;87-121.
60. Mercy JA. Assaultive violence and war. In Levy BS, Sidel VW, eds. *Social Injustice and Public Health.* New York: Oxford University Press, 2006;294-317.
61. Hayward RF. *Breaking the Earthenware Jar: Lessons from South Asia to End Violence Against Women and Girls.* Kathmandu, Nepal: UNICEF, 2000.
62. Bennet L, Manderson L, Astbury J. *Mapping a Global Pandemic: Review of Current Literature on Rape, Sexual Assault and Sexual Harassment of Women.* Melbourne, Australia: University of Melbourne, 2000.
63. Dobash RE, Dobash RP. *Violence Against Wives: A Case Against the Patriarchy.* New York: Free Press, 1979.

64. Levinson D. *Family Violence in a Cross-Cultural Perspective*. Thousand Oaks, CA: Sage Publications, 1989.
65. Sanday P. The socio-cultural context of rape: a cross-cultural study. *Journal of Social Issues* 1981;37:5-27.
66. Hosken F. *The Hosken Report: Genital and Sexual Mutilation of Females*. Lexington, MA: Women's International Network, 1993.
67. Walker A, Parmar P. *Warrior Marks: Females Genital Mutilation and the Sexual Blinding of Women*. New York: Harcourt Brace & Company, 1993.
68. United Nations Centre for Human Rights. *Fact sheet No. 23, Harmful traditional practices affecting the health of women and children*. Geneva, Switzerland: United Nations High Commission for Human Rights, 1996.
69. Mercy JA, Abdel Megid LAM, Salem EM, et al. Intentional injuries. In: Mashaly AY, Graitcer PL, Youssef ZM, eds. *Injury in Egypt*. Cairo, Egypt: United States Agency for International Development (PASA #263-0102-P-HI-1013-00; Project # E-17-C), 1993.
70. Johnson K. The politics of the revival of infant abandonment in China, with special reference to Hunan. *Population and Development Review* 1996;22:77-99.
71. The People's Review. *Scourge of Dowry Raising Its Head*. August 12, 1997 (Nepal). http://www.yomari.net/p-review/august97//august-21/scourge.html.
72. Phillips MR, Xianyun L, Yanping Z. Suicide rates in China, 1995-99. *Lancet* 2002;359:835-840.
73. Heise L, Raikes A, Watts CH, et al. Violence against women: a neglected health issue in less developed countries. *Social Science & Medicine* 1994;39:1165-1171.
74. Jewkes R, Nduna M, Jama PN. *Stepping Stones, South African Adaptation*, 2nd Edition. Pretoria, South Africa: Medical Research Council, 2002.
75. Jewkes R, Nduna M, Levin J, Jama N, Dunkle K, Khuzwayo N, Koss M, Puren A, Wood K, Duvvury N. A cluster randomized controlled trial to determine the effectiveness of Stepping Stones in preventing HIV infections and promoting safer sexual behavior amongst youth in the rural Eastern Cape, South Africa: trial design, methods, and baseline findings. *Tropical Medicine and International Health* 2006;11:3-16.
76. Pronyk PM, Hargreaves JR, Kim JC, Morison LA, Phetla G, Watts C, Busza J, Porter JDH. Effect of a structural intervention for the prevention of intimate-partner violence and HIV in rural South Africa: a cluster randomised trial. *Lancet* 2006;368:1973-1983.
77. WHO-ISPCAN. *Preventing Child Maltreatment: A Guide to Taking Action and Generating Evidence*. Geneva, Switzerland: WHO, 2006.
78. Reproductive health effects of gender-based violence. In: United Nations Population Fund. *Annual Report 1998*; 20-21. Available at http://www.unfpa.org/about/report/report98/ppgenderbased.htm (accessed November 1, 2002), 1998.
79. Centre for Women's Global Leadership. Available at http://www.cwgl.rutgers.edu/16days/about.html (accessed April 11, 2007).
80. Usdin S et al. Achieving social change on gender-based violence: a report on the impact evaluation of Soul City's fourth series. *Social Science and Medicine* 2005;61:2434-2445.
81. Pampel FC, Gartner R. Age structure, socio-political institutions, and national homicide rates. *European Sociological Review* 1995;11:243-260.
82. Messner SF, Rosenfeld R. Political restraint of the market and levels of criminal homicide: a cross-national application of institutional-anomie theory. *Social Forces* 1997;75:1393-1416.
83. Noronha CV, Machado EP, Tapparelli G, Cordeiro TR, Laranjeira DH, Santos CA. Violência, etnia e cor: um estudo dos diferenciais na região metropolitana de Salvador, Bahia, Brasil [Violence, ethnic group, and skin color: a study of disparities in the metropolitan region of Salvador, Bahia, Brazil]. *Rev Panam Salud Publica* 1999;5:268-277.

84. Mercy JA, Krug EG, Dahlberg LL, Zwi AB. Violence and health: the United States in a global perspective. *American Journal of Public Health* 2003;93(2):256-261.
85. Black D. *Violent Structures.* Paper prepared for a Workshop on Theories of Violence. Washington, DC: National Institute of Violence, 2002.
86. Senechal de la Roche R. Collective violence as social control. *Sociological Forum* 1996;11:97-128.
87. Senechal de la Roche R. Why is collective violence collective? *Sociological Theory* 2001;19:126-144.
88. Black D. *The Social Structure of Right and Wrong.* San Diego, CA: Academic Press, 1998.
89. Varshney A. *Ethnic Conflict and Civic Life: Hindus and Muslims in India.* New Haven, CT: Yale University Press, 2002.
90. Sampson RJ, Lauritsen JL. Violent victimization and offending: individual-, situational-, and community-level risk factors. In: Reiss AJ, Roth JA, eds. *Understanding and Preventing Violence, Volume 3, Social Influences.* Washington, DC: National Academy Press, 1994;1-114.
91. Reiss AJ, Roth JA, eds. *Understanding and Preventing Violence.* Washington, DC: National Academy Press, 1993.
92. Sampson RJ, Raudenbush S, Earls F. Neighborhoods and violent crime: a multilevel study of collective efficacy. *Science* 1997;277:918-924.
93. Gartner R. The victims of homicide: a temporal and cross-national comparison. *American Sociological Review* 1990;55:92-106.
94. Fajnzylber P, Lederman D, Loayza N. *Inequality and Violent Crime.* Regional Studies Program, Office of the Chief Economist for Latin America and the Caribbean. Washington, DC: The World Bank, December 1999.
95. Unnithan NP, Whitt HP. Inequality, economic development and lethal violence: a cross-national analysis and suicide and homicide. *International Journal of Comparative Sociology* 1992;33:182-196.
96. Wilson WJ. *The Truly Disadvantaged: The Inner City, the Underclass, and Public Policy.* Chicago, IL: University of Chicago Press, 1987.
97. Ludwig J, Duncan GJ, Hirschfield P. Urban poverty and juvenile crime: evidence from a randomized housing-mobility experiment. *Quarterly Journal of Economics* 2001;16:655-680.
98. Centers for Disease Control and Prevention. Community interventions to promote healthy social environments: early childhood development and family housing. *Morbidity and Mortality Weekly Report* 2002;51 RR-1.
99. Barancik JI, Chatterjee YC, Greene E, Michenzi M, Fife D. Northeastern Ohio trauma study. I. Magnitude of the problem. *American Journal of Public Health* 1983;73:746-751.
100. Cohen S, De Vos E, Newberger E. Barriers to physician identification and treatment of family violence: lessons from five communities. *Academic Medicine* 1997;72(1): S19-S25.
101. Wolf R, Daichman L, Bennett G. Abuse of the elderly. In: Krug E, Dahlberg LL, Mercy JA, Zwi AB, Lozano R, eds. *World Report on Violence and Health.* Geneva, Switzerland: World Health Organization, 2002;125-145.
102. Jewkes R, Sen P, Garcia-Moreno C. Sexual violence. In: Krug E, Dahlberg LL, Mercy JA, Zwi AB, Lozano R, eds. *World Report on Violence and Health.* Geneva, Switzerland: World Health Organization, 2002;149-181.
103. Bross DC et al. *World Perspectives on Child Abuse: The Fourth International Resource Book.* Denver, CO: Kempe Children's Center, University of Colorado School of Medicine, 2000.

104. Committee on Trauma Research, National Research Council, Institute of Medicine. *Injury in America: A Continuing Public Health Problem*. Washington, DC: National Academy Press, 1985.

105. Harris AR, Thomas SH, Fisher GA, Hirsch DJ. Murder and medicine: the lethality of criminal assault 1960-1999. *Homicide Studies* 2002;6(2):128-166.

106. U.S. Department of Health and Human Services. *Youth Violence: A Report of the Surgeon General*. Rockville, MD: U.S. Department of Health and Human Services, Centers for Disease Control and Prevention, National Center for Injury Prevention and Control; Substance Abuse and Mental Health Services Administration, Center for Mental Health Services; and National Institutes of Health, National Institute of Mental Health, 2001.

107. Lipsey MW, Wilson DB. Effective intervention for serious juvenile offenders: a synthesis of research. In Loeber R, Farrington DP, eds. *Serious and Violent Juvenile Offenders: Risk Factors and Successful Interventions*. Thousand Oaks, CA: Sage Publications, 1998;313-345.

108. Hahn RA, Bilukha O, Lowy J, Crosby A, Fullilove MT, Liberman A, Moscicki E, Snyder S, Tuma F, Corso P, Schofield A, Task Force on Community Preventive Services. The effectiveness of therapeutic foster care for the prevention of violence: a systematic review. *American Journal of Preventive Medicine* 2005;28(2S1):72-90.

# THE INTERSECTION OF VIOLENCE AGAINST WOMEN AND HIV/AIDS

*Jacquelyn C. Campbell, PhD, RN, FAAN*[1]
*Marguerite L. Baty, PhD student, MSN, MPH, RN*[1]
*Reem Ghandour, DrPH student, MPA*[2]
*Jamila Stockman, PhD Candidate, MPH*[2]
*Leilani Francisco, PhD Candidate, MA*[2]
*Jennifer Wagman, MHS*[2]

## Introduction

Nearly half of the 40 million people living with HIV/AIDS in the world today are women, and women all around the world make up the fastest growing group of persons newly infected with HIV. In sub-Saharan Africa, women represent the majority of those infected and the majority of those dying. A critical aspect of this trend is the intersection of HIV/AIDS and violence against women (VAW), which has been recognized and documented with persuasive and rigorous research (e.g., Dunkle et al. 2004; Gielen et al. 1997; Greenwood et al. 2002; Maman et al. 2000, 2002; Relf 2001; Wingood 2001; Wingood and DiClemente 1997; Wyatt et al. 2002). While VAW can take on many forms including sexual violence that occurs during times of conflict, the scope of this paper primarily is a focus on intimate partner violence and the associated research regarding the overlap with HIV risk. Although men are also victims of violence, women in low- and middle-income countries are most frequently the victims of intimate partner violence (IPV), and therefore, they are most affected by this intersection.

This association between IPV and risk for HIV infection has been the focus of a growing body of evidence that has begun to shed light on the complexities of this intersection. Existing research has demonstrated several important interfaces, which are discussed further in this paper. They include the following: (1) epidemiological studies showing significant overlap in

[1] Johns Hopkins University School of Nursing.
[2] Johns Hopkins University Bloomberg School of Public Health.

prevalence; (2) studies showing IPV as a risk factor for HIV infection among women and men; (3) studies showing both past and current violent victimization increasing HIV risk behaviors; (4) studies showing violence or fear of violence from an intimate as an impediment or as a consequence of HIV testing; (5) studies showing partner violence as a risk factor for sexually transmitted infections (STIs), which increases the rate of HIV infection; (6) studies showing the difficulties of negotiating safe sex behavior for abused partners; (7) data suggesting that various adverse health effects related to IPV compromise women's immune systems in a way that increases their risk of HIV; and (8) data indicating that abusive men are more likely to have other sexual partners unknown to their wives.

As critical as it is to address this global epidemic, the issues of IPV and gender inequality remain inadequately addressed by most policy, research, and prevention and intervention initiatives in the United States and globally. The World Health Organization began the call for action in several publications highlighting aspects of the intersection of IPV and HIV (WHO 2000, 2004). More recently, the Institute of Medicine sought to extend this effort through a 2007 Workshop on Violence Prevention in Low- and Middle-Income Countries. As background for this most recent effort, this paper will provide a review of the existent literature, both in the United States and internationally; highlight the areas of new research; and propose directions for initiatives by which the complex interface of HIV and IPV can be addressed.

## Review Process

### Search Strategy

Pubmed, PsychINFO, and Scopus databases were searched using the following key words: domestic violence, intimate partner violence, relationship abuse, physical abuse, sexual abuse, HIV/AIDS, condom use, sexual negotiation, sexual risk reduction, intervention, and prevention. Searches were restricted to those conducted with women during the past decade (1998-2007) and submitted to or published in peer-reviewed journals in English.

### Inclusion Criteria

Studies were eligible for inclusion in the review if they met at least one of following criteria: (1) addressed HIV/AIDS as a risk factor for violence against women; (2) addressed violence against women as a risk factor for HIV/AIDS. All studies also had to present original data (i.e., review articles and opinion pieces were excluded). Additionally, studies had to focus on heterosexual relationships among populations aged 12 and older.

*Selection of Articles*

Articles were excluded if they did not meet the study inclusion criteria, only addressed child abuse, included multiple forms of violence such that results for IPV could not be discerned, or the analyses were not gender specific. Relevant studies were also identified by the authors based on their previous research and knowledge of the topic, and a scan of citations in the selected articles. A total of 82 articles were ultimately selected for full article review. All authors then participated in the review, summarizing and synthesizing the selected articles.

## Epidemiology of the Problem

VAW is defined as IPV (physical and/or sexual assault or threats thereof between married, romantically involved partners or former partners) and sexual assault. For the purposes of this paper, we will focus primarily on aspects of IPV (including sexual assault by an intimate) unless otherwise noted.

In the United States, approximately 1.3 million women are physically assaulted by an intimate partner compared to 835,000 men (CDC 2006). According to the 2005 United States National Violence Against Women Survey, 64 percent of the women who reported being raped, physically assaulted, or stalked since age 18 were victimized by a current or former husband, cohabitating partner, boyfriend, or date. In addition, one in six women have experienced an attempted or completed rape, defined as a forced or threatened vaginal, oral, and anal penetration, in their lifetime, and many are raped at an early age (CDC 2006). Of the 18 percent of all women surveyed who said they had been the victim of a completed or attempted rape at some time in their life, 22 percent were younger than age 12 when they were first raped, and 32 percent were ages 12 to 17 years (CDC 2006). For a global perspective of VAW, the World Health Organisation conducted a multicountry study on women's health and domestic violence. In the majority of settings, over 75 percent of women physically or sexually abused since the age of 15 years reported abuse by a partner (Garcia-Moreno et al. 2005). Lifetime prevalence estimates of physical violence by partners ranged from 13 percent in Japan city to 61 percent in Peru province, with African countries such as Namibia and Tanzania reporting estimates of 31 and 47 percent, respectively. The range of reported lifetime prevalence of sexual violence by partners was between 6 percent (city sites in Japan, Serbia, and Montenegro) and 59 percent (Ethiopia province). Namibia and Tanzania had lifetime sexual violence estimates of

17 and 31 percent, respectively. Japan city consistently reported the lowest prevalence of all forms of violence, whereas the provinces of Bangladesh, Ethiopia, Peru, Tanzania, and Namibia reported the highest estimates (Garcia-Moreno et al. 2005). Lifetime prevalence estimates of forced sex by an intimate partner varied from 4 percent in Serbia and Montenegro to 46 percent in Bangladesh and Ethiopia provinces (Garcia-Moreno et al. 2005). The high rates of forced sex is particularly alarming in light of the HIV/AIDS epidemic and the difficulty that women often face with protecting themselves from HIV infection.

Concurrently, the number of women with HIV infection and AIDS has increased steadily worldwide. By the end of 2005, according to the World Health Organisation, 17.5 million women worldwide were infected with HIV. Similarly, the Centers for Disease Control and Prevention estimated that between 2000 through 2004, the number of AIDS cases in the United States increased 10 percent among females and 7 percent among males. In the United States, women account for more than 25 percent of all new HIV/AIDS diagnoses (CDC 2004). HIV disproportionately affects African American and Hispanic women. Together they represent less than 25 percent of all U.S. women, yet they account for more than 79 percent of AIDS cases in women (NIH NIAID 2006). Sub-Saharan Africa remains the worst affected region in the world by the HIV epidemic on women. Women, ages 15 to 49 years, account for the majority (59 percent) of those estimated to be living with HIV/AIDS in the region (UNAIDS 2006). The impact on women is even more pronounced in some countries within the region. In Kenya, for example, 56 percent of all people living with HIV/AIDS are women; in Tanzania, it is 49 percent (WHO 2006). Young women, ages 15 to 24 years, are especially vulnerable because they comprise 76 percent of all young people estimated to be living with HIV/AIDS in sub-Saharan Africa. In some countries within the region, infection rates are up to 6 times higher among young women compared to men (CDC 2004). The impact on young women is exacerbated by the fact that the population of sub-Saharan Africa is quite young relative to other regions in the world, with 44 percent of the population below the age of 15 (compared to 29 percent globally) (UNAIDS 2006).

## Overlapping Prevalence of HIV and IPV

Studies conducted in the United States, Europe, Asia, and sub-Saharan Africa found prevalence of lifetime experience of IPV to be as high as 67 percent among women who were HIV seropositive or at risk of HIV (Cohen et al. 2000; Chandrasekaran et al. 2007) and current exposure to be as high as 64 percent (Gielen et al. 2000). However, estimates of the prevalence of

IPV among HIV-positive women vary by the definition of IPV and study population in question.

Of the emerging research that addresses the intersection of IPV and HIV, 18 studies specifically focused on the overlapping prevalence in the United States (Bogart et al. 2005; Burke et al. 2005; Cohen et al. 2000; El-Bassel et al. 2005, 2007; Gielen et al. 2000; Henny et al. 2007; McDonnell et al. 2003, 2005; Molitor et al. 2000; Newcomb and Carmona 2004; Whetten et al. 2006) Tanzania, South Africa, Kenya (Brown et al. 2006; Dunkle et al. 2004; Fonck et al. 2005; Jewkes et al. 2006a; Maman et al. 2002), and Ukraine in Europe (Dude 2007).

## Studies Comparing HIV-Positive and HIV-Negative Women

Results from studies examining the overlapping prevalence of HIV and violence using HIV-negative women as a comparison group were not consistent among studies conducted within the United States. McDonnell and colleagues (2003, 2005) found rates of emotional abuse by an intimate approximately equal among HIV-seropositive women and their seronegative counterparts (55 and 53 percent, respectively), while physical abuse by a partner was experienced *less* frequently among seropositive women than seronegative (56 vs. 64 percent, respectively). Cohen et al. (2000) found a similar, statistically significant difference between HIV-positive and HIV-negative women experiencing physical or sexual intimate partner violence in the past year (21 vs. 28 percent, respectively). On the other hand, El-Bassel et al. (2007) and Burke et al. (2005) did not find significant differences between HIV-positive and HIV-negative groups with regard to physical and sexual intimate partner violence.

More consistent results in the opposite direction have been found in international studies. Four of five sub-Saharan African studies (Dunkle et al. 2004; Fonck et al. 2005; Jewkes et al. 2006a; Maman et al. 2002) have showed that HIV-positive women report more lifetime partner violence compared to HIV-negative women, with the greatest difference reported in Tanzania (52 vs. 29 percent, respectively). Differences in definitions and measurement may help explain the discrepancies in results with past year and multiple types of abuse more often measured in the U.S. studies, while in Africa, lifetime IPV was more often measured using fewer questions about a narrow range of types of violence. Overall, less research has been conducted (to date) on the links between violence and HIV in Africa, although the greater prevalence of HIV among African women results in greater effect sizes when differences are found.

*Studies Among HIV-Positive Women*

Of the U.S. studies that focused on violence among HIV-positive women only, the prevalence of IPV in the past 6 months ranged from 18.1 to 19.8 percent (Bogart et al. 2005; Henny et al. 2007), while lifetime exposure to IPV (physical) ranged from 62 to 68 percent and adult sexual abuse ranged from 32 to 46 percent (Geilen et al. 2000; Henny et al. 2007). Additionally, prevalence of child sexual abuse among HIV-positive women was 31 percent (Whetten et al. 2006), and Gielen et al. (2000) found a prevalence of 13 percent for combined intimate partner and other perpetrator physical and sexual abuse after receiving an HIV diagnosis.

*Studies with Abused Women*

Only three studies assessed the prevalence of HIV among abused and nonabused women (Dude 2007; Molitor et al. 2000; Wingood et al. 2000a,b). Molitor et al. (2000) found that women with a history of forced sex were less likely to have been tested than nonabused women but if tested were more likely to self-report HIV infection. Other studies have studied prevalence of other STIs or STIs in general among abused versus nonabused women. Wingood and colleagues found that women who had experienced both physical and sexual violence, compared to women who reported sexual abuse alone, were more likely to have had a recent STI and to have been threatened when negotiating condom use (Wingood et al. 2000a). Similarly, Dude (2007) reported that Ukrainian women who have been physically abused by a sexual partner, whether recently or less recently, were significantly more likely to report having had an STI. Abused women have been found to be more likely to self-report STIs than nonabused women in a number of U.S. controlled investigations (e.g., Champion et al. 2004; Coker et al. 2002; Laughon et al. 2007; Martin et al. 1999).

*Studies with Adolescents*

In the United States, adolescent girls account for a growing number of new cases of HIV and AIDS. In 2003, adolescent girls (13-19 years) accounted for 50 percent of HIV cases (CDC 2004) and AIDS diagnoses among women and adolescent girls rose from 8 percent in 1995 to 27 percent in 2004 (CDC 2005). Evidence suggests that the majority of adolescents in this age group are dating (Wolfe and Feiring, 2000) and unfortunately, a significant number of these young relationships include partner-perpetrated violence (Foshee et al. 1996; Fredland et al. 2005; Wekerle and Wolfe 1999). Research investigations into prevalence estimates of partner violence have noted that between 6 and 46 percent of adolescents have experienced some form of IPV (Ackard et al. 2003; CDC 2006; Coker et al. 2000; Foshee et al. 1996; Glass et al. 2003; Spencer and Bryant 2000; Valois et al. 1999; Watson et al. 2001). In a recent review, Teitelman and colleagues explored the relationship between the experience of IPV victimization among heterosexually active adolescent girls, condom use, and the implications for HIV prevention (Teitelman et al. in press). Using gender and power theories to evaluate existing research, the authors conclude that physical and verbal IPV by male intimate partners is associated with condom nonuse and therefore an increased risk of HIV infection among their adolescent partners. The review highlights the need for additional research to better understand the direction of causality and the context of both abuse among teen partners and HIV risk behavior.

### IPV and HIV: Mutual Risk Factors

Prevalence studies have called attention to the overlap in HIV and IPV in women's lives and have demonstrated that women in abusive relationships are at a compounded risk for HIV infection. Further research has examined several mechanisms that may explain how exposure to IPV increases a woman's risk of STIs. Due to the multifaceted, complex nature of the two issues, exact causal relationships have been difficult to ascertain. Maman and colleagues hypothesized that exposure to IPV can increase women's risk for HIV infection in three ways: (1) through forced sex with an infected partner, (2) through limited or compromised negotiation of safer sex practices, and (3) through increased sexual risk-taking behaviors (Maman et al. 2000). These mechanisms may operate in tandem or individually and have particular significance for adolescent girls in sexual relationships with older men (Garcia-Moreno et al. 2005).

### Biology and Forced Sex

Current evidence suggests that women are biologically more vulnerable than men to contracting STIs, including HIV. Research has shown that abuse in a relationship places a woman at a fourfold higher risk for contracting STIs, including HIV, than her nonabused counterpart (Campbell and Soeken 1999; Dude 2007; Koenig et al. 2004; Wingood et al. 2000a,b). The apparent female biological susceptibility may be explained partially or completely by the sexually coercive behaviors of abusive partners (Miller et al. 1999; Raj et al. 2004; Wu et al. 2003). Forced sex occurs in approximately 40 to 45 percent of physically violent intimate relationships and increases a woman's risk for STIs by 2 to 10 times over that of physical abuse alone (Campbell and Soeken 1999; Wingood et al. 2000a). As a result of forced sex, genital injuries, such as vaginal lacerations, facilitate

disease transmission (Liebschutz et al. 2000). Lichtenstein and others found
that abusive partners used deliberate HIV infection, lack of disclosure about
known serostatus, and forced injection drug use as mechanisms to control
and endanger their intimate partners (Lichtenstein 2005; Neundorfer et al.
2005).

*IPV, Substance Use, and HIV*

The relationship among violence against women, HIV risk, and substance use is a particularly complex one. Studies in the United States have
found that women exposed to abuse during childhood or adulthood are
more likely to abuse alcohol and illicit substances, potentially as a coping mechanism (Beadnell et al. 2000; Gilbert et al. 2000; Wingood et
al. 2000a). Substance abuse, in turn, has been associated with high risk
behaviors for HIV and other STI infection (Collins et al. 2005; El-Bassel
2000). Unfortunately, because many studies of gender-based violence and
HIV risk are cross-sectional in design, it is not possible to determine the
temporal relationship between factors. For example, exposure (as a witness
or victim) to abuse during childhood has been documented as a risk factor
for victimization by an intimate partner later in life (Tjaden and Thoennes
2000). Similarly, children who experience maltreatment are at increased
risk for a wide range of negative health consequences, including substance
abuse (Felitti et al. 1998). Viewed from a lifecourse perspective, the precise
relationship between substance use, a known risk factor for sexual risk-
taking behavior, and IPV, a known precursor for substance use, is difficult
to ascertain. Finally, STI risk, including HIV risk, may also be indirectly
exacerbated by the victim's psychological trauma of violence and abuse
leading to impaired decision making, substance abuse, and greater risk
taking (Campbell and Lewandowski 1997; Miller et al. 1999). In spite of
the role that substance abuse plays in HIV and VAW in the United States,
substance abuse is rarely part of the HIV transmission picture in low- and
middle-income countries.

*Sexual Decision Making and IPV*

IPV also impairs open communication between partners regarding safe
sex practices including condom negotiation, monogamy, or HIV status disclosure. Kalichman and colleagues (1998) found that women with abusive
partners were more likely to fear negotiating condom use, believing that her
insistence may be seen as implying unfaithfulness or untrustworthiness of
either partner. The fear of retributive violence is real among abused women
at risk for HIV. Studies have shown that a woman's fear of her partner's
potentially violent reaction to suggesting condom use hinders her ability

to negotiate safe sexual health practices, which is a critical component to enhancing women's health, particularly in the area of HIV prevention (e.g., Champion et al. 2004; Davila 2002; Davila and Brackley 1999). Additionally, this fear of violence can influence whether a woman utilizes voluntary counseling and testing services (Karamagi et al. 2006).

Communication about sexual and reproductive health is also impacted by cultural norms. In the United States, Davila and colleagues found that males were the primary decision makers regarding safe sexual practices, particularly among married women who reported less ability to negotiate condom use than single/dating women (Davila 2002; Davila and Brackley 1999). Similarly, several studies have demonstrated the impact of relationship status and power on sexual health practices. In South Africa, Pettifor et al. (2004) found that low relationship power is significantly associated with inconsistent condom use among women. In the same region, Dunkle and colleagues (2004) found that pregnant women with low relationship power are at a twofold risk for never using a condom as compared to those women who feel they have high levels of power in the relationship.

Further, a history or diagnosis of an STI may be an initiating factor for partner violence (Gielen et al. 2000; Koenig et al. 2002; Medley et al. 2004; Zierler et al. 2000). Studies by Maman et al. (2002) and Kiarie and colleagues (2006) found that this fear was substantiated, as HIV-positive women were up to two times more likely to experience immediate violence after disclosure than HIV-negative women. Fear of violence from an intimate partner may also serve as a barrier to HIV-positive women seeking and obtaining needed health care (Lichtenstein 2005).

## Male Behavior, IPV, and HIV

Several studies conducted in international settings have found that male perpetrators of intimate partner violence engage in behavior that puts their partners at greater risk for HIV. As discussed earlier, studies have found that among women, there is an association between being a victim of IPV and having STIs, which puts women at greater risk for HIV. In addition, recent studies have established that among women, there is an association between being a victim of IPV and having a confirmed HIV-positive status. These studies have emphasized the need to conduct research on the specific HIV risk behaviors engaged in by male abusers.

Most research to date has utilized self-report by women regarding their partner's behavior within their relationship. In these studies measuring the victims' perceptions of their partners' HIV risk behaviors, abused women report more high-risk behaviors among their partners than nonabused women (Garcia-Moreno et al. 2005). This adds a level of complexity to the woman's risk for HIV infection within the context of intimate relationships.

Yet few studies explore the HIV risk behaviors among perpetrators versus nonperpetrators, as reported by men themselves. Five recent studies have addressed this gap. Although they are limited by their cross-sectional designs, limited measurement of violent behaviors, and potential underreporting of sensitive behaviors, they consistently reflect an association between male engagement in HIV risk behavior and perpetration of IPV.

The first study by Abrahams et al. (2005) was conducted in three Cape Town municipalities and explored risk factors for male sexual intimate partner violence perpetration. Data were collected from 1,368 randomly selected males. The study found an association between the perpetration of sexual violence and two HIV risk behaviors, including problematic alcohol use and having more than one current partner (adjusted OR = 2.87, 95 percent CI 2.08–2.96).

A second study by Dunkle et al. (2006), conducted in rural South Africa, explored the associations between HIV risk behaviors and the perpetration of IPV. Data were collected from 1,275 males in 70 communities as part of a baseline assessment for a randomized controlled trial of the Stepping Stones HIV prevention program. The study found that perpetrators of violence are significantly more likely to engage in HIV risk behaviors, such as casual partners, transactional sex, use of drugs and alcohol, and non-IPV sexual assault, than nonperpetrators. The level of risk behavior was correlated with level of violence severity.

Also in sub-Saharan Africa, Andersson and colleagues (2007) explored the relationship between male perpetration of physical violence and the HIV risk behavior of having multiple partners. The sample consisted of 8,767 men (and 11,872 women) from Botswana, Lesotho, Swaziland, Malawi, Mozambique, Namibia, Zambia, and Zimbabwe. Men who had multiple partners were two times more likely to also be perpetrators of violence, except in Mozambique.

The fourth study by Silverman et al. (2007) explored the association between violence against women and sexual risk behaviors among men in Bangladesh. The sample consisted of 3,096 married men, who participated in the MEASURE Demographic Health Survey. Violent behaviors included physical and/or sexual violence, while HIV risk behaviors included having premarital and extramarital sex partners, having STI symptoms or an STI diagnosis in the past year, and failing to disclose their infection status to their wives. Perpetrators of physical and sexual violence were 1.8 times more likely to report both premarital and extramarital partners than their nonabusing counterparts. Those using physical violence were 1.68 times more likely to report STI symptoms or diagnosis than nonperpetrators. Perpetrators of physical violence who had an STI diagnosis were somewhat less likely to disclose their infection status to their wives (OR = 1.58, 95 percent CI 0.93–2.70) than infected men not perpetrating physical violence.

A final study conducted by Lary et al. (2004) explored the associations between HIV and violence among young people in Dar es Salaam, Tanzania. Data reflecting HIV risk behaviors among male abusers were gathered via qualitative semistructured interviews with 40 young men between the ages of 16 and 24. Men who reported using violence against their partners also often reported sexual infidelity.

These recent data as well as evidence from the WHO Multi-Country Study of Violence Against Women (Garcia-Moreno et al. 2005) provide evidence that men who perpetrate violence against their intimate partners are also more likely to engage in HIV risk behaviors than men who do not perpetrate intimate partner violence. This is of particular note given that data on such behaviors among male abusers is available from the perspective of the female survivors, as well as from the male abusers themselves.

### Compromised Immunofunction Among Abused Women

Women who experience IPV suffer a wide and well-documented range of adverse health consequences, including increased prevalence of stress, depression, and chronic anxiety (Campbell 2002; Golding 1999; Pico-Alfonso et al. 2004, 2006; Woods et al. 2000). A few recent U.S.-based studies have explored the impact of violence victimization on immune system functioning in women. Significant associations have been found between intimate partner abuse and altered red blood cell and decreased T-cell function (Brokaw 2002; Constantino et al. 2000). Further research has revealed associations between violence and hypothalamic-pituitary-adrenal axis functioning, such that women in abusive relationships had greater occurrence of altered levels of cortisol and dehydroepiandrosterone (Griffin et al. 2005; Pico-Alfonso et al. 2004; Seedat et al. 2003) compared to nonabused women. Other studies have found that partner violence alters neuropsychological functioning (Stein et al. 2002) and negatively impacts immune responses related to HSV-1 infection (Garcia-Linares et al. 2004). Woods et al. (2000) explored the interrelationship of IPV, psychopathology, and immune system functioning to determine if posttraumatic stress disorder (PTSD) symptoms mediate the effect of violence on cytokine levels. Their findings indicate that cytokine values were higher among women who were abused and experiencing PTSD, suggesting mediation and a partial explanation for comorbidities of mental and physical health symptoms in victims of violence.

A similar body of existent literature demonstrates a strong relationship between stress and other psychosocial factors with disease progression in HIV-infected persons. Specifically, HIV-infected people have been found to suffer from adverse mental health sequalae (including stress and depression) which, in turn, have been associated with increased morbidity (Ickovics et al. 2001) and faster progression to AIDS (Kimerling et al. 1999; Leserman et al. 1999, 2002). A rapidly growing body of literature indicates the impact of PTSD and depression in HIV biomarkers, including decreased CD4 counts and immune decrements (Boarts et al. 2006; Delahanty et al. 2004; Sledjeski et al. 2005).

Despite increasing attention being paid to how stress and immune function relate to IPV and HIV, no known research has investigated the hypotheses that an association exists between abuse and reduced immunity to HIV acquisition or that intimate partner violence might be associated with increased disease progression (reduction of CD4 levels) among HIV-infected women. A striking commonality does exist, however, in the above referenced findings on IPV and immune function and HIV and immune function, namely that the depressive episodes described in both associations have the same effects on the immune system. These findings indicate an important direction for future research on the intersections of IPV and HIV. Research is warranted to examine the impact of violence-related PTSD and comorbid depression on immunity to HIV acquisition and disease progression in HIV-infected women.

## Conclusions

The research reviewed clearly indicates complex but real relationships between two epidemics threatening the health and safety of women in the United States and around the world, particularly among low- and middle-income countries. The increased risk for HIV/AIDS related to violence against women, particularly IPV, works through both male and female behavior, through physiological consequences of violence, and affects both adult women and adolescents. There is now evidence that all three behavioral areas proposed by Maman and colleagues (2000) as mechanisms by which the risk is increased: forced sex with an infected partner, limited or compromised negotiation of safer sex practices, and increased sexual risk-taking behaviors (Maman et al. 2000). Another mechanism found to be important is the increase in other STIs that accompany abuse and facilitate HIV transmission. There is beginning to be evidence of a connection between abuse-related immunocompromised states which may have implications for both HIV infection, conversion from HIV to AIDS, or AIDS-related infections such as tuberculosis, also potentially fatal. All of these connections need further investigation of the precise mechanisms of enhanced transmission (e.g., forced anal sex) in order to design effective prevention strategies. Further epidemiological studies are needed, but even more important is the need for studies that combine physiological and qualitative data with self-report so that these complex relationships can be better elucidated. Prospective studies are critical to address issues of causality and time ordering, as almost all studies to date have been cross-sectional. Also imperative are studies that indicate how women who are being abused can protect themselves from HIV safely, and even more importantly, how to reduce abusive behavior toward women by men (e.g., Jewkes et al. 2006b; Pronyk et al. 2006). Finally, although similar risk factors for HIV and IPV have been identified among women around the world, significant differences exist in the quantity and quality of research conducted to date in various settings. Future efforts should target multiple low- and middle-income countries where the AIDS epidemic is widespread or emerging so that the effects of culture and context on the ways that HIV/AIDS risk is increased by violence against women can be both better explicated and contextually understood.

*Implications for Prevention*

Given the evidence related to men's behavior, efforts to prevent HIV need to focus on the reduction of male use of violence against women as well as reduction of male HIV risk behaviors in intimate partnerships. The need to focus specifically on the reduction of multiple and concurrent partners to prevent HIV was one of two major recommendations at a recent meeting on preventing AIDS in high-HIV-prevalence countries in southern Africa convened by the Southern African Development Community and UNAIDS in 2006. After reviewing evidence reflecting the limited success of current HIV efforts and calls for revised HIV prevention strategies, two recommendations were made: one focused on male circumcision, and the second on the reduction of multiple and concurrent partners (Halperin and Epstein 2007). What was missing was a recommendation about reducing violence in intimate partner relationships. Future policy and programmatic efforts must address this area of primary prevention in order to effectively reduce women's risk of HIV infection.

## References

Abrahams, N. et al. 2005. Sexual violence against intimate partners in Cape Town: Prevalence and risk factors reported by men. *Bulletin of the World Health Organization* 82:330-337.

Ackard, D. M., D. Neumark-Sztainer, and P. Hannan. 2003. Dating violence among a nationally representative sample of adolescent girls and boys: associations with behavioral and mental health. *Journal of Gender-Specific Medicine* 6(3):39-48.

Andersson, N. et al. 2007. Risk factors for domestic physical violence: National cross-sectional household surveys in eight southern African countries. *BMC Women's Health* 7:11.

Beadnell, B, S. A. Baker, and D. M. Morrison. 2000. HIV/STD risk factors for women with violent male partners. *Sex Roles* 42(7-8):661-689.

Boarts, J. M. et al. 2006. The differential impact of PTSD and depression on HIV disease markers and adherence to HAART in people living with HIV. *AIDS and Behavior* 10(3):253-261.

Bogart, L. et al. 2005. The association of partner abuse with risky sexual behaviors among women and men with HIV/AIDS. *AIDS and Behavior* 9(3):325-333.

Brokaw, J. 2002. Health status and intimate partner violence: A cross-sectional study. *Annals of Emergency Medicine* 39(1):31-38.

Brown, L. et al. 2006. Sexual violence in Lesotho. *Studies in Family Planning* 37(4): 269-280.

Burke, J. et al. 2005. Intimate partner violence, substance use, and HIV among low-income women: Taking a closer look. *Violence Against Women* 11:1140-1161.

Campbell, J. C. 2002. Health consequences of intimate partner violence. *Lancet* 359(9314): 1331-1336.

Campbell, J. C., and K. Soeken. 1999. Forced sex and intimate partner violence: Effects on women's health. *Violence Against Women.* 5:1017-1035.

Campbell, J. C., and L. A. Lewandowski. 1997. Mental and physical health effects of intimate partner violence on women and children. *Psychiatric Clinics of North America,* 20:353-374.

CDC (Centers for Disease Control and Prevention). 2004. *HIV/AIDS surveillance in adolescents: L265 slide series.* http://www.cdc.gov/hiv/graphics/adolesnt.htm (accessed October 9, 2005).

CDC. 2005. *HIV/AIDS surveillance report*, 2004. Atlanta, GA: US Department of Health and Human Services. 16:1-46.

CDC. 2006. Extent, nature, and consequences of rape victimization: Findings from the National violence against women survey. Washington DC: U.S. Department of Justice, National Institute of Justice.

Champion, J. D., J. Piper, and R. N. Shain. 2004. Minority adolescent women with sexually transmitted diseases and a history of sexual or physical abuse. *Issues in Mental Health Nursing* 25(3):293-316.

Chandrasekaran, V. et al. 2007. Determinants of domestic violence among women attending an human immunodeficiency virus voluntary counseling and testing center in Bangalore, India. *Indian Journal of Medical Science* 61(5):253-262.

Cohen, M. et al. 2000. Domestic violence and childhood sexual abuse in HIV-infected women and women at risk for HIV. *American Journal of Public Health* 90:560-565.

Coker, A. L. et al. 2000. Severe dating violence and quality of life among South Carolina high school students. *American Journal of Preventive Medicine* 19(4):220-227.

Coker, A. L. et al. 2002. Physical health consequences of physical and psychological intimate partner violence. *Archives of Family Medicine* 9:451-456.

Collins, R. L. et al. 2005. Isolating the nexus of substance use, violence and sexual risk for HIV infection among young adults in the United States. *AIDS and Behavior* 9(1):73-87.

Constantino, R. E. et al. 2000. Negative life experiences, depression, and immune function in abused and nonabused women. *Biological Research for Nursing* 1(3):190-198.

Davila, Y. R. 2002. Influence of abuse on condom negotiation among Mexican-American women involved in abusive relationships. *Journal of the Association of Nurses in AIDS Care* 13(6):46-56.

Davila, Y. R., and M. H. Brackley. 1999. Mexican and Mexican American women in a battered women's shelter: Barriers to condom negotiation for HIV/AIDS prevention. *Issues in Mental Health Nursing* 20(4):333-355.

Delahanty, D. L. et al. 2004. Posttraumatic stress disorder symptoms, salivary cortisol, medication adherence, and CD4 levels in HIV-positive individuals. *AIDS Care* 16(2):247-260.

Dude, A. 2007. Intimate partner violence and increased lifetime risk of sexually transmitted infection among women in Ukraine. *Studies in Family Planning* 38(2):89-100.

Dunkle, K. et al. 2004. Gender-based violence, relationship power, and risk of HIV infection in women attending antenatal clinics in South Africa. *Lancet* 363:1415-1421.

Dunkle, K. et al. 2006. Perpetration of partner violence and HIV risk behaviour among young men in the rural Eastern Cape, South Africa. *AIDS*, 20:1-8.

El-Bassel, N. et al. 2000. Fear and violence: Raising the HIV stakes. *AIDS Education and Prevention* 12(2):154-170.

El-Bassel, N. et al. 2005. HIV and intimate partner violence among methadone-maintained women in New York City. *Social Science Medicine* 61:171-183.

El-Bassel, N. et al. 2007. Intimate partner violence prevalence and HIV risks among women receiving care in emergency departments: Implications for IPV and HIV screening. *Emergency Medicine Journal* 24:255-259.

Felitti, V. J. et al. 1998. Relationship of childhood abuse and household dysfunction to many of the leading causes of death in adults. The Adverse Childhood Experiences (ACE) Study. *American Journal of Preventive Medicine* 14(4):245-258.

Fonck, K. et al. 2005. Increased risk of HIV in women experiencing physical partner violence in Nairobi, Kenya. *AIDS and Behavior* 9(3):335-339.

Foshee, V. A. et al. 1996. The Safe Dates Project: theoretical basis, evaluation design, and selected baseline findings. *American Journal of Preventive Medicine* 12(5 Suppl):39-47.

Fredland, N. M. et al. 2005. The meaning of dating violence in the lives of middle school adolescents: a report of focus group study. *Journal of School Violence* 4(2):95-114.

Garcia-Linares, M. I. et al. 2004. Intimate male partner violence impairs immune control over herpes simplex virus type 1 in physically and psychologically abused women. *Psychosomatic Medicine* 66(6):965-972.

Garcia-Moreno, C. et al. 2005. WHO multi-country study on women's health and domestic violence against women. Geneva, Switzerland: World Health Organization.

Gielen, A. C. et al. 1997. Women's disclosure of HIV status: experiences of mistreatment and violence in an urban setting. *Women and Health* 25(3):19-31.

Gielen, A. C. et al. 2000. Women's lives after an HIV-positive diagnosis: disclosure and violence. *Maternal and Child Health Journal* 4(2):111-119.

Gilbert, L. et al. 2000. The converging epidemics of mood-altering drug use, HIV, HCV, and partner violence: A conundrum for methadone maintenance treatment. *Mt Sinai Journal of Medicine* 67(5-6):452-464.

Glass, N. et al. 2003. Adolescent dating violence: prevalence, risk factors, health outcomes, and implications for clinical practice. *Journal of Obstetric, Gynecological, and Neonatal Nursing* 32(2):227-238.

Golding, J. M. 1999. Intimate partner violence as a risk factor for mental disorders: A meta-analysis. *Journal of Family Violence* 14(2):99-132.

Greenwood, G. L. et al. 2002. Battering victimization among a probability-based sample of men who have sex with men (MSM). *American Journal of Public Health* 92(12):1964-1969.

Griffin, M.G., P.A. Resick, and R. Yehuda. 2005. Enhanced cortisol suppression following dexamethasone administration in domestic violence survivors. *American Journal of Psychiatry* 162:1192-1199.

Halperin, D. T., and H. Epstein. 2007. Why is HIV prevalence so severe in southern Africa? The role of multiple concurrent partnerships and lack of male circumcision: Implications for AIDS prevention. *The Southern African Journal of HIV Medicine* 26:19-25.

Henny, K. et al. 2007. Physical and sexual abuse among homeless and unstably housed adults living with HIV: Prevalence and associated risks. *AIDS and Behavior* 11(6): 842-853.

Ickovics, J. R. et al. 2001. Mortality, CD4 cell count decline, and depressive symptoms among HIV-seropositive women: Longitudinal analysis from the HIV Epidemiology Research Study. *JAMA* 285:1460-1465.

Jewkes, R. et al. 2006a. Factors associated with HIV sero-status in young rural South African women: Connections between intimate partner violence and HIV. *International Journal of Epidemiology* 35(6):1461-1468.

Jewkes, R. et al. 2006b. A cluster randomized-controlled trial to determine the effectiveness of Stepping Stones in preventing HIV infections and promoting safer sexual behaviour amongst youth in the rural Eastern Cape, South Africa: Trial design, methods and baseline findings. *Tropical Medicine and International Health* 2(1):3-16.

Kalichman, S. C. et al. 1998. Sexual coercion, domestic violence, and negotiating condom use among low-income African American women. *Journal of Women's Health* 7:371-378.

Karamagi, C. A. et al. 2006. Intimate partner violence against women in eastern Uganda: Implications for HIV prevention. *BMC Public Health* 20(6):284.

Kiarie, J. N. et al. 2006. Domestic violence and prevention of mother-to-child transmission of HIV-1. *AIDS* 20(13):1763-1769.

Kimerling, R. et al. 1999. Traumatic stress in HIV-infected women. *AIDS Education and Prevention* 11:321-330.

Koenig, L. J. et al. 2002. Perinatal Guidelines Evaluation Project Group. Violence during pregnancy among women with or at risk for HIV infection. *American Journal of Public Health* 92(3):367-370.

Koenig, M. A. et al. 2004. Coercive sex in rural Uganda: Prevalence and associated risk factors. *Social Science & Medicine* 58(4):787-798.

Lary, H. et al. 2004. Exploring the association between HIV and violence: Young people's experiences with infidelity, violence and forced sex in Dar es Salaam, Tanzania. *International Family Planning Perspectives* 30(4):200-206.

Laughon, K. et al. 2007. The relationship among sexually transmitted infection, depression and lifetime violence in a sample of predominantly African American women. *Research in Nursing and Health* 30(4):413-428.

Leserman, J. et al. 1999. Progression to AIDS: The effects of stress, depressive symptoms, and social support. *Psychosomatic Medicine* 61:397-406.

Leserman, J. et al. 2002. Progression to AIDS, a clinical AIDS condition, and mortality: psychosocial and physiological predictors. *Psychological Medicine* 32:1059-1073.

Lichtenstein, B. 2005. Domestic violence, sexual ownership, and HIV risk in women in the American deep south. *Social Science and Medicine* 60(4):701-711.

Liebschutz, J. M. et al. 2000. Physical and sexual abuse in women infected with the human immunodeficiency virus: increased illness and health care utilization. *Archives of Internal Medicine* 160:1659-1664.

Maman, S. et al. 2000. The intersections of HIV and violence: Directions for future research and interventions. *Social Science & Medicine* 50(4):459-478.

Maman, S. et al. 2002. HIV-positive women report more lifetime partner violence: Findings from a voluntary counseling and testing clinic in Dar es Salaam, Tanzania. *American Journal of Public Health* 92(8):1331-1337.

Martin, S. L., L. S. Matza, L. L. Kupper, J. C. Thomas, M. Daly, and S. Cloutier. 1999. Domestic violence and sexually transmitted diseases: The experience of prenatal care patients. *Public Health Reports* 114:262-268.

McDonnell, K. et al. 2003. Does HIV status make a difference in the experience of lifetime abuse? Descriptions of lifetime abuse and its context among low-income urban women. *Journal of Urban Health* 80(3):494-509.

McDonnell, K. et al. 2005. Abuse, HIV status and health-related quality of life among a sample of HIV positive and HIV negative low income women. *Quality of Life Research* 14:945-957.

Medley, A. et al. 2004. Rates, barriers and outcomes of HIV serostatus disclosure among women in developing countries: implications for prevention of mother-to-child transmission programmes. *Bulletin of the World Health Organization* 82(4):299-307.

Miller, H. G. et al. 1999. Correlates of sexually transmitted bacterial infections among U.S. women in 1995. *Family Planning Perspectives* 31(1):4-9, 23.

Molitor, F. et al. 2000. History of forced sex in association with drug use and sexual HIV risk behaviors, infection with STDs, and diagnostic medical care: results from the Young Women Survey. *Journal of Interpersonal Violence* 15(3):262-278.

Neundorfer, M. M., P. B. Harris, and P. J. Britton. 2005. HIV-risk factors for midlife and older women. *Gerontologist* 45(5):617-625.

Newcomb, M., and J. Carmona. 2004. Adult trauma and HIV status among Latinas: Effects upon psychological adjustment and substance use. *AIDS and Behavior* 8(4):417-428.

NIH (National Institutes of Health), NIAID (National Institute of Allergy and Infectious Diseases). 2006. *HIV infection in women factsheet.* Bethesda, MD: U.S. Department of Health and Human Services, NIH.

Pettifor, A. E. et al. 2004. Sexual power and HIV risk, South Africa. *Emerging Infectious Disease* 10(11):1996-2004.

Pico-Alfonso, M. A. et al. 2004. Changes in cortisol and dehydroepiandrosterone in women victims of physical and psychological intimate partner violence. *Biological Psychiatry* 56(4):233-240.

Pico-Alfonso, M. A. et al. 2006. The impact of physical, psychological, and sexual intimate male partner violence on women's mental health: Depressive symptoms, posttraumatic stress disorder, state anxiety, and suicide. *Journal of Womens Health (Larchmt)* 15(5):599-611.

Pronyk, P. M., J. R. Hargreaves, J. C. Kim, L. A. Morison, G. Phetla, C. Watts, J. Busza, and J. D. H. Porter. 2006. Eff ect of a structural intervention for the prevention of intimate-partner violence and HIV in rural South Africa: A cluster randomised trial. *Lancet* 368:1973-1983.

Raj, A., J. G. Silverman, and H. Amaro. 2004. Abused women report greater male partner risk and gender-based risk for HIV: Findings from a community-based study with Hispanic women. *AIDS Care* 16(4):519-529.

Relf, M. V. 2001. Battering and HIV in men who have sex with men: A critique and synthesis of the literature. *Journal of the Association of Nurses in AIDS Care* 12(3):41-48.

Seedat, S. et al. 2003. Plasma cortisol and neuropeptide Y in female victims of intimate partner violence. *Psychoneuroendocrinology* 28(6):796-808.

Silverman, J. G. et al. 2007. Violence against wives, sexual risk and sexually transmitted infection among Bangladeshi men. *Sexually Transmitted Infections* 83:211-215.

Sledjeski, E. M. et al. 2005. Incidence and impact of posttraumatic stress disorder and comorbid depression on adherence to HAART and CD4+ counts in people living with HIV. *AIDS Patient Care and STDs* 19(11):728-736.

Spencer, G. A., and S. A. Bryant. 2000. Dating violence: A comparison of rural, suburban, and urban teens. *Journal of Adolescent Health* 27(5):302-305.

Stein, M. B., C. M. Kennedy, and E. W. Twamley. 2002. Neuropsychological function in female victims of intimate partner violence with and without posttraumatic stress disorder. *Biological Psychiatry* 52(11):1079-1088.

Teitelman, A.M. et al. In press. A review of the literature on intimate partner violence, condom use and HIV risk for adolescent girls: Implications for research and prevention. *Journal of HIV/AIDS Prevention in Children and Youth.*

Tjaden, P. G., and N. Thoennes. 2000. *Full report of the prevalence, incidence, and consequences of violence against women* (Rep. No. NCJ-183781). Washington, DC: National Institute of Justice.

UNAIDS (Joint United Nations Programme on HIV/AIDS). 2006. *Report on the global AIDS epidemic.* Geneva, Switzerland: UNAIDS.

Valois, R. F. et al. 1999. Relationship between number of sexual intercourse partners and selected health risk behaviors among public high school adolescents. *Journal of Adolescent Health* 25(5):328-335.

Watson, J. M. et al. 2001. High school students' responses to dating aggression. *Violence and Victims* 16(3):339-348.

Wekerle, C., and D. A. Wolfe. 1999. Dating violence in mid-adolescence: Theory, significance, and emerging prevention initiatives. *Clinical Psychology Review* 19(4):435-456.

Whetten, K. et al. 2006. Prevalence of childhood sexual abuse and physical trauma in an HIV-positive sample from the deep south. *American Journal of Public Health* 96:1028-1030.

WHO (World Health Organisation). 2000. *Violence against women and HIV/AIDS: Setting the research agenda.* Meeting Report. Geneva, Switzerland.

WHO. 2004. *Violence against women and HIV/AIDS: Critical intersections.* Information Bulletin Series, number 1. Geneva, Switzerland.

WHO. 2006. *Epidemiological fact sheets on HIV/AIDS and sexually transmitted infections.* Geneva, Switzerland.

Wingood, G. M. 2001. Adverse consequences of intimate partner abuse among women in non-urban domestic violence shelters. *American Journal of Preventive Medicine* 19(4):270-275.

Wingood, G. M., and R. J. DiClemente. 1997. The effects of an abusive primary partner on the condom use and sexual negotiation practices of African-American women. *American Journal of Public Health* 87:1016-1018.

Wingood, G. M., R. J. DiClemente, and A. Raj. 2000a. Adverse consequences of intimate partner abuse among women in non-urban domestic violence shelters. *American Journal of Preventive Medicine* 19(4):270-275.

Wingood, G. M., R. J. DiClemente, and A. Raj. 2000b.Identifying the prevalence and correlates of STDs among women residing in rural domestic violence shelters. *Women and Health* 30(4):15-26.

Wolfe, D. A., and C. Feiring. 2000. Dating violence through the lens of adolescent romantic relationships. *Child Maltreatment* 5(4):360-363.

Woods, S. J. et al. 2000. Prevalence and patterns of posttraumatic stress disorder in abused and postabused women. *Issues in Mental Health Nursing* 21(3):309-324.

Wyatt, G. E. et al. 2002. Does a history of trauma contribute to HIV risk for women of color? Implications for prevention and policy. *American Journal of Public Health* 92(4):660-665.

Wu, E. et al. 2003. Intimate partner violence and HIV risk among urban minority women in primary health care settings. *AIDS and Behavior* 7(3):291-301.

Zierler, S. et al. 2000. Violence victimization after HIV infection in a U.S. probability sample of adult patients in primary care. *American Journal of Public Health* 90(2):208-215.

# A LOGICAL FRAMEWORK FOR PREVENTING INTERPERSONAL AND SELF-DIRECTED VIOLENCE IN LOW- AND MIDDLE-INCOME COUNTRIES

Susan Zaro[1]
Mark L. Rosenberg[2]
James A. Mercy[3, 4]

Presentation on next page.

[1]Susan Zaro, MPH.

[2]Mark L. Rosenberg is Executive Director of the Task Force for Child Survival and Development, Decatur, Georgia, USA.

[3]James A. Mercy is with the Division of Violence Prevention National Center for Injury Prevention and Control (NCIPC), Centers for Disease Control and Prevention (CDC), Atlanta, Georgia, USA.

[4] The findings and conclusions of this paper are those of the authors and do not necessarily represent the views of the CDC.

# A Logical Framework for Preventing Interpersonal and

| ACTIVITIES |
|---|

**Leadership**

- Develop participatory, multisectoral, and multidisciplinary collaborations and a coordinating mechanism
- Develop, implement, and monitor a global action plan as well as national action plans
- Strengthen and fully utilize those agencies and organizations with comparative advantage vis-à-vis global violence prevention (GVP)
- Advocate for, communicate about, and build political will to expand resources and funding
- Promote adherence to existing international laws, treaties, and protection of human rights and sponsor new ones as needed

**Research and Data Collection**

- Create a country-driven, collaborative process to develop data standards, including elements, definitions, and methods for data collection, sharing, and dissemination
- Identify data providers, users, needs, and gaps
- Develop comprehensive, multisectoral data collection systems, including surveillance systems, at the country, regional, and national levels
- Collect and analyze data that will illuminate the root causes, risk factors, costs, and interrelationships among different types of violence

**Capacity Building and Dissemination**

- Develop information, technical assistance, and training systems to support implementation of evidenced-based prevention strategies and victim services
- Develop prevention and treatment delivery systems that integrate key sector involvement in implementation of evidenced-based strategies
- Translate and disseminate information on violence, evidenced-based prevention, and treatment and their successful implementation strategies
- Assure the needed management capacity and human resources to effectively implement, manage, and evaluate violence prevention interventions and treatment services

**Intervention Development**

Develop and test interventions to:
- Increase safe, stable, and nurturing relationships between children and their parents/caretakers
- Reduce availability and misuse of alcohol
- Reduce access to lethal means
- Promote gender equality
- Change cultural norms that support violence
- Reduce recidivism among perpetrators
- Improve criminal justice and social welfare systems
- Reduce social distance between conflicting groups
- Reduce economic inequality and concentrations of poverty

**Victim Services**

Develop and test strategies to:
- Engage the health sector in violence prevention to identify victims and help them prevent future violence
- Educate health care providers about intersection of violence and other health problems
- Link health care, social services, and police services
- Provide culturally appropriate mental health and social services for victims of violence
- Improve emergency response to injuries from violence

# Self-Directed Violence in Low- and Middle-Income Countries

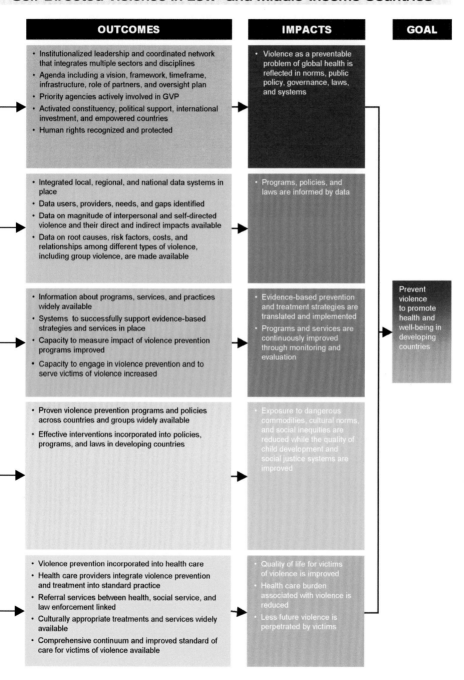

**OUTCOMES**

- Institutionalized leadership and coordinated network that integrates multiple sectors and disciplines
- Agenda including a vision, framework, timeframe, infrastructure, role of partners, and oversight plan
- Priority agencies actively involved in GVP
- Activated constituency, political support, international investment, and empowered countries
- Human rights recognized and protected

- Integrated local, regional, and national data systems in place
- Data users, providers, needs, and gaps identified
- Data on magnitude of interpersonal and self-directed violence and their direct and indirect impacts available
- Data on root causes, risk factors, costs, and relationships among different types of violence, including group violence, are made available

- Information about programs, services, and practices widely available
- Systems to successfully support evidence-based strategies and services in place
- Capacity to measure impact of violence prevention programs improved
- Capacity to engage in violence prevention and to serve victims of violence increased

- Proven violence prevention programs and policies across countries and groups widely available
- Effective interventions incorporated into policies, programs, and laws in developing countries

- Violence prevention incorporated into health care
- Health care providers integrate violence prevention and treatment into standard practice
- Referral services between health, social service, and law enforcement linked
- Culturally appropriate treatments and services widely available
- Comprehensive continuum and improved standard of care for victims of violence available

**IMPACTS**

- Violence as a preventable problem of global health is reflected in norms, public policy, governance, laws, and systems

- Programs, policies, and laws are informed by data

- Evidence-based prevention and treatment strategies are translated and implemented
- Programs and services are continuously improved through monitoring and evaluation

- Exposure to dangerous commodities, cultural norms, and social inequities are reduced while the quality of child development and social justice systems are improved

- Quality of life for victims of violence is improved
- Health care burden associated with violence is reduced
- Less future violence is perpetrated by victims

**GOAL**

Prevent violence to promote health and well-being in developing countries

## COLLECTIVE VIOLENCE:
## HEALTH IMPACT AND PREVENTION

*Victor W. Sidel, MD*[1]
*Barry S. Levy, MD, MPH*[2]

### Introduction

Collective violence, especially in the form of armed conflict, accounts for more death and disability than many major diseases worldwide. Collective violence destroys families, communities, and sometimes entire cultures. It diverts scarce resources away from the promotion and protection of health, medical care, and other health and social services. It destroys that health-supporting infrastructure of society. It limits human rights and contributes to social injustice. It leads individuals and nations to believe that violence is the only way to resolve conflicts. And it contributes to the destruction of the physical environment and the overuse of nonrenewable resources. In sum, collective violence threatens much of the fabric of our civilization.

### Definition of "Collective Violence"

In 1996 the World Health Assembly, the governing body of the World Health Organisation (WHO), adopted Resolution WHA49.25, which declared violence "a major and growing public health problem across the world" (World Health Assembly, 1996). The Assembly asked the WHO

---

[1]Distinguished University Professor of Social Medicine, Montefiore Medical Center and Albert Einstein College of Medicine, Bronx, New York; Adjunct Professor of Public Health, Weill Medical College of Cornell University, New York, New York.
[2]Adjunct Professor of Public Health, Tufts University School of Medicine, Boston, Massachusetts.

Director-General to develop public health activities to deal with the problem. The resulting *World Report on Violence and Health*, published by WHO in 2002, was the first comprehensive report by WHO on violence as a public health problem (Krug et al., 2002). The WHO report presents a typology of "violence" that defines three broad categories based on characteristics of those committing the violent acts: self-directed violence, interpersonal violence, and collective violence. This paper deals with elements of the third category, collective violence, with a primary focus on collective violence that involves "armed conflict."

The three forms of violence in some ways overlap. Those engaged in collective violence may engage in self-directed violence as a symptom of posttraumatic stress syndrome or as a result of self-hatred because of acts committed in war. Collective violence may also be associated with interpersonal violence. For example, individuals and groups engaged in armed conflict may commit interpersonal violence, sometimes fueled by ethnic tensions or in the military by conflict with superior officers or with fellow servicemembers in the midst of war. Soldiers may return from war with a battlefield mindset in which they commit interpersonal violence to address interpersonal conflicts that might have been addressed in nonviolent ways. And children raised in the midst of war may come to believe that violence is an appropriate way to settle interpersonal conflicts.

Collective violence has been characterized as "the instrumental use of violence by people who identify themselves as members of a group—whether this group is transitory or has a more permanent identity—against another group or set of individuals, in order to achieve political, economic, ideological, or social objectives" (Zwi et al., 2002). The WHO report gives, as examples of collective violence, "violent conflicts between nations and groups, state and group terrorism, rape as a weapon of war, the movement of large numbers of people displaced from their homes and gang warfare." As noted in the report, "all of these occur on a daily basis in many parts if the world" and "the effects of these different types of events on health in terms of deaths, physical illness, disabilities and mental anguish, are vast." This paper includes extensive discussion of war and other military activities and brief discussion of "terrorism" and the "war on terror" (Levy and Sidel, 2008a).

### Definition of "Armed Conflict"

Conflict is a common characteristic of most societies but rarely escalates into the use of physical force and even more rarely into the use of weapons. When weapons are used in "collective violence," they are usually termed "arms." This paper concentrates on collective violence in which weapons are used, for which we use the term "armed conflict." These weapons range from knives, bayonets, and machetes to nuclear weapons. In this paper, we are primarily concerned with "small arms and light weapons," since these are the weapons most often used in armed conflict in low- and middle-income countries, but we will also include discussion of bombs (both airborne and land-based, such as "improvised explosive devices"), landmines, and artillery shells, which are also commonly used. Nuclear, chemical, and biologic weapons, sometimes termed WMD (weapons of mass destruction), are also discussed since these are weapons that pose the risk of indiscriminate and widespread devastation, injury, and death.

*Definition of "Low- and Middle-Income Countries"*

The World Bank classifies countries into economic groupings based mainly on the country's gross national income (GNI) per capita (World Bank, 2007). Based on its GNI per capita, every economy is classified as low income, middle income (subdivided into lower middle and upper middle), or high income. The World Bank's tables classify all 185 member countries, and all other economies with populations of more than 30,000 (208 total). Low-income and middle-income economies, the Bank comments, are sometimes referred to as "developing countries," a term we use in this background paper. The use of the term is convenient; it is not intended to imply that all countries in the group are experiencing similar development or that other economies have reached a preferred or final stage of development. Classification by income does not necessarily reflect development status. The World Bank currently classifies economies according to 2006 GNI per capita, calculated using the World Bank Atlas method. The groups are as follows: low income, $905 or less; lower-middle income, $906 to $3,595; upper-middle income, $3,596 to $11,115; and high income, $11,116 or more. The countries in the low-income, lower-middle-income, and upper-middle-income groups can be found on the World Bank website. Examples of low-income economies include those of the Democratic Republic of Congo (DRC), Haiti, India, Nigeria, Pakistan, Vietnam, and Zimbabwe. Examples of lower-middle-income economies include those of China, Cuba, Egypt, Iran, Iraq, the Philippines, Thailand, and Ukraine. Examples of upper-middle-income economies include those of Argentina, Brazil, Hungary, Mexico, Poland, South Africa, and Turkey.

World Bank data demonstrate a striking relationship between the wealth of a nation and its chances of having a civil war. For example, a country with a gross domestic product (GDP) per capita of US$250 has a 15 percent probability of war onset in the next 5 years, and this probability reduces by approximately half for a country with a GDP of $600 per person. In contrast, countries with per capita income of more than US$5,000 have less than a 1 percent probability of having a civil conflict, all else being equal. In addition to poverty, risk factors for armed conflict may be associated with poor health and poor access to quality medical care, low status of women, large gaps between the rich and the poor, weak development of a civil society within a country, people not having the right to vote or otherwise participate in decisions that affect their lives, limited education and employment opportunities, increased access to small arms and light weapons, and the basic needs of civilians not being met (deSoysa and Neumayer, 2005).

## The Health Impacts of Collective Violence

There are profound direct and indirect health consequences of armed conflict (Levy and Sidel, 2008a,b,c). These are described below.

### Direct Consequences of War and Military Operations

Armed conflicts in the 21st century largely consist of the civil wars (conflicts within countries, to which other countries sometimes contribute military troops) that continue to rage in many parts of the world. For example, at the beginning of 2007 it was reported that there were 15 significant armed conflicts (1,000 or more reported deaths) and another 21 "hot spots" that could slide into or revert to war (Smith, 2007). During the post–Cold War period of 1990-2001, there were 57 major armed conflicts in 45 locations—all but three of which were civil wars (Stockholm International Peace Research Institute, 2002).

Some of the impacts of war on public health are obvious, while others are not. The direct impact of war on mortality and morbidity is apparent. Many people, including an increasing percentage of civilians, are killed or injured during war. An estimated 191 million people died directly or indirectly as a result of conflict during the 20th century, more than half of whom were civilians (Rummel, 1994). The exact figures are unknowable because of generally poor recordkeeping in many countries and its disruption in time of conflict.

War has direct, immediate, and deadly impact on human life and health. The "body counts" and the data on those with war-caused injuries and disabilities, both physical and psychological, while woefully incomplete, document the many people tragically killed and wounded as a direct result of military activities. Through the early 20th century, up to the start of World War II, the vast preponderance of the direct casualties of war were uniformed combatants, usually members of national armed forces. Although noncombatants suffered social, economic, and environmental consequences of war and may have been the victims of what is now termed "collateral damage" of military operations, "civilians" were generally not

directly targeted and were largely spared direct death and disability resulting from war (Zwi et al., 1999; Levy and Sidel, 2008a).

But since 1937, when Nazi forces bombed the city of Guernica, a
non-military target in the Basque region of Spain, military operations have
increasingly killed and maimed civilians through purposeful targeting of
non-military targets. The use of "carpet bombing" and the collateral damage of heavy attacks on military targets have caused many civilian casualties. The percentage of civilian deaths as a proportion of all deaths directly
caused by war has therefore increased dramatically (Levy and Sidel, 2008a).
Many of these civilian deaths may have been indirectly rather than directly
caused by war.

## Indirect Effects of War and Other Military Activities

Along with the direct impacts of war and other military activities
on health, collective violence may also cause serious health consequences
through its impact on the physical, economic, social, and biologic environments in which people live. The environmental damage may affect people
not only in nations directly engaged in collective violence but in all nations.
Much of the morbidity and mortality during war, especially among civilians, has been the result of devastation of societal infrastructure, including
destruction of food and water supply systems, health care facilities and
public health services, sewage disposal systems, power plants and electrical
grids, and transportation and communication systems. Destruction of infrastructure has led to food shortages and resultant malnutrition, contamination of food and of drinking water and resultant foodborne and waterborne
illness, and health care and public health deficiencies and resultant disease
(Levy and Sidel, 2005).

Preparation for war also can adversely affect human health. Some of
the impacts are direct, such as injuries and deaths during training exercises; others are indirect. As with war itself, preparation for war can divert
human, financial, and other resources that otherwise might be used for
health and human services. Not only is the actual use of arms a problem,
but also the threat to use them. This is especially true of WMD but also
applies to spending on other weapons, from small arms and light weapons
to warplanes and warships. The resources used for preparation for war are
frequently diverted from the resources a country needs for education, housing, and medical and social services. Preparation for war is also destructive
to the environment, including the use of nonrenewable resources and the
use of bombs and shells in military training and military exercises. Perhaps
most important, preparation for war may incite preparation for war by
potential enemies and may make war more likely.

Damage to the physical environment—water, land, air, and space—and use of nonrenewable resources may be the result of preparation for war as well as war itself. Lakes, rivers, streams and aquifers, land masses, and the atmosphere may be polluted through testing and use of weaponry. Outer space could be damaged by placement of weapons. Significant amounts of nonrenewable resources may be used in weapons production, testing, and use (Renner, 2000; Levy and Sidel, 2005; Westing, 2008).

The economic environment may also be adversely affected by the diversion of resources from education, housing, nutrition, and other human and health services to military activities and through an increase in national debt and/or taxation. These economic impacts affect both developed and developing countries (National Priorities Project, 2007).

Governmental and societal preoccupation with preparation for wars— often known as "militarism"—may lead to massive diversion and subversion of efforts to promote human welfare. This preoccupation may lead to policies that promote "preemptive war" (when an attack is allegedly imminent) and to "preventive war" (when an attack may be feared sometime in the future). Diversion of resources to war is a problem worldwide but is especially important in developing countries. Many developing countries spend substantially more on military expenditures than on health-related expenditures; for example, in 1990, Ethiopia spent $16 per capita for military expenditures and only $1 per capita for health, and Sudan spent $25 per capita for military expenditures and only $1 per capita for health (Foege, 2000). The social environment may be affected by increasing militarism, by encouragement of violence as a means of settling disputes, and by infringement on civil rights and civil liberties. In addition, preparation for war, like war itself, can promote violence as a means for settling disputes.

Another indirect impact of war is the creation of many refugees and internally displaced persons. Many of the world's 12 million refugees have left their native countries as a result of war. Refugees often flee to neighboring less-developed countries, which often face significant challenges in addressing the public health needs of their own populations. In addition, the vast majority of the 22 to 25 million internally displaced persons worldwide have left their homes to escape war. The vast majority of refugees and internally displaced persons as a result of war are women, children, and elderly people who may be highly vulnerable not only to disease and malnutrition, but also to threats of their security. These internally displaced persons are often worse off than refugees who have left their countries because internally displaced persons often do not have easy access to food, safe water, health care, shelter, and other necessities. Approximately 8 million of these internally displaced persons live in the DRC, Uganda, and Sudan—all in Africa (Roberts and Muganda, 2008). In West Darfur, Sudan, hundreds of thousands of people have been internally displaced and hundreds of thousands have fled to refugee camps in neighboring Chad as a result of bitter ethnic conflict (Sirkin, 2008). Refugees and internally displaced persons experience much higher rates of mortality and morbidity, much of it due to malnutrition and infectious diseases (Associated Press, 2007; Toole, 2008).

The biological environment may be disrupted: by conventional weapons during use in training, in conflict or from their disposal; by ionizing radiation from nuclear weapons production, testing, use, and disposal and from use or testing of radioactive weapons, including depleted uranium; by toxic substances from production, testing, use, and disposal of chemical or toxin weapons and from "conventional" weapons during their use in training or in combat or from their disposal. Spread of infectious diseases may occur as a result of degradation of protective factors, such as safe sewage disposal and water treatment, or possibly by the production, testing, and use of bioweapons.

Hazardous wastes from military operations represent potential contaminants of air, water, and soil. For example, groundwater was contaminated with trichloroethylene, a probable human carcinogen, and other toxins at the Otis Air Force Base in Massachusetts; 125 chemicals were dumped over 30 years at the Rocky Mountain Arsenal in Colorado; and benzene, a definite human carcinogen, was found in extremely high concentrations at the McChord Air Force Base in the state of Washington (Renner, 2000).

During both war and the preparation for war, military forces consume huge amounts of fossil fuels and other nonrenewable materials. Energy consumption by military equipment can be substantial. For example, an armored division of 348 battle tanks operating for 1 day consumes more than 2.2 million liters of fuel, and a carrier battle group operating for 1 day consumes more than 1.5 million liters of fuel. In the late 1980s, the U.S. military annually consumed 18.6 million tons of fuel (more than 44 percent of the world's total) and emitted 381,000 tons of carbon monoxide, 157,000 tons of oxides of nitrogen, 78,000 tons of hydrocarbons, and 17,900 tons of sulfur dioxide (Renner, 2000).

### Specific Wars

*Civil Wars in Africa*

According to data from the Stockholm International Peace Research Institute, for the 1990-2005 period, the regions that had the largest number of armed conflicts were Asia and Africa. For example, in 1998, when there were 26 major armed conflicts reported, 11 were in Africa and 8 were in Asia, and in 2005, when there were 16 armed conflicts reported, there were 6 in Asia and 3 in Africa. There has been a progressive decline in armed conflicts in Africa since 1990, with most of these conflicts being civil wars.

For example, in 1990, there were 19 conflicts in 17 locations in the region, only one of which was an interstate conflict (between Eritrea and Ethiopia). The three armed conflicts reported in Africa in 2005 were the lowest number for the region in the period after the end of the Cold War. Like in Africa, most of the recent armed conflicts in Asia have been within states as opposed to between states. In the 1990-2005 period, there were four conflicts in Africa that were active in all 16 years in this period: those in India (Kashmir), Myanmar (Karen), Sri Lanka (Eelam), and the Philippines. One conflict in the region was fought between states, that between India and Pakistan (Stockholm International Peace Research Institute, 2006).

A civil war in the DRC, which began in 1996 and involved forces from other countries between 1998 and 2002, accounted for almost 4 million deaths, primarily of civilians (Roberts and Muganda, 2008). Most of the deaths in this war, in one analysis approximately 98 percent, were not directly due to warfare, but rather due to malnutrition, infectious disease, and other indirect effects due to damage to the health-supporting infrastructure of society (Roberts and Muganda, 2008). The impact of this war on civilians was documented by epidemiologic surveys conducted by the International Rescue Committee, the results of which were widely publicized in the news media and then in peer-reviewed journals. Although foreign armies formally withdrew in 2002, when a peace accord was signed, there have been difficulties in establishing a functional central government, especially in the eastern section of the DRC. Lessons that can be learned from this war include the following:

1. This war resulted from the unwillingness of the international community to arrest and control the perpetrators of the Rwandan genocide who had fled to neighboring countries.
2. The international community did little to respond to Rwanda and Uganda invading the DRC in 1996 to overthrow the government.
3. This war demonstrated the importance of recognizing and preventing the public health and human rights consequences that generally accompany armed conflict.
4. Even intrastate conflicts can cross national boundaries and these conflicts can be harder to control since most conflict control machinery is aimed at interstate conflicts.

*The Iraq War*

An important current example of the direct and the indirect effects of armed conflict in a lower-middle-income country is the impact on Iraq of war from 1980 to the present. In the Iran-Iraq War from 1980 to 1988, between 500,000 and 1 million people were killed, and another 1 to 2 million people were wounded. The Iran-Iraq War uprooted 2.5 million people and destroyed whole cities. It cost over $200 billion (Levy and Sidel, 2008c).

In the 1991 Persian Gulf War, tens of thousands of people died, many were injured, and many became chronically ill. But the numbers of deaths and illnesses during the Persian Gulf War were far exceeded by those that occurred in the several years after the war. UNICEF estimated that between 350,000 and 500,000 excessive children's deaths occurred in Iraq from 1991 to 1998, largely due to postwar sanctions imposed by the United States and other countries (Levy and Sidel, 2008c). These sanctions restricted food and medicine from getting into Iraq for several years until the Oil-for-Food Program began.

In March 2003, U.S. and other Coalition forces invaded Iraq. Two months after the invasion, President Bush declared that most hostilities were over. Most of the health consequences of this war, however, have occurred since then. There have been more than 3,200 deaths among U.S. military personnel, and more than 24,000 U.S. military personnel have been wounded (as of July 2007). An additional 30,000 U.S. military personnel have suffered significant injuries or illnesses during the war. There has been a high incidence of mental health disorders among U.S. troops; the Surgeon General of the U.S. Army has estimated that 30 percent of returning troops have stress-related mental health problems. The toll on Iraqis has been many times greater than that on U.S. military personnel. A study in 2006 based on a systematic sample of approximately 2,000 households found that since the start of the war approximately 650,000 Iraqis have died, approximately 600,000 as a result of violence, most commonly gunfire (Roberts et al., 2004; Burnham et al., 2006). The Iraq War has had profound effects on health services and the health-supporting infrastructure in Iraq, including water treatment facilities, sewage treatment plants, the food supply, and transportation and communication systems. In addition, there have been many violations of human rights, including cruel punishment and torture of detainees. The war has diverted a huge amount of resources that might otherwise have been spent for health and other human services in Iraq, the United States, and elsewhere. And there have been many adverse impacts of the war on the physical, sociocultural, and economic environments, especially within Iraq (Levy and Sidel, 2008c).

Eight million Iraqis—nearly one in three—are now in need of emergency aid, states a report, "Rising to the Humanitarian Challenge in Iraq," by Oxfam International and the NGO Coordination Committee in Iraq (NCCI), a network of aid organizations working in Iraq (Oxfam International, 2007). According to the report,

* Four million Iraqis—15 percent—regularly cannot buy enough to eat.

- 70 percent are without adequate water supplies, compared to 50 percent in 2003.
- 28 percent of children are malnourished, compared to 19 percent before the 2003 invasion.
- 92 percent of Iraqi children suffer learning problems, mostly due to the climate of fear.
- More than 2 million people—mostly women and children—have been displaced inside Iraq.
- A further 2 million Iraqis have become refugees, mainly in Syria and Jordan.

## Weapons Systems

### Conventional Weapons

Conventional weapons consist of explosives, incendiaries, and weapons of various sizes, ranging from small arms and light weapons (SALWs) to heavy artillery and bombs. SALWs, which include pistols, rifles, machine guns, and other hand-held or easily transportable weapons, are the weapons most often used in wars. While some restrictions have been placed on their use in war, such as the outlawing of the use of "dum-dum bullets," which cause extensive injuries when striking a human, there has been little effective effort to outlaw their use (Cukier and Sidel, 2006). In the Millennium Report of the UN Secretary-General to the General Assembly, Kofi Annan stated that small arms could be described as WMD because of the fatalities they produce. "The death toll from small arms dwarf that of all other weapons systems—and in most years greatly exceeds the toll of the atomic bombs that devastated Hiroshima and Nagasaki. In terms of the carnage they cause, small arms, indeed, could be described as 'weapons of mass destruction.' Yet there is still no global non-proliferation regime to limit their spread" (Taljaard, 2003).

Conventional weapons have accounted for the overwhelming majority of adverse environmental consequences due to war. During World War II, for example, extensive carpet bombing of cities in Europe and Japan accounted not only for many deaths and injuries, but also widespread devastation of urban environments. As another example, the more than 600 oil well fires in Kuwait during the Persian Gulf War accounted for widespread environmental devastation as well as acute, and possibly chronic, respiratory ailments among people who were exposed to the smoke from these fires. As a further example, bombing of mangrove forests during the Vietnam War led to destruction of these forests, and the resultant bomb craters remain several decades afterward, often filling with stagnant water that is a breeding ground for mosquitoes that transmit malaria and other mosquito-borne diseases (Allukian and Atwood, 2008; Westing, 2008).

*Nuclear Weapons*

Nuclear weapons have been increasingly widespread since their development in the 1940s. There are now an estimated 27,000 nuclear warheads in at least eight nations—the United States, Russia, the United Kingdom, France, China, Israel, India, and Pakistan—and possibly also North Korea (Sutton and Gould, 2007). The historic high in explosive capacity of the world nuclear weapons stockpiles was reached in 1960 with an explosive capacity equivalent to 20 thousand megatons (20 billion tons or 40 trillion pounds) of TNT, equivalent to that of 1.4 million of the nuclear bombs dropped on Hiroshima (Yokoro and Kamada, 2000). In the United States in 1967, the nuclear stockpile had reached approximately 32,000 nuclear warheads of 30 different types. In 2003, the U.S. stockpile was about 10,400 warheads, totaling about 2,000 megatons—equivalent to 140,000 Hiroshima-size bombs. Five thousand of the nuclear weapons in the United States, Russia, and possibly other countries are on "hair-trigger" alert, ready to fire on a few minutes notice.

The detonation of nuclear bombs over Hiroshima and Nagasaki in August 1945 during World War II led to the immediate deaths of approximately 200,000 people, primarily civilians, as well as lasting injury and later death of many others and massive devastation—and widespread radioactive contamination—of the environment in these two cities (Yokoro and Kamada, 2000). Atmospheric testing of nuclear weapons by the United States, the Soviet Union, and other countries has also led to environmental contamination, with increased rates of leukemia and other cancers among populations who were downwind from these tests. The carcinogenic effects on children of exposure to iodine-131, a radioactive isotope of iodine produced by the testing, have been well documented (Institute of Medicine and National Research Council, 1999). In addition to the potential for the use of nuclear weapons by national armed forces, such as that described in the recent U.S. Nuclear Posture Review, which threatened use of nuclear weapons under a wider range of circumstances, there is an increasing threat of their use by individuals and groups (Gordon, 2002; Sutton and Gould, 2008).

*Radiologic Weapons*

"Dirty bombs," consisting of conventional explosive devices mixed with radioactive materials, or attacks on nuclear power plants with explosive weapons could widely scatter highly radioactive materials. Another example of a radioactive substance used in weapons is depleted uranium (DU), uranium from which the isotope usable for nuclear weapons or as fuel rods for nuclear power plants has been removed. DU is used militarily as a casing for armor-penetrating shells. An extremely dense material, uranium used as a casing increases the ability of the shell to penetrate the armor of tanks; uranium is also pyrophoric and bursts into flame on impact. DU-encased shells were used by the United States during the Persian Gulf War and the Iraq War and the war in Kosovo; similar shells were used by the United Kingdom in the Iraq War. DU, which is both radioactive and extremely toxic, has been demonstrated to cause contamination of the soil and groundwater. Use of DU is considered legal by the nations using it, but its use is considered by others to be illegal under the Geneva Conventions and other international treaties (Hindi et al., 2005; Bertell, 2006).

*Chemicals*

A variety of chemical weapons and related materials have the potential for direct health effects during collective violence and also for contaminating the physical environment during war and the preparation for war. The potential for exposure exists not only for military and civilian populations who may be exposed during the use of chemical weapons in wartime, but also for workers involved in the development, production, transport, and storage of these weapons and community residents living near facilities where these weapons are developed, produced, transported, and stored. In addition, disposal of these weapons, including their disassembly and incineration, can be hazardous.

During the Vietnam War, the U.S. military used defoliants on mangrove forests and other vegetation, which not only defoliated and killed trees and other plants, but may also have led to excessive numbers of birth defects and cases of cancer among nearby residents in Vietnam (Levy and Sidel, 2005). In addition, development and production of conventional weapons involve the use of many chemicals that are toxic and can contaminate the environment. Furthermore, there is now a plausible threat of nonstate agents using chemical weapons. A Japanese cult, Aum Shinrikyo, used sarin in the subway system of two Japanese cities in the mid 1990s, accounting for the death of 19 people and injuries to thousands (Spanjaard and Khabib, 2007).

The Chemical Weapons Convention (CWC), which entered into force in 1997, prohibits all development, production, acquisition, stockpiling, transfer, and use of chemical weapons. It requires each state party to destroy its chemical weapons and chemical weapons production facilities, and any chemical weapons it may have abandoned on the territory of another state party. The verification provisions of the CWC affect not only the military sector but also the civilian chemical industry worldwide through certain restrictions and obligations regarding the production, processing, and consumption of chemicals that are considered relevant to the objectives of the convention. These provisions are to be verified through a combination of reporting requirements, routine onsite inspection of declared sites, and short-notice challenge inspections. The Organization for the Prohibition of Chemical Weapons (OPCW) in The Hague, established by the CWC, ensures the implementation of the provisions of the CWC. The disposal of chemical weapons required by the CWC has raised controversy about the safety of two different methods of disposal: incineration and chemical neutralization. The controversy about safety and protection of the environment has delayed completion of the disposal by the date required by the CWC (Lee and Kales, 2008).

*Biological Agents*

Biological agents consist of bacteria, viruses, other microorganisms, and their toxins, which can not only directly produce illness in humans, but can be used against other animals or plants, thereby adversely affecting human food supplies or agricultural resources and indirectly affecting human health. Biological agents have been used relatively infrequently during warfare, but there has long been a potential for their use. These agents have been used as weapons, albeit sporadically, since ancient times. In the 6th century BCE, Persia, Greece, and Rome tried to contaminate drinking water sources with diseased corpses. In 1346 AD, Mongols beseeching the Crimean seaport of Kaffa placed cadavers of plague victims on hurling machines and threw them into Kaffa. In the mid-18th century, during the French and Indian War, a British commander sent blankets infected with smallpox to Native Americans. During World War I, Germany dropped bombs that contained plague bacteria over British positions and used cholera in Italy. During the 1930s, Japan contaminated the food and water supplies of several cities and sprayed the cities with cultures of microorganisms. In subsequent years, a number of nations, including the United States and the Soviet Union, continued to develop and test biological weapons, but there is no evidence that they were used in war (Harris and Paxman, 1982; Cole, 1988; Meselson, 1994; Levy and Sidel, 2008b).

There is concern that biological agents could be used as terrorist weapons. In the fall of 2001, anthrax spores were disseminated through the U.S. mail, ultimately causing 23 cases of inhalational and skin anthrax, 5 of which were fatal. The Centers for Disease Control and Prevention has identified three categories of diseases caused by biological agents, according to its level of concern that they may be used as terrorist weapons. Category A consists of the agents that cause anthrax, botulism, plague, smallpox, tularemia, and several viral hemorrhagic fevers. Category B consists of the agents that cause brucellosis, glanders, melioidosis, psittacosis, Q fever, and food safety threats (such as *Salmonella* and *Shigella* species, and *Escherichia coli* O157:H7), as well as epsilon toxin of *Clostridium perfringens*, ricin toxin from castor beans, and Staphylococcyl enterotoxin B. Category C consists of the agents that cause emerging infectious diseases such as Nipah virus and hantavirus (Levy and Sidel, 2008b).

## Antipersonnel Landmines

There are now approximately 80 million landmines still deployed worldwide in at least 78 countries. These landmines have been termed "weapons of mass destruction, one person at a time." They have often been placed in rural areas, posing a threat to residents of these areas and often disrupting farming and other activities. Civilians are the most likely to be injured or killed by landmines, which continue to injure and kill 15,000 to 20,000 people annually. It is estimated that half of all landmine victims die of their injuries before they reach appropriate medical care. More than 90 percent of landmine victims are civilians, primarily poor people living in rural areas. One-fourth of landmine victims are children, putting landmines among the six most preventable major causes of death to children throughout the world. Although a mine may cost as little as $3 to produce, it may cost as much as $1,000 to remove and its adverse economic impact on human health and well-being is substantially higher. Mines, in addition to maiming and killing people, also make large areas of land uninhabitable. Remaining in place for many years, they pose long-term threats to people, including refugees and internally displaced persons returning to their homes after long periods of war. Since the entry into force of the Anti-Personnel Landmine Convention in 1997, production of landmines has been markedly reduced and a number of those that had been implanted in the ground have been removed. Many of the mines are still buried and additional resources will be required to continue unearthing and destroying them, tasks that pose inherent risks to demining personnel (International Campaign to Ban Landmines, 2006; Sirkin et al., 2008).

## Genocide

Genocide has been formally defined by the Convention on the Prevention and Punishment of the Crime of Genocide, which was explained by the United Nations, and entered into force on January 12, 1951. That convention defines genocide as any of the following acts committed with intent to destroy, in whole or in part, a national, ethical, racial, or religious group:

- Killing members of the group
- Causing serious bodily or mental harm to members of the group
- Deliberately inflicting on the group conditions of life calculated to bring about its physical destruction in whole or in part
  - Imposing measures intended to prevent births within the group
  - Forcibly transferring children of the group to another group

Acts of genocide are generally difficult to establish for prosecution since intent and demonstrating a chain of accountability has to be established. International criminal courts and tribunals function primarily because the states involved are incapable or unwilling to prosecute crimes of this magnitude themselves. An International Criminal Court (ICC) was established in 2002 for jurisdiction when international courts are unwilling or unable to investigate or prosecute genocide. The United States refused to ratify the Statute establishing the ICC (Sewall and Kaysen, 2000).

Groups that are widely considered to have suffered genocide include people in Armenia, in Nazi Germany before and during World War II, in former Yugoslavia, in Rwanda, and in Darfur (Power, 2002; Sirkin, 2008). Genocide in Germany during World War II, commonly known as the Holocaust, involved the systematic murder of primarily Jews as well as gypsies, those accused of being homosexuals, and others. Trials in which one of the charges was genocide were held in Nuremberg from 1945 to 1949. The first of these was the trial of major war criminals, which was conducted by all four of the powers occupying Germany. The second trial is known as "the doctors trial" and was conducted by the United States.

Genocide in former Yugoslavia since 1991 has been investigated by the International Criminal Tribunal for the Former Yugoslavia, which is located in The Hague. Among those found guilty of genocide or crimes against humanity was Radislav Kristic, a general in the Bosnian Serb Army, sentenced to 35 years in prison for genocide in Srebrenica, crimes against humanity, and violation of the laws or customs of war (Milanovic, 2007).

Widespread murders in Rwanda that have been termed "genocide" began in April 1994. The International Criminal Tribunal for Rwanda, a court under the auspices of the United Nations, has finished 19 trials and convicted 25 people accused of genocide and related crimes.

In 2004, the U.S. Secretary of State declared that the conflict in Darfur, Sudan, which started in 2003, was genocidal. Although the application of the term to Darfur is still controversial, it is estimated that 2 million people have been displaced and between 200,000 and 400,000 people have died (Sirkin, 2008).

## Terrorism and the "War on Terror"

Since September 11, 2001, there has been increasing concern in the United States and other countries about violence conducted by individuals and groups to create fear and advance a political agenda—a form of violence commonly called "terrorism" (Levy and Sidel, 2007). Terrorism is often defined in a partisan fashion: those called "terrorist" by one side in a conflict may be viewed as "patriots," "freedom fighters," or "servants of God" by the other. The term *terrorist* is "generally applied to one's enemies and opponents, or to those with whom one disagrees and would otherwise prefer to ignore" (Hoffmann, 1998). Groups that have been relatively powerless, in contrast to very powerful foes, have often used terrorist tactics, believing that these tactics represented effective weapons against superior forces. The use of the term, therefore, depends on one's point of view. The term *terrorist* implies a moral judgment; if one group can attach the term to its opponent, then it may persuade others to adopt its moral perspective (Jenkins, 1980).

Terrorism is intended to have psychological effects that go beyond the immediate victims to intimidate a wider population, such as a rival ethnic or religious group, a national government or political party, or an entire country (Hoffmann, 1998). It is often intended to establish power where there is none or to consolidate power where there is little. Although many nations, including the United States, differentiate terrorism from war, especially a war formally declared by a nation, we perceive little difference between terrorism and a war directed largely against civilian populations.

U.S. law defines terrorism as "premeditated, politically motivated violence perpetrated against non-combatant targets by subnational groups or clandestine agents" (22 U.S.C. 2656 (d)(2)). Based on this definition, the National Counterterrorism Center reported that, during 2006, there were 14,352 terrorist attacks worldwide that resulted in 20,573 deaths (13,340 in Iraq), with an additional 36,214 people wounded. There were nearly 300 incidents that resulted in 10 or more deaths, 90 percent of which were in the Near East and South Asia. Armed attacks and bombings led to 77 percent of the fatalities during 2006. The bombings of the World Trade Center in 1993, the Alfred P. Murrah Federal Building in Oklahoma City in 1995, and U.S. military and diplomatic facilities abroad in the late 1990s, the September 11, 2001, attacks on the World Trade Center and the Pentagon, and the letters contaminated with anthrax spores that were mailed to two U.S. senators and several news organizations have all been considered "terrorist acts" (National Counterterrorism Center, 2007).

Some analysts, on the other hand, construe the term terrorism to encompass the use by countries of weapons designed to cause mass casualties among civilian populations, sometimes termed "state terrorism." Attacks cited above as examples of attacks during war designed to cause mass casualties among civilian populations, including the bombing of Guernica and the carpet bombing of urban centers during World War II, are in our view also examples of state terrorism. We have therefore defined terrorism as "politically motivated violence or the threat of violence, especially against civilians, with the intent to instill fear." (Levy and Sidel, 2007). This definition includes violent acts against civilians with the intent to instill fear conducted by nation-states as well as acts committed by individuals and subnational groups. The term "terrorism" has considerable overlap with the term "war" and many actions conducted during war fit our definition of terrorism. The initiation of a *war* on terror, in contrast to use of education, law enforcement, economic aid, and other methods to prevent such acts, has led some analysts to include the "war on terror" as an example of collective violence.

Since the September 11, 2001, attacks, billions of dollars have been spent by federal, state, and local governments in the United States on emergency preparedness and response capabilities for potential terrorist attacks, part of the "war on terror." Although some of this money has been used to improve public health capabilities, work to prepare for low-probability events has diverted much attention and many resources from widespread existing public health problems (Rosner and Markowitz, 2006). In addition, the "war on terror" has generated attacks on civil rights and civil liberties which impact well-being, a public health concern (Sidel, 2004; Levy and Sidel, 2007).

We believe that there needs to be a balanced approach to strengthening systems and protecting people in response to the threat of terrorism, an approach that strengthens a broad range of public health capacities and preserves civil liberties. Public health workers, in our view, need to support measures to ensure emergency preparedness, not only for potential terrorist attacks but also for chemical emergencies, radiation emergencies, natural disasters, severe weather events, and large outbreaks of disease. The Centers for Disease Control and Prevention (CDC) website provides useful information on emergency preparedness (CDC, 2007).

As part of its "war on terror," the United States has taken actions that endanger not only civil liberties within the United States but also human rights and peace worldwide. It has indiscriminately attacked civilians whom it labels "terrorists" in Afghanistan, Iraq, and Somalia; has denied *habeas corpus* (a legal action or writ by which detainees can seek relief from unlawful imprisonment) and the right to counsel and a speedy trial to detainees at Abu Ghraib and at Guantanamo Bay; and has "renditioned" detainees to other countries for torture. These actions violate human rights and threaten peace.

## Public Health Approaches

The health and environmental problems created by collective violence can appear to be overwhelming. However, standard public health principles and implementation measures can be successfully applied in addressing these problems, including (1) surveillance and documentation, (2) education and awareness raising, (3) advocacy for sound policies and programs, and (4) implementation of programs aimed at both prevention and the provision of acute and long-term care.

### Surveillance and Documentation

Surveillance and other activities can document the health problems caused by war and terrorism. While the numbers of deaths, wounds, and injuries among uniformed combatants are generally well documented, deaths, wounds, and injuries among civilians are more difficult to document. Household cluster surveys have been used during the Iraq War and the civil war in the DRC to estimate the civilian casualties. Technical approaches to surveillance can include environmental monitoring and biological monitoring to document and assess the human burden of environmental contaminants and their adverse health consequences. Nontechnical approaches can include information from physician reports, reports in the mass media, and assessments by government agencies.

### Education and Awareness Raising

Much can be accomplished by educating and raising the awareness of health professionals, policy makers, and the general public about the problems caused by war and terrorism. A multifaceted approach that incorporates publications by citizens groups and professional organizations, communications of the mass media, and personal communication is often valuable. In addition, efforts should be made to assist people in distinguishing between accurate and inaccurate information and in setting priorities.

### Advocacy for Sound Policies and Programs

Advocating for improved policies and programs can help prevent collective violence and minimize the public health impact of war and terrorism. Public health workers can address the underlying causes of war and terrorism and promote a greater understanding of these issues. These causes include historical, political, economic, social, philosophical, and ideological roots of war and terrorism. Public health workers should promote programs and other activities that support better understanding and tolerance among people of different backgrounds and nations. They should work to ensure that basic human needs are met and human rights are protected. They can address the threat to freedom posed by the curtailment of civil rights and civil liberties imposed by governments (Annas and Geiger, 2008).

## Levels of Prevention

Those concerned with the promotion and protection of health classify preventive measures into four basic categories: pre-primary (or primordial) prevention, primary prevention, secondary prevention, and tertiary prevention. Pre-primary prevention consists of measures to prevent adverse health consequences by removing the conditions that lead to them. Primary prevention consists of measures to prevent the health consequences of a specific illness or injury by preventing its occurrence in a specific individual or among a specific group. Secondary prevention consists of measures to prevent or limit the health consequences of an illness or injury, or to limit the spread of an infectious disease to others, after the disease process has begun. Tertiary prevention consists of efforts to rehabilitate those injured and to reintegrate them into society or, in the case of prevention of collective violence, to prevent the resumption of violence.

### Pre-Primary Prevention

In general, pre-primary prevention requires political and social will. Pre-primary and primary prevention may be difficult to accomplish because the causes of the disease or injury may be unknown and, when they are known, the preventive methods may be difficult to implement technically or politically. Acts of war or terrorism and their health consequences can be prevented or ameliorated through pre-primary prevention, but this will require alliances among civil society (nongovernmental) organizations and governmental or intergovernmental units.

The underlying causes of collective violence include poverty, social inequities, adverse effects of globalization, and shame and humiliation. Persistence of socioeconomic disparities and other forms of social injustice are among the leading underlying causes of war and terrorism. The rich-poor divide is growing. In 1960, in the 20 richest countries, the per-capita GDP was 18-fold that in the 20 poorest countries; by 1995, this gap had increased to 37-fold. Between 1980 and the late 1990s, inequality increased in 48 of 73 countries for which there are reliable data, including China, Russia, and the United States (Marmot and Bell, 2006). Inequality is not restricted to personal income but also applies to other important areas of life, including health status, access to health care, education, and employment opportunities. In addition, abundant national resources, such as oil, minerals, metals, gemstones, drug crops, and timber, have fueled many wars in developing countries.

Globalization is similarly a two-edged sword. Insofar as globalization leads to good relations among nation-states and reductions in poverty and disparities within and among nations, it may play a powerful role in prevention of collective violence. Conversely, if globalization leads to exploitation of people, of the environment, and of other resources, it may be among the causes of war.

The Carnegie Commission on Preventing Deadly Conflict has identified the following factors that put nations at risk of violent conflict, including the following:

- Lack of democratic processes and unequal access to power, particularly in situations where power arises from religious or ethnic identity, and leaders are repressive or abusive of human rights
- Social inequality characterized by markedly unequal distribution of resources and access to these resources, especially where the economy is in decline and there is, as a result, more social inequality and more competition for resources
- Control by one group of valuable natural resources, such as oil, timber, drugs, or gems
- Demographic changes that are so rapid that they outstrip the capability of the nation to provide basic necessary services and opportunities for employment (Carnegie Commission, 2007)

Wealthy nations can play an important role in preventing collective violence by increasing funding for humanitarian and sustainable development programs that address the root causes of collective violence, such as hunger, illiteracy, and unemployment.

### Promoting Multilateralism

Since its founding in 1946, the United Nations has attempted to live up to the goal stated in its charter: "to save succeeding generations from the scourge of war." Its mandate, along with preventing war, includes protecting human rights, promoting international justice, and helping the people of the world to achieve a sustainable standard of living. Its affiliated programs and specialized agencies include, among many others, the United Nations Children's Fund (UNICEF), WHO, the Food and Agriculture Organization, the International Labor Organization (ILO), the United Nations Development Program, and the Office of the UN High Commissioner for Refugees. These UN-related organizations, and the UN itself, have made an enormous difference in the lives of people over the past half-century.

The resources allocated to the UN by its member states are grossly inadequate. The annual budget for the core functions—the Secretariat operations in New York, Geneva, Nairobi, Vienna, and five Regional Commissions—is $1.25 billion. This is about 4 percent of New York City's annual budget—and nearly a billion dollars less than the yearly cost of Tokyo's Fire Department. The entire UN system (excluding the World Bank and International Monetary Fund) spends $12 billion a year. By comparison, annual world military expenditures—$1 trillion—would pay for the entire UN system for more than 65 years.

The UN has no army and no police. It relies on the voluntary contribution of troops and other personnel to halt conflicts that threaten peace and security. The United States and other Member States on the Security Council decide when and where to deploy peacekeeping troops. Long-term conflicts, such as those in the Sudan and Kashmir, and the Israeli-Palestinian conflict, fester while conflicting national priorities deadlock the UN's ability to act. In fact, if stymied by the veto, the organization has little power beyond the bully pulpit. The United States and the United Kingdom have severely weakened the UN's ability to prevent collective violence by their unauthorized and illegal invasion of Iraq in 2003. The United States also failed to support the International War Crimes Tribunal through signature and ratification of the Statute of the International Criminal Court (Sewall and Kaysen, 2000).

## Ending Poverty and Social Injustice

Poverty and other manifestations of social injustice contribute to conditions that lead to collective violence. Growing socioeconomic and other disparities between the rich and the poor within countries, and between rich and poor nations, also contribute to the likelihood of armed conflict. By addressing these underlying conditions through policies and programs that redistribute wealth within nations and among nations, and by providing financial and technical assistance to less-developed nations, countries like the United States can minimize poverty and other forms of social injustice that lead to collective violence. The Commission on Social Determinants of Health was established in 2005 to spearhead action on the social causes that underlie ill health and will recommend the best ways to address health's social determinants and safeguard to help the poor and marginalize the population (Commission, 2007; Marmot and Bell, 2006).

## Creating a Culture of Peace

People in the health and environment sectors can do much to promote a culture of peace, in which nonviolent means are utilized to settle conflicts.

A culture of peace is based on the values, attitudes, and behaviors that form the deep roots of peace. They are in some ways the opposite of the values, attitudes, and behaviors that reflect and inspire collective violence, but should not be equated with just the absence of war. A culture of peace can exist at the level of the family, workplace, school, and community as well as at the level of the state and in international relations. Health and environment professionals and others can play important roles in encouraging the development of a culture of peace at all these levels.

The Hague Appeal for Peace Civil Society Conference was held in 1999 on the 100th anniversary of the 1899 Hague Peace Conference. The 1899 conference, attended by governmental representatives, was devoted to finding methods for making war more humane. The 1999 conference, attended by 1,000 individuals and representatives of civil-society organizations, was devoted to finding methods to prevent war and to establish a "culture of peace." The document adopted at the 1999 conference, *The Hague Appeal for Peace and Justice for the 21st Century*, has been translated by the UN into all its official languages and distributed widely around the world. Its 10-point action agenda addressed education for peace, human rights, and democracy; the adverse effects of globalization; sustainable and equitable use of environmental resources; elimination of racial, ethnic, religious, and gender intolerance; protection of children; reduction of violence; and other issues (Hague Appeal, 2007).

## Primary Prevention

Primary prevention includes preventing specific elements of collective violence and sharply reducing preparation for war. This includes not only wars between nations but wars within nations as well.

## Strengthening of Nuclear Weapons Treaties

Unlike the implementation of treaties banning chemical weapons and biological weapons, there is no comprehensive treaty banning the use or mandating the destruction of nuclear weapons. Instead a series of overlapping incomplete treaties have been negotiated. The Partial Test Ban Treaty (PTBT) of 1963, promoted in part by concerns about radioactive environmental contamination, banned nuclear tests in the atmosphere, underwater, and in outer space. The expansion of the PTBT, the Comprehensive Nuclear-Test-Ban Treaty (CTBT), a key step toward nuclear disarmament and preventing proliferation, was opened for signature in 1996 but has not yet received sufficient signatures or ratifications to enter into force. It bans nuclear explosions, for either military or civilian purposes, but docs not ban computer simulations and subcritical tests, which some nations rely on to maintain the option of developing new nuclear weapons. The CTBT has been signed and ratified by 140 nations. Entry into force requires ratification by the 44 nuclear-capable nations, which has not yet been achieved. The United States has not yet ratified the CTBT.

The Treaty on the Non-Proliferation of Nuclear Weapons (the "Nuclear Non-Proliferation Treaty," or NPT) was opened for signature in 1968 and entered into force in 1970. A total of 189 states parties (nations) have ratified the treaty. The five nuclear-weapon states recognized under the NPT— China, France, Russia, the United Kingdom, and the United States—are parties to the treaty. The NPT attempts to prevent the spread of nuclear weapons by restricting transfer of certain technologies. It relies on a control system carried out by the International Atomic Energy Agency, which also promotes nuclear energy. In exchange for the non-nuclear-weapons states' commitment not to develop or otherwise acquire nuclear weapons, the NPT commits the nuclear-weapon states to good-faith negotiations on nuclear disarmament. Every 5 years since 1970 the states parties have held a review conference to assess implementation of the treaty. The review conference in 2000 identified and approved practical steps toward the total elimination of nuclear arsenals. The International Court of Justice (the World Court) in 2006 in an advisory opinion urged that the nations possessing nuclear weapons move expeditiously toward nuclear disarmament, as is required by Article VI of the NPT (Weapons of Mass Destruction Commission, 2006).

The Anti-Ballistic Missile (ABM) Treaty between the United States and the Soviet Union was signed and entered into force in 1972. The ABM Treaty, by limiting defensive systems that would otherwise spur an offensive arms race, has been seen as the foundation for the strategic nuclear arms reduction treaties. In late 2001, President Bush announced that the United States would withdraw from the ABM Treaty within 6 months and gave formal notice, stating that it "hinders our government's ability to develop ways to protect our people from future terrorist or rogue-state missile attacks." The United States in 2007 announced plans to establish a ballistic missile defense system in Eastern Europe, which led Russia to threaten to increase its armory of nuclear weapons.

Nuclear-weapons states should help stop the spread of nuclear weapons by actively supporting and adhering to these treaties and by setting an example for the rest of the world by renouncing the first use of nuclear weapons and the development of new nuclear weapons. It should work with Russia to dismantle nuclear warheads and increase funding for programs to secure nuclear materials so they will not fall into the hands of individuals and groups.

*Strengthening the Chemical Weapons Convention*

The CWC is the strongest of the arms control treaties outlawing a single class of weapons. Inspection and verification of compliance with its provisions lies in the hands of the OPCW in The Hague, established by the CWC (Spanjaard and Khabib, 2007). The CWC has been signed and ratified by 182 nations. Controversies about safety and protection of the environment during the disposal of chemical weapons required by the CWC has delayed completion of the disposal, and large stockpiles still remain in a number of the world's nations that pose a continuing threat to health and to the environment. The United States and other nations have failed to fully support the OPCW in its difficult tasks of inspection and in urging nations to comply with CWC (Lee and Kales, 2008).

*Strengthening the Biological and Toxin Weapons Convention*

While the development, production, transfer, or use of biological weapons was prohibited by the 1975 Biological and Toxin Weapons Convention (BWC), which has been signed and ratified by 158 nations, several nations are believed to retain stockpiles of such weapons. The verification measures included in the BWC are weak and attempts to strengthen them have been unsuccessful. During 2002, the United States blocked attempts to strengthen the verification measures of the BWC, announcing that such measures might lead to exposure of U.S. industrial or military secrets. The United States and other nations must be urged to agree to support the international community's attempts to develop strong inspection and verification protocols for the BWC. Efforts must be made to convince all nations to support strengthening of the BWC and all nations must refrain from secret activities, often termed "defensive," that may fuel a biological arms race.

Perhaps even more important, global public health capacity to deal with all infectious disease must be strengthened. The best individual and collective efforts at diagnosing and treating disease outbreaks can be overwhelmed by any natural or intentionally induced epidemic. Consequently, support for strong global preventive public health capabilities provides the best ultimate defense against ever-evolving threats. The significant vulnerabilities to persistent global reservoirs of endemic illness in impoverished and underserved populations can provide the source of future pandemics. For example, in India during 1999 there were 2 million new cases of tuberculosis, causing about 450,000 deaths. An investment of $30 million annually over a few years, compared to the current U.S. contribution to India of $1 million for this purpose, could virtually wipe out the disease. In addition, the UN has estimated that $10 billion invested in safe water supplies could cut by up to one-third the current 4 billion cases of diarrhea worldwide that result in 2.2 million annual deaths. Strengthening the BWC and preventing suspicion of human-cost infection will help to eliminate the fear that at times prevents action to prevent naturally cost infection.

### Promoting the Support of the Anti-Personnel Landmines Convention (Ottawa Mine Ban Treaty)

A total of 157 nations have signed or ratified the 1997 Ottawa Mine Ban Treaty, also known as the Anti-personnel Landmines Convention. Regrettably, over 30 nations have not signed, including China, India, Iran, Iraq, Israel, Russia, and the United States. Resources are desperately needed to clear the landmines currently deployed. All the nations of the world must be urged to contribute more resources to this task (Hindi et al., 2005; Bertell, 2006; Sirkin, 2008).

### Secondary Prevention

The consequences of collective violence can also be prevented or diminished by secondary prevention: if war occurs, by preventing casualties among military personnel and civilians and preventing environmental destruction and by seeking an end to the war. Secondary prevention methods include strengthening adherence to the Geneva Conventions and other treaties that lessen the effects of war; reducing military activities, including preparation for war; and negotiating effective treaties to lessen environmental damage.

### Tertiary Prevention

Efforts after the end of an armed conflict to reconstruct the damage and to prevent new conflicts and new collective violence are extremely important. The initiation of World War II was in part caused by the failure by the Allies to deal with the problems of defeated Germany after World War I. Tertiary prevention methods include providing appropriate aid to countries damaged by war, such as the Marshall Plan after World War II; requiring environmental reconstruction after the war has ended; and demanding appropriate reparations for physical and environmental damage.

## The Role of Nongovernmental Organizations

Important roles for public health workers in prevention and alleviation of the consequences of collective violence lie in work with nongovernmental organizations (NGOs) (Loretz, 2008). These organizations are increasingly being called "civil society organizations" and focus on war from a medical and public health perspective in a variety of ways:

- Intervening to mitigate the consequences of armed conflict
- Researching the effects of war
- Educating the public and decision makers about its impact on health and the environment
- Advocating for changes in global attitudes and policies toward war and the most dangerous weapons and practices of war
- Changing the social, economic, and political determinants of collective violence

Other NGOs provide direct humanitarian assistance to the victims of collective violence. These organizations generally participate in secondary and tertiary prevention but some, such as the Red Cross, have also in recent years begun to play a role in primary prevention. Humanitarian assistance organizations may also play a role in primary prevention of specific acts of violence and atrocities. They may be strong advocates on behalf of civilian populations among whom they live and for whom they provide humanitarian assistance (Waldman, 2008).

As the Preamble to the Constitution of the United Nations Educational, Scientific, and Cultural Organization (UNESCO) states, "Since wars begin in the minds of men, it is in the minds of men that the defenses of peace must be constructed" (UNESCO, 2007).

## Acknowledgments

The authors are grateful to Mark Rosenberg and James Mercy for their perceptive comments on the draft of this paper and their cogent suggestions for its improvement.

## References

Allukian, M. Jr., and P. L. Atwood. 2008. The Vietnam War. In *War and public health*. 2nd ed., edited by B. S. Levy and V. W. Sidel. New York: Oxford University Press. Pp. 313-336.

Annas, G.J., and H.J. Geiger. 2008 war and human rights. In *War and public health*. 2nd ed., edited by B.S. Levy and V. W. Sidel. New York: Oxford University Press. Pp. 37-50.

Associated Press. 2007. *U.N.: Malnutrition on the rise in Darfur*. http://enews.earthlink.net/channel/news/print?guid=20070831/36d8e3c0_3ca6_1552620070 (accessed September 2, 2007).

Bertell, R. 2006. Depleted uranium: All the questions about DU and Gulf War syndrome are not yet answered. *International Journal of Health Services* 36(3):503-520.

Burnham, G., R. Lafta, S. Doocy, and L. Roberts. 2006. Mortality after the 2003 invasion of Iraq: A cross-sectional cluster sample survey. *Lancet* 368:1421-1428.

Carnegie Commission. 2007. *Carnegie Commission on preventing deadly conflict*. http://www.wilsoncenter.org/subsites/ccpdc/index.htm (accessed September 3, 2007).

CDC (Centers for Disease Control and Prevention). 2007. http://www.bt.cdc.gov (accessed June 4, 2007).

Cole, L. A. 1988. *Clouds of secrecy: The Army's germ warfare tests over populated areas.* Totowa, NJ: Rowman & Littlefield.

Commission on Social Determinants of Health. 2007. http://www.who.int/social_determinants/en/ (accessed August 31, 2007).

Cukier, W., and V. W. Sidel. 2006. *The global gun epidemic: From Saturday Night Specials to AK-47s.* Westport, CT: Praeger Security International.

deSoysa, I., and E. Neumayer. 2005. *Resource wealth and the risk of civil war onset: Results from a new data set of natural resource 1970-1999.* Revised version, November. Presented at the European Consortium for Political Research Conference in Budapest, Hungary, September 2005.

Foege, W. H. 2000. Arms and public health: a global perspective. In *War and public health.* Updated ed., edited by B. S. Levy and V. W. Sidel. Washington, DC: American Public Health Association. P. 7.

Gordon, M. 2002. U.S. nuclear plan sees new weapons and new targets. *New York Times,* March 10.

Hague Appeal. 2007. *Hague Appeal for Peace.* http://www.haguepeace.org (accessed September 3, 2007).

Harris, R., and J. Paxman. 1982. *A higher form of killing: The secret story of chemical and biological weapons.* New York: Hill and Wang.

Hindi, R, D. Brugge, and B Panikkar. 2005. Teratogenicity of depleted uranium aerosols: A review from and Epidemiologic perspective. *Environmental Health* 4:17

Hoffman, B. 1998. *Inside terrorism.* New York: Columbia University Press.

Institute of Medicine and National Research Council. 1999. *Exposure of the American people to iodine-131 from Nevada nuclear-test: Review of the National Cancer Institute report and public health implications.* Washington, DC: National Academy Press. P. 193.

International Campaign to Ban Landmines. 2006. www.icbl.org (accessed March 8, 2006).

Jenkins, B. M. (December) 1980. *The study of terrorism: Definitional problems.* P-6563. Santa Monica, (CA: RAND Corporation.

Krug, E. G., et al. (eds.). 2002. *World report on violence and health.* Geneva, Switzerland: World Health Organization. http://www.who.int/violence_injury_prevention/violence/world_report/en/full_en.pdf (accessed on November 15, 2007).

Lee, E. C., and S. N. Kales. 2008. Chemical weapons. In *War and public health.* 2nd ed., edited by B. S. Levy and V. W. Sidel. New York: Oxford University Press. Pp. 117-134.

Levy, B. S., and V. W. Sidel. 2005. War. In *Environmental health: From local to global.* Edited by H. Frumkin. New York: Jossey-Bass. Pp. 269-287.

Levy, B. S., and V. W. Sidel (eds.). 2007. *Terrorism and public health: A balanced approach to strengthening systems and protecting people.* Updated ed. New York: Oxford University Press.

Levy, B. S., and V. W. Sidel. 2008a. War and public health: An overview. In *War and public health.* 2nd ed., edited by B. S. Levy and V. W. Sidel. New York: Oxford University Press. Pp. 3-20.

Levy, B. S., and V. W. Sidel. 2008b. Biological weapons. In *War and public health.* 2nd ed., edited by B. S. Levy and V. W. Sidel. New York: Oxford University Press. Pp. 135-151.

Levy, B. S., and V. W. Sidel. 2008c. The Iraq War. In *War and public health.* 2nd ed., edited by B. S. Levy and V. W. Sidel. New York: Oxford University Press. Pp. 243-263.

Loretz, J. 2008. The role of nongovernmental organizations. In *War and public health.* 2nd ed., edited by B. S. Levy and V. W. Sidel. New York: Oxford University Press. Pp. 381-392.

Marmot, M., and R. Bell. 2006. The socioeconomically disadvantaged. In *Social injustice and public health.* Edited by B. S. Levy and V. W. Sidel. New York: Oxford University Press. Pp. 25-45.

Meselson, M., J. Guillemin, M. Hugh-Jones, et al. 1994. The Sverdlovsk anthrax outbreak of 1979. *Science* 266:1202-1208.

Milanovic, M. 2007. State responsibility for genocide. *European Journal of International Law* 18.

National Counterterrorism Center. 2007. *Report of terrorist incidents—2006.* http://wits.nctc. gov/reports/crot2006nctcannexfinal.pdf (accessed July 20, 2007).

National Priorities Project. 2007. http://www.nationalpriorities.org/costsofwar/index-public-education.html (accessed July 11, 2007).

Oxfam International. 2007. *Rising to the humanitarian challenge in Iraq.* http://www.oxfam. org/en/policy/briefingpapers/bp105_humanitarian_challenge_in_Iraq0707 (accessed August 30, 2007).

Power, S. 2002. *A problem from hell: America and the age of genocide.* New York: Basic Books.

Renner, M. 2000. Environmental and health effects of weapons production, testing, and maintenance. In *War and public health.* Updated ed., edited by B. S. Levy and V. W. Sidel. Washington, DC: American Public Health Association. Pp. 117-136.

Roberts, L., and C. L. Muganda. 2008. War in the Democratic Republic of Congo. In *War and public health.* 2nd ed., edited by B. S. Levy and V. W. Sidel. New York: Oxford University Press.

Roberts, L., R. Lafta, R. Garfield, et al. 2004. Mortality before and after the 2003 invasion of Iraq: cluster sample survey. *Lancet* 364:1857-1864

Rosner, D., and G. Markowitz. 2006. *Are we ready? Public health since 9/11.* Berkeley: University of California Press.

Rummel, R. J. 1994. *Death by government: Genocide and mass murder since 1900.* New Brunswick, NJ, and London, UK: Transaction Publications.

Sewall, S. B., and C. Kaysen. 2000. *The United States and the International Criminal Court.* Lanham, MD: Rowman and Littlefield.

Sidel, M. 2004. *More secure, less free?: Antiterrorism policy and civil liberties after September 11.* Ann Arbor, MI: University of Michigan Press.

Sirkin, S. 2008. Darfur. In *War and public health.* 2nd ed., edited by B. S. Levy and V. W. Sidel. New York: Oxford University Press. Pp. 211-212.

Sirkin, S., J. Cobey, and E. Stover. 2008. Landmines. In *War and public health.* 2nd ed., edited by B. S. Levy and V. W. Sidel. New York: Oxford University Press. Pp. 102-116.

Smith, D. 2007. World at war. *The Defense Monitor* 36(1):1-9.

Spanjaard, H., and O. Khabib. 2007. Chemical weapons. In *Terrorism and public health: A balanced approach to strengthening systems and protecting people.* Updated ed., edited by B. S. Levy and V. W. Sidel. New York: Oxford University Press. Pp. 199-219.

Stockholm International Peace Research Institute. 2002. *SIPRI yearbook 2002: Armaments, disarmament and international security.* New York: Oxford University Press.

Stockholm International Peace Research Institute. 2006. *SIPRI yearbook 2006: Armaments, disarmament and international security.* New York: Oxford University Press.

Sutton, P. M., and R. M. Gould. 2007. Nuclear, radiological, and related weapons. In *Terrorism and public health: A balanced approach to strengthening systems and protecting people.* Updated ed., edited by B. S. Levy and V. W. Sidel. New York: Oxford University Press. Pp. 220-242.

Sutton, P. M., and R. M. Gould. 2008. Nuclear weapons. In *War and public health.* 2nd ed., edited by B. S. Levy and V. W. Sidel. New York: Oxford University Press. Pp. 152-176.

Taljaard, R. 2003. *The bigger problem: Weapons of individual destruction (WID).* Daily Times, Pakistan. http://www.dailytimes.com.pk/default.asp?page=story_19-10-2003_pg3_6 (accessed August 29, 2007).

Toole, M. J. 2008. Displaced persons and war. In *War and public health*. 2nd ed., edited by B. S. Levy and V. W. Sidel. New York: Oxford University Press.

UNESCO (United Nations Educational, Scientific, and Cultural Organization). 2007. *Constitution*. http://www.jcomos.org/unesco/unesco_constituion.html (accessed September 2, 2007).

Waldman, R. 2008. The roles of humanitarian assistance. In *War and public health*. 2nd ed. edited by B. S. Levy and V. W. Sidel. New York: Oxford University Press.

Weapons of Mass Destructions Commission. 2006. *Weapons of terror: Freeing the world of nuclear, biological and chemical arms*. Stockholm, Sweden: Fitzef. http://www.wmdcommidsion.org (accessed August 21, 2006).

Westing, A. H. 2008. The impact of war in the environment. In *War and public health*. 2nd ed. edited by B. S. Levy and V. W. Sidel. New York: Oxford University Press. Pp. 69-84.

World Bank. 2007. www.worldbank.org (accessed September 3, 2007).

World Health Assembly. 1996. Resolution WHA49.25.

Yokoro, K., and N. Kamada. 2000. The health effects of the use of nuclear weapons. In *War and public health*. Updated ed., edited by B. S. Levy and V. W. Sidel. Washington, DC: American Public Health Association. Pp. 65-83.

Zwi, A., A. Ugalde, and P. Richards. 1999. The effects of war and political violence on health services. In *Encyclopedia of violence, peace and conflict*. Edited by L. Kurtz. San Diego, CA. Academic Press. Pp. 679-690.

Zwi, A. B., R. Garfield, and A. Lorreti. 2002. Collective violence. In *World report on violence and health*. Edited by J. E. Krug, L. L. Dahlberg, J. A. Mercy, and R. Lozano. Geneva, Switzerland: World Health Organization. Pp. 213-239.

# VIOLENCE, HEALTH, AND DEVELOPMENT

Richard Matzopoulos[1]
Brett Bowman[2]
Alexander Butchart[3, 4]

## Executive Summary

The burden of violence-related deaths is heaviest in low- to middle-income countries (LMICs). Less than 10 percent of all violence-related deaths occur in high-income countries (HICs), and LMICs have a mortality rate due to violence that is almost two-and-a-half times greater than for high-income countries. Over and above the substantial contribution of violence as a cause of death and physical injuries, victims of violence are also more vulnerable to a range of mental and physical health problems.

---

[1]Richard Matzopoulos is a Researcher at the the University of Cape Town School of Public Health and Family Medicine, and a Specialist Scientist at the MRC/UNISA Crime, Violence and Injury Lead Programme in South Africa.

[2]Brett Bowman is a Senior Researcher in the Discipline of Psychology at the School of Human and Community Development of the University of the Witwatersrand, Johannesburg, South Africa.

[3]Alexander Butchart is the Coordinator, Prevention of Violence in the Department of Injuries and Violence Prevention of the World Health Organization, Geneva, Switzerland.

[4]The findings and conclusions of this paper are those of the author and do not necessarily represent the views of the World Health Organization.

**Terms of reference**

The following paper was prepared as a scoping document for participants of the two-day workshop hosted by the Institute of Medicine in Washington DC from 26 to 27 June 2007: Preventing Violence in Low- and Middle-Income Countries: Finding a Place on the Global Health Agenda. The contents are those of the autho(s) and do not necessarily reflect the opinions or positions of the Institute of Medicine.

Although the effects of violence on other health outcomes are less well documented, some highly prevalent forms, such as child maltreatment, intimate partner violence (IPV), and abuse of the elderly, have been shown to have numerous noninjury health consequences. These consequences include high-risk behaviors such as alcohol and substance misuse, smoking, unsafe sex, eating disorders, and the perpetration of violence. These behaviors in turn contribute to such leading causes of death as cardiovascular disorders, cancers, depression, diabetes, and HIV/AIDS. The social toll of violence is further exacerbated by economic costs that represent formidable threats to fiscal growth and development.

Several studies describe the deleterious impact of different types of violence on a range of health outcomes, but no review has yet been undertaken that presents a composite overview of the current state of knowledge. This paper aims to review the scientific literature describing the nature, magnitude, and impact of violence on health and development in LMICs. It has the following specific objectives:

• To review the literature on violence in LMICs according to the typology commonly used by international agencies such as the World Health Organisation (WHO)
• To describe what is known about the negative impacts of violence on health and human development in LMICs
• To examine available information about the economic costs and impacts on economic development of violence in LMICs
• To describe violence prevention policy developments within the global health and development agenda

The paper includes a review of recent research on violence in LMICs around seven subtypes of violence: (1) child abuse and neglect, (2) youth violence, (3) intimate partner violence (IPV), (4) sexual violence, (5) abuse of the elderly, (6) self-directed violence, and (7) collective violence, and discusses its broader implications and macro-level impacts on health and development.

## Child Maltreatment and Other Violence Directed at Children

Homicide rates are considerably higher in LMICs than in HICs among older children: 2.6 times higher among boys aged 5 to 9 years, 3.6 times higher among girls aged 5 to 9, and more than 4 times higher among children aged 10 to 14 for both sexes. Sexual and physical abuse experienced during childhood are just some of the numerous psychological and behavioral factors endemic in many LMIC settings that may predispose children and young adults to display violent and aggressive behavior later in life and have been shown to have substantial long-term effects on health.

## Youth Violence

Countries with the highest adolescent homicide rates are either developing countries or those experiencing rapid social changes. Among children aged 15 to 17 years male homicide rates in LMICs were three times higher than in HICs, and female rates in LMICs more than double those in HICs. There is an increased risk of violence in populations where adolescents and young adults are overrepresented and, as is the case in LMICs, may include a large percentage of "marginalized youth" with poor prospects of education and employment.

## Intimate Partner Violence

Many of the risks associated with a man's likelihood of abusing a female intimate partner are prevalent in low-income settings and some of the highest rates of IPV have been recorded in LMICs.

## Sexual Violence

The true extent of sexual violence is difficult to gauge within HICs as well as in LMICs, as statistics on rape and indecent assaults are typically underreported. Nevertheless, there are indications that rates of sexual violence in LMICs are substantial.

## Abuse of the Elderly

Most research on violence against the elderly has been conducted in HICs. While more descriptive work in the area is required, there is growing evidence to suggest that the elderly are also frequently victims of violence in LMICs.

## Self-Directed Violence

Suicide was the leading cause of death due to violence in LMICs in 2002, although it accounted for a smaller percentage of all deaths due to violence in LMICs than in HICs.

## Collective Violence

Collective violence is an endemic and enduring feature of many LMICs. The hallmark of countries that have been at war is a combination of poverty, strained economic and social infrastructure, and severely eroded health services. Collective violence is restricted almost entirely to LMICs, with particularly high rates experienced in Africa followed by the Eastern Mediterranean and LMICs in the European region.

## The Impact of Violence on Health

Violence has numerous impacts on health and these can be measured in a variety of ways. The most common and direct ways of measuring its impact are in terms of the numbers and rates of deaths and injuries it causes. Although less easy to measure, violence also has important impacts on a range of mental and physical health problems. It is important and useful to quantify these various impacts in both health and economic terms.

## The Burden of Injury

Estimated mortality rates compiled by WHO for 2002 suggested that overall mortality rates due to violence in LMICs were on average more than double those of HICs. Violence is also projected to increase in rank from the 15th to the 13th leading cause of death between 2002 and 2030 with middle-income countries likely to bear most of this burden.

## The Burden of Violence on Other Causes of Ill Health

The impact of violence on other health outcomes is clearly reflected in comparative risk assessment studies, which show that standard burden of disease measures underrepresent the impact of interpersonal violence by at least 26 percent for deaths and 30 percent for disability-adjusted life-years (DALYs) when its contribution to other health outcomes resulting from child sexual abuse and IPV are taken into account.

## The Economic Impact of Violence on Health

The direct costs (or impacts) of violence include the medical costs related to the treatment of the victims of violence and nonmedical costs associated with prevention. Indirect costs include those that are tangible such as the impact of violence on the broader macro economy and those that are intangible such as those relating to quality of life. Based on existing estimates primarily calculated in South Africa, the Caribbean, and Latin America, it is clear that the costs of violence are enormous in LMICs. Overall, WHO reports that health care expenditure related to violence consumes a significant portion of gross domestic product (GDP) in LMICs. These direct health expenditures represent just a fraction of violence-related costs and impacts.

## The Impact of Violence on Development

Collective, interpersonal, and self-directed violence all have extensive and pervasive long-term implications for development as well as health. These effects are themselves multilayered and can therefore undermine development at individual, communal, or national levels. This paper describes the impact of violence in relation to all eight goals of the Millennium Development Plan. The impact of violence on the Millennium Development Goals (MDGs) must also be read alongside growing evidence that demonstrates the negative, enduring effects of exposure to violence in childhood.

## The Economic Impact of Violence on Development

Violence in whatever form absorbs sizeable amounts of health care expenditure that could be better used to prevent other forms of health threat. Although data are limited, health economic research on violence has begun to demonstrate the substantial economic impacts of violence in LMICs. National spending on collective violence in the form of "defense" budgetary allocations and investment in postconflict recovery have been shown to lead to drastic reductions in national investment in health care services.

## The Emergence of Violence Prevention as Part of the Health and Development Agenda

There are clear indications that violence prevention is an emerging priority in the global health and development agenda, particularly in LMICs. Since the publication of the *World Report on Violence and Health*, there have been two World Health Assembly resolutions calling on countries to invest in violence prevention, and by 2006 three out of six WHO regional committees (Africa, the Americas, and Europe) had adopted similar resolutions.

## Conclusion

Violence is a pressing global health concern and is inextricably linked with a range of other health indicators. Yet despite the fact that early projections indicate that violence is on the increase, vigorous and concerted violence prevention efforts can turn this trend around. International development partners may have an important role to play in providing financial and technical support for intersectoral collaboration, multilateral research cooperation, and the development of research capacity in LMICs.

## Background and Overview

Violence is a global problem. In 2002, violence claimed approximately 1.6 million human lives and caused at least another 16 million injuries severe enough to warrant medical attention. These consequences burden health systems, cripple communities, and are responsible for immeasurable human suffering. The burden of violence-related deaths is heaviest in LMICs. Less than 10 percent of all violence-related deaths occur in HICs (Krug et al., 2002; Mathers et al., 2002), and LMICs have a mortality rate due to violence that is almost two-and-a-half times greater than for HICs (see Figure C-1). Over and above the substantial contribution of violence as a cause of death and physical injuries, victims of violence are also more vulnerable to a range of mental and physical health problems.

The size of the violence problem can be better appreciated when it is compared to other major health threats. The estimated 1.6 million deaths due to violence in 2002 was around half the number of deaths due to HIV/AIDS, roughly equal to deaths due to tuberculosis, greater than the number of road traffic deaths, and 1.5 times the number of deaths due to malaria. Suicide was the leading cause, accounting for 870,000 or 54 percent of violent deaths; homicide accounted for 560,000 deaths (35 percent) and the remaining 170,000 deaths (11 percent) were the direct result of war (Krug et al., 2002).

Although the effects of violence on other health outcomes are less well documented, some highly prevalent forms, such as child maltreatment, IPV, and abuse of the elderly, have been shown to have numerous noninjury health consequences. These consequences include high-risk behaviors such as alcohol and substance misuse, smoking, unsafe sex, eating disorders, and the perpetration of violence. These behaviors in turn contribute to such leading causes of death as cardiovascular disorders, cancers, depression, diabetes, and HIV/AIDS. The social toll of violence is further exacerbated by economic costs that represent formidable threats to fiscal growth and development (Krug et al., 2002; Felitti et al., 1998; Waters et al., 2005).

### Aim and Objectives

Because a composite review of the literature on the relationships between various types of violence and health and development in LMICs has not yet been undertaken, this paper aims to review the scientific literature dealing with the magnitude and impact on health and development of violence in LMICs, and has the following specific objectives:

- To review the literature on violence in LMICs according to the typology commonly used by international agencies such as WHO

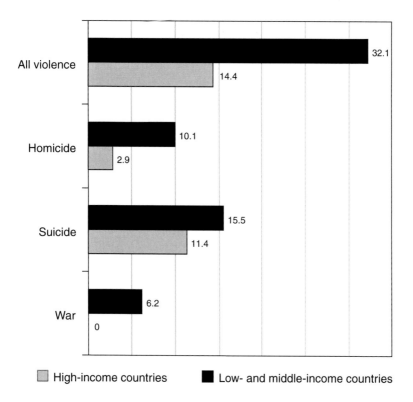

FIGURE C-1 Estimated mortality rate per 100,000 population from violence by income level, 2000.
SOURCE: Mathers et al., 2002.

- To describe what is known about the negative impacts of violence on health and human development in LMICs
- To examine available information about the economic costs and impacts on economic development of violence in LMICs
- To describe violence prevention policy developments within the global health and development agenda

*Scope and Limitations of This Paper*

The review of literature is limited primarily to English language publications and the authors welcome suggestions regarding additional texts and resources that may be relevant.

# The Nature of Violence in LMICs

The *World Report on Violence and Health* (Krug et al., 2002, p. 5) defines violence as

> The intentional use of physical force or power, threatened or actual, against oneself, another person, or against a group or community, that either results in or has a high likelihood of resulting in injury, death, psychological harm, maldevelopment or deprivation.

The following subsections review recent research on violence in LMICs according to seven subtypes of violence also identified in the *World Report on Violence and Health*, namely (1) child abuse and neglect, (2) youth violence, (3) IPV, (4) sexual violence, (5) abuse of the elderly, (6) self-directed violence, and (7) collective violence. The broader implications of violence and its macro-level impacts on health and development are discussed in Sections 3 and 4.

It is noted that while this categorization is useful for describing violence and identifying prevention opportunities, the different subcategories are not mutually exclusive and there are strong links between different types of violence. For example, child maltreatment victims are more likely than nonvictims to experience IPV, sexual violence, and youth violence, while perpetrators of homicide where the victim is another family member are at substantially increased risk of later committing suicide. Similarly, the collective violence of war and civil unrest may be precipitated by overwhelming levels of severe interpersonal violence; and some effects of collective violence, such as increased access to firearms and erosion of nonviolent value systems, increase the risk of interpersonal violence. Crosscutting these causal links between the different subtypes of violence are shared risk factors—such as alcohol and substance misuse, parental loss, crime, household poverty, and social and economic inequalities—that underlie most of the subtypes.

## Child Maltreatment and Other Violence Directed at Children

Among children younger than 4 years of age, death rates due to violence in LMICs are comparable with rates in HICs, although closer analysis shows that, whereas rates of homicide among boys in this age category are 10 percent lower in LMICs, the homicide rate among girls is 20 percent higher. There are also distinct regional differences, with homicide rates among African children more than double the global average for both boys and girls (Krug et al., 2002, p. 357). However, homicide rates are considerably higher in LMICs than in HICs among older children: 2.6 times higher among boys aged 5 to 9 years, 3.6 times higher among girls aged 5 to 9, and more than 4 times higher among children aged 10 to 14 for both sexes.

Data on nonfatal child maltreatment in LMICs are, unfortunately, limited, as they are derived from studies that use different definitions and assessment methods. Nevertheless, there is growing consensus on the definition of child maltreatment (Leeb et al., 2007; WHO and ISPCAN, 2006) and the development of recent surveillance guidelines for child maltreatment should ensure better comparability between future studies (Leeb et al., 2007).

Despite the current methodological challenges, what we can deduce from the available data is that child maltreatment is indeed a widespread and serious problem. Physical child maltreatment often associated with punishment by parents or other caregivers has been examined in a number of LMICs. In a study of students aged 11 to 18 in the Kurdistan Province of the Islamic Republic of Iran, 38.5 percent reported experiencing mild to severe physical injuries from abuse at home (Stephenson et al., 2006). In a survey of households in Romania 4.6 percent of children reported suffering severe and frequent abuse and nearly half of Romanian parents admitted to beating their children regularly (Browne et al., 2002). In Ethiopia 21 percent of urban and 64 percent of rural school children reported bruises or swellings on their bodies from being physically punished by their parents (Ketsela and Kedebe, 1997). Among younger children, serious injuries most frequently arise as a consequence of head injuries or injuries to the internal organs, often at the hand of a caregiver. Shaken infant or shaken impact syndrome is a potentially devastating form of child abuse.

The physical, medical, and emotional neglect of children is also an important dimension of child maltreatment. In many countries it is the most frequently reported form of maltreatment. In Kenya, for example, the forms of abuse most commonly cited by adults in selected communities were abandonment and neglect (African Network for the Prevention and Protection Against Child Abuse and Neglect, 2000).

Young children and infants may also be the victims of sexual abuse, but findings from descriptive studies point to the increased risk of sexual abuse among girls with the onset of adolescence, whereas among boys this vulnerable period is marked by a much increased likelihood of engaging in physical violence. Data from a children's hospital in Cape Town, South Africa, for example, show that whereas boys accounted for a greater percentage of cases presenting for violence-related injuries (63 percent), sexual assaults were the cause of injury among 48 percent of girls compared to only 3 percent of boys (Matzopoulos and Bowman, 2006).

However, such findings cannot be generalized. Another South African study, this time among secondary school students in the Limpopo Province, reported a prevalence rate of 54 percent of the total sample reporting contact sexual abuse before the age of 18 years with similar rates for males and females (Madu and Pelzer, 2001). Lalor (2004) points to rapid social change, the patriarchal nature of society, and HIV/AIDS as both a cause and consequence of sexual exploitation of children in sub-Saharan Africa. In other LMIC settings many studies reveal lower rates. For example, in a study across three Latin American countries (El Salvador, Guatemala, and Honduras), the percentage of women reporting being sexually assaulted before the age of 15 years ranged from 4.6 to 7.8 percent (Speizer et al., n.d.). However, the intimate nature of child sexual abuse, which often involves close family members and acquaintances as victims and perpetrators, along with cultural norms and taboos that may discourage disclosure, compromises the collection and comparison of data across different settings.

Sexual and physical abuse experienced during childhood are just some of the numerous psychological and behavioral factors endemic in many LMIC settings that may predispose youths and young adults to display violent and aggressive behavior later in life (Karr-Morse and Wiley, 1997), and have been shown to have substantial long-term effects on health (see Section 3.2). In addition to these impacts of direct victimization, children exposed to violence as witnesses and bystanders may also be psychologically traumatized. In South Africa, for example, a study of Xhosa-speaking youth in a township with high levels of community violence showed that all of the 60 respondents had been exposed to community violence, while 56 percent had been victims and 45 percent had witnessed at least one murder. The psychological imprint of these experiences manifested in 22 percent of these children fitting the diagnosis for posttraumatic stress disorder, 32 percent for dysthymia, and 7 percent for major depression (Ensink et al., 1997). Domestic violence also has direct effects on children, with one study suggesting that a substantial proportion of unintentional injuries in young children may have occurred in the course of their being used as "shields" by women attempting to protect themselves from physical attack by their male partners (Fieggen et al., 2004).

*Youth Violence*

Age and sex are important risk factors for interpersonal violence, with males in particular being more likely to engage in physical violence during adolescence and young adulthood. Consequently there is a sharp increase in the rate of aggressive behavior and victimization from the age of about 15 years. In LMICs this is compounded by underresourced educational systems and the fragility of traditional family and community structures that create an enabling environment for violence within homes and communities. Invariably, the countries with the highest adolescent homicide rates are either developing countries or those experiencing rapid social changes (Pinheiro, 2006, p. 287).

Among children aged 15 to 17 years, male homicide rates in LMICs were three times higher than in HICs, and female rates in LMICs more than double those in HICs. In every region homicide rates among children aged 15 to 17 compared to those aged 10 to 14 are at least three times greater among males and nearly double among female children (Pinheiro, 2006, p. 287). Nevertheless, there are sharp regional differences, with Africa recording the highest rates among girls across all age categories and among boys aged 10 to 14 years, whereas the highest fatality rates among boys aged 15 to 17 were recorded in the Latin American and Caribbean regions, followed closely by Africa (Pinheiro, 2006, p. 357).

The Latin American, Caribbean, and African regions have a large population under the age of 25, many of whom are raised in poverty, and rates of interpersonal violence are among the highest in the world (see Figures C-2 and C-3). Living off the informal economy and without family structures there is little hope of these children being integrated into formal society (Maddaleno et al., 2006). It is estimated that adolescents from 10 to 19 years of age comprise a third of all homicides in the Americas (PAHO, 2003) and globally rates of fatal violence are higher among 15- to 19-year-olds than in other 4-year age groups (Pinheiro, 2006, p. 287).

In South Africa, a cross-sectional study revealed that more than 50 percent of all boys and girls had experienced violence, either as victims or perpetrators (Swart et al., 2002). In the Lavender Hill and Steenberg areas in Cape Town, over 70 percent of a sample of primary school children

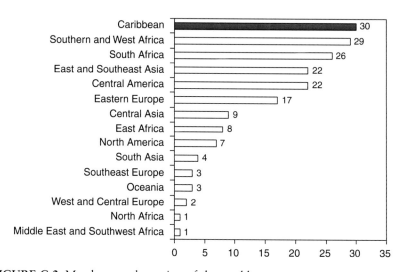

FIGURE C-2 Murder rates by region of the world.
SOURCE: UN Crime Trends Survey and Interpol, 2002.

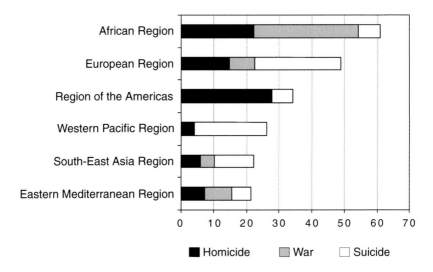

**FIGURE C-3** Estimated mortality rates per 100,000 population from violence in LMICs by health region, 2000.
SOURCE: Adapted from WHO's *World report on violence and health* by Mathers et al., 2002.

reported exposure to violence (Van der Merwe and Dawes, 2000). A youth risk behavior study conducted among a representative sample of in-school youth revealed that approximately 17 percent of pupils carried weapons and that approximately 30 percent of pupils had been involved in a physical assault in the past 6 months (MRC, 2002).

These findings suggest there is an increased risk of violence in populations where adolescents and young adults are overrepresented and, as is the case in LMICs, may include a large percentage of "marginalized youth" with poor prospects of education and employment. Therefore sound educational and macro-economic policies applied at a societal and structural level to address the existential needs and long-term prospects of vulnerable youth and young adults may have important violence prevention effects.

*Intimate Partner Violence*

Among the numerous risk factors associated with a man's likelihood of abusing a female intimate partner are young age, heavy drinking, depression, personality disorders, low academic achievement, low income, marital conflict, marital instability, male dominance in the family, economic stress, and poor family functioning. Some studies have shown that boys who are exposed to conflict in early childhood are at increased risk to be violent as adults. Correspondingly the community and societal factors for IPV include weak community sanctions against domestic violence, poverty and low social capital (Heise and Garcia-Moreno, 2002), and, at a societal level, cultural norms and values such as those that support gender inequality are particularly important.

As many of these factors are prevalent in low-income settings it is not surprising that some of the highest rates of IPV have been recorded in LMICs: 27 percent of all women who have ever had an ongoing sexual partnership in Leon, Nicaragua, and 52 percent of currently married Palestinian women in the West Bank and Gaza Strip reported ever having experiencing IPV. A WHO multicountry study on women's health and domestic violence against women in sampled country sites found that 37 percent of respondents in Brazil, 56 percent of women in Tanzania, and 62 percent of women in Bangladesh reported having ever experienced physical or sexual violence by an intimate partner (WHO, 2005). In South Africa, women aged 14 and older were killed by an intimate partner at a rate of 8.8 per 100,000, accounting for approximately half of all women murdered in a single year, the highest recorded rate in the world (Mathews et al., 2004).

*Sexual Violence*

Sexual violence encompasses a wide range of sexually violent acts perpetrated by family members, acquaintances, strangers in the community, and, particularly in LMICs, the perpetrators of collective violence. The true extent of sexual violence is difficult to gauge within HICs as well as in LMICs, as statistics on rape and sexual assaults are typically underreported. Nevertheless, there are indications that rates of sexual violence in LMICS may be higher. For example, in an address to parliament in September 2005, the South African Minister of Safety and Security reported that during the period April 1, 2004, through March 31, 2005, 55,184 rapes were reported at a rate of more than 250 per 100,000 women compared to 80 per 100,000 in the United States for the same period (also see Section 2.3). Another South African study in Cape Town reported that 32 percent of pregnant adolescents and 18 percent of matched controls had been forced into their first sexual experience (Jewkes et al., 2001).

Comparing data across countries and national reports from the international crime victim survey between 1992 and 1997 indicated that LMICs in Latin America, Africa, and Eastern Europe have among the highest percentage of women aged 16 years and older who report having been sexually assaulted (United Nations, 1998). Similarly, countries in these regions accounted for some of the highest percentages of adult women reporting sexual victimization by an intimate partner and forced sexual initiation.

*Abuse of the Elderly*

Elder abuse encompasses acts of physical, psychological, or sexual violence or neglectful financial and material maltreatment of older persons (Wolf et al., 2002). In Africa, the extent of elder abuse remains largely unknown, although it has been linked to practices such as persecutions of women suspected of witchcraft (Wolf et al., 2002) and the ostracism of tribal elders (Lachs and Pillemer, 2004). More systematic measurement has, however, been undertaken. There is growing evidence that the elderly are becoming increasingly at risk for violence in Africa (Gorman, 2000). In South Africa, the homicide rate among men aged older than 60 years was 6.4 times higher than the global rate in 2000, whereas it was 6.9 times the global rate among women (Norman et al., 2007a). Another South African study found that the elderly are frequently the victims of physical, psychological, and sexual violence in townships on the periphery of Cape Town (Keikelame and Ferreira, 2000). In South America, elderly women represented 2 percent of the victims of violence in an Argentinean study. This figure matches estimates of violence against the elderly in Denmark (Aalund et al., 1989). A study of mortality and morbidity patterns in Brazil showed that violence resulted in a significant number of hospitalizations in the elderly (Minayo, 2003). A survey study by Bezerra-Flanders and Clark (2006) in Brazil found that psychological abuse and abandonment, followed by physical abuse, were the most cited forms of elderly abuse in the sample. A multicountry qualitative study of perceptions of elder abuse found that violence against the elderly was identified as significant problem in Kenya, India, Brazil, Lebanon, and Argentina (WHO/INPEA, 2002). In combination, these studies have begun to identify violence against the elderly as a significant problem in LMICs, although far more descriptive work is required.

*Self-Directed Violence*

Suicide was the leading cause of death due to violence in LMICs in 2002, although it accounted for a smaller percentage of all deaths due to violence than in HICs (50 versus 68 percent, respectively; WHO, n.d.). However, as self-inflicted injuries are more frequently fatal, interpersonal violence imposed a greater burden in LMICs when nonfatal outcomes such as disabilities and other long-term effects were considered, accounting for 46 percent of DALYs, compared to 40 percent for suicide (WHO, n.d.).

As with the other subtypes of violence there are wide regional variations, and in a substantial number of LMICs in 2000 the suicide rate was considerably higher than the global average (13.5 per 100,000 population), particularly in Eastern Europe (28.2 per 100,000 population) and China

(23 per 100,000 population). Whereas the suicide rate in India has been estimated at 13.6 per 100,000 (Peden et al., 2002), the rate in Sri Lanka in 1995 was estimated at 47.7 per 100,000 (Eddleston et al., 1998).

In Africa, which as a region had one of the lowest estimated suicide rates at 4.3 per 100,000 population in 2000 (Peden et al., 2002), there is a paucity of data on the burden of self-inflicted violence (Bertolote and Fleischmann, 2002), which makes regional and international comparisons difficult (Kinyanda, 2006). As with certain other types of violence socio-political and cultural factors may increase vulnerability and also inhibit the collection of comprehensive and reliable data. Nevertheless, there is growing concern about suicide as a public health priority in the region.

*Collective Violence*

Following the *World Report on Violence and Health*, collective violence is defined as "the instrumental use of violence by people who identify themselves as members of a group—whether this group is transitory or has a more permanent identity—against another group or set of individuals, in order to achieve political, economic or social objectives" (Zwi et al., 2002). Collective violence is an endemic and enduring feature of many LMICs, which bear what Sidel (1995) described as the hallmark of countries that have been at war: poverty, destroyed economic and social infrastructure, and severely eroded health services. Collective violence is restricted almost entirely to LMICs, with particularly high rates experienced in Africa followed by the Eastern Mediterranean and LMICs in the European Regions (see Figure C-3).

Muggah (in press) maintains that the health implications of collective violence for civilians in LMICs are dramatic, as conflicts are frequently characterized by multiple armed groups, the targeting of civilians, the use of rape as a weapon of war, the involvement of child soldiers, and ultimately state fragility and even collapse (Duffield, 2001; Kaldor, 1999). The human costs extend well beyond death, physical injuries, and disabilities, and may lead to intergenerational "collective trauma" as many civilians witness shootings, killings, rapes, and the loss of family members.[1] Interviews with 301 former child soldiers abducted by the northern Ugandan rebellion movement, the "Lord's Resistance Army," provide some insight. On average the children had been exposed to six different traumatic events, with 77 percent witnessing someone being killed during their abduction; 6 percent witnessing their own father, mother, brother, or sister being killed; 39 percent killing another person themselves; and 2 percent killing their

---

[1] See, for example, Abramowitz (2005), De Jong et al. (2000), Miles and Medi (1994), and Mollica (1999).

own relatives. Most of the children (64 percent) were forced to participate in fights and 27 percent had to drink their own urine (Derluyn et al., 2004). It is estimated that 300,000 children younger than 18 years are currently serving as soldiers, guerrilla fighters, or in supporting roles in conflicts around the world (Machel, 2001).

Furthermore, collective violence in LMICs fundamentally influences many of the structural factors such as migration and rapid urbanization that stress the social fabric of families and communities, which in turn fuel a range of social ills that may give rise to interpersonal and self-directed violence. Hence, unfavorable living conditions, family characteristics, and perceptions among youths that they will derive economic benefit, social rec-

---

**BOX C-3**
**The Economic and Health Costs of War in Iraq**

The cumulative economic costs of war in Iraq are staggering and the economic impacts of the war are experienced daily across the global economy. According to a comprehensive report released by the Institute for Policy Studies in 2005, total U.S. expenditure amounted to $204.4 billion. In September 2006, the revised report calculated total U.S. spending at $321 billion and projected total long-term spending to be US$ 1.3 trillion (Bennis and Lever, 2005). A paper presented at the Allied Social Sciences Association Congress of 2006 reported total costs of the war in Iraq to be US$ 251 billion as of December 30, 2005, and projected a total cost in excess of US$ 1 trillion, assuming U.S. troops return by 2010 (Bilmes and Stiglitz, 2006).

As astounding as these costs may appear, they are nonetheless relatively meaningless without some form of comparison with missed opportunity costs for global development. Drawing on the earliest 2005 figure, war spending by the U.S. government could have cut world hunger in half and covered HIV/AIDS medicine, childhood immunization, and clean water and sanitation needs of the developing world for almost 3 years (Bennis and Lever, 2005).

Although the country had not yet fully recovered from the effects of the first Gulf War of 2001, there were relatively few deaths as a result of violence prior to the 2003 invasion. Burnham et al. (2006) surmise that as deaths due to violence rose sharply after coalition forces entered Iraq, all postinvasion violent deaths can be considered "excess violent deaths" as these would presumably not have occurred in the absence of the invasion. Postinvasion crude mortality rose from 5.5 to 13.2 per 1,000. Deaths due to violence accounted for approximately three-quarters of the increase and were primarily responsible for the escalating mortality toll that has resulted in approximately 600,000 Iraqi deaths. There are indications that the incidence of interpersonal violence has increased, as sampled households have attributed fewer and fewer deaths to coalition forces as the war has continued. Between June 2005 and June 2006, over 74 percent of all violent deaths were attributed to sources other than the coalition forces.

The effects of the war on the social and health infrastructure of Iraq clearly illustrate

ognition, and easier access to drugs are among the frequently cited as risk factors for the emergence of gangs in the Americas, essentially a manifestation of collective violence at a micro level (PAHO, 2002). Frequently these groups of young men, drawn together for purposes of criminal activities, companionship, or protection, develop their own social norms in the absence of traditional family or community support structures and violence is a frequent means of resolving conflict and acting out social justice or revenge.

As a case study, the war in Iraq, which has received widespread international media coverage from its onset, also provides a comprehensive yet tragic example of the social costs and consequences of sustained conflict (Box C-3).

the developmental consequences of collective violence. Increases in overall mortality have strained the health system in many ways and have hampered access to health services. Access to health care in central Iraq and Baghdad in particular is constrained by constant security threats, and health services for vulnerable groups such as pregnant women and the elderly are severely compromised. Collective violence in Iraq has thus produced collective health effects by driving increases in overall mortality and morbidity due to other forms of violence and communicable diseases. This is exacerbated by a systematic deterioration at all levels of health care services. It is estimated that over one-third of the country's doctors have emigrated since conflict erupted.

There has also been no significant improvement in food and water security as well as a marked decrease in standards of sanitation, which has multiple effects on population health. WHO (2007) reports that 80 percent of people lack effective sanitation, 70 percent lack access to regular clean water, and only 60 percent have access to the public food distribution system. Diarrhea and acute respiratory infections are worsened by these barriers to nutrition and essential health care services and so account for about two-thirds of deaths among children under age 5 years. According to the report, the chronic child malnutrition rate is estimated at 21 percent and the successes of the country's polio immunization program in keeping Iraq polio free for some 6 years could be undermined by disruptions related to violence.

It must be emphasized that the accuracy and validity of some of the research that has been conducted in Iraq can be disputed from a scientific standpoint. There are very real difficulties in conducting research and collecting accurate and representative data in countries in constant turmoil, such as Iraq and Afghanistan. As well as concerns about safety, there are also powerful forces that can restrict access to information, not only as a result of overt (or even covert) action, but also by shaping the social and political climate that enables the free flow of information. Hence there is a clear need for the development of guidelines for the collection of credible information in similar circumstances.

## The Impact of Violence on Health

The definition of violence encompasses a wide range of actions and possible deleterious health and developmental outcomes (see *The Impact of Violence on Other Causes of Ill Health* section below). These health impacts can be measured in a variety of ways. The most common and direct ways of measuring its impact are in terms of the numbers and rates of deaths and injuries it causes. Although less easy to measure, violence also has important impacts on a range of mental and physical health problems. It is important and useful to quantify these various impacts in both health and economic terms. The paucity of accurate and detailed data, however, make it difficult to fully measure all of these impacts in LMICs. Furthermore, as many of the impacts of violence present within the health sector as major risk factors and causes for a range of other health conditions and outcomes, it could be said that violence foments a vicious cycle. For example, the adverse impacts of violence on quality of life may lead to the deterioration of mental health and well-being that may in turn impose a direct (and measurable) burden on the health system, while at the same time driving rates of violence even higher within afflicted communities.

Hence the impacts of violence on health and development in LMICs are addressed in separate subsections. With regard to health impacts, the burden of violence relating specifically to the physical effects of violence-related injuries is first described, followed by a review of how violence impacts upon other noninjury health outcomes. Available data on the direct costs of violence on the health system are then reviewed. The impact of violence on development, which mirrors the WHO/Centers for Disease Control (CDC) typology with respect to the nonmedical and many of the tangible and intangible indirect costs, is described in more detail below.

### The Burden of Injury

The most commonly used measures to describe the health impact of violence are mortality rates to describe its direct consequences (i.e., deaths as a result of physical injuries). Typically expressed as homicide (or murder[2]) and suicide rates, the uncommonly high rates in LMICs are apparent in the mortality rates cited by health (Figure C-1) and criminal justice agencies (Figure C-2). Data from the UN Crime Trends Survey and Interpol (Figure C-1) point to a considerable variation in regional murder

---

[2]The term homicide refers to the intentional use of force resulting in the death of another person. "Murder" is a criminal justice term that may exclude certain categories of homicide where a crime is not perceived to have been committed. Although the terms refer to marginally different subsets, for the purposes of this report they are essentially interchangeable.

rates, but the highest rates invariably occur in LMICs, particularly in South and Central America, and South and West Africa.

Estimated mortality rates compiled by the WHO for 2000 also suggested that overall mortality rates due to violence in LMICs were on average more than double those of HICs (Mathers et al., 2002). This was mainly attributable to higher homicide rates and deaths resulting from wars and conflict, which almost exclusively afflicted LMICs in 2000.

Among LMICs, there was considerable regional variation with regard to the type of violence. Mortality rates due to injuries arising from interpersonal violence were highest in the Americas followed by the African and the European regions,[3] whereas suicide rates were highest in the European and Western Pacific regions. At 32 per 100,000 population, injury mortality rates from war and conflicts were far higher in Africa in 2000 than in any other region and almost four times higher than the next most afflicted region, the Eastern Mediterranean, with an injury mortality rate of 8.2 per 100,000 population.

Violence is also projected to increase in rank from 15th to 13th position among the leading causes of death between 2002 and 2030 and middle-income countries will likely bear most of this burden. This will mainly be attributable to increases in the rate of interpersonal violence as rates of suicide are projected to decrease over the next 30 years (Mathers and Loncar, 2006).

Although these data clearly show a substantial injury burden in LMICs directly attributable to violence, there are a number of reasons why they are likely to underrepresent the actual magnitude of the problem. First, injuries from violence afflict a younger population cohort than most non-communicable diseases (e.g., chronic conditions associated with diseases of lifestyle) and some infectious diseases and, consequently, account for a larger percentage of premature deaths than evinced by mortality rates. Second, as mortality rates only reflect the number of people who die from a specific cause, they ignore the often significant burden imposed on survivors living with physical disabilities or mental illnesses and their next of kin. Third, whereas the mortality rates cited above reflect only violence-related deaths, violence affects health and development broadly and may contribute to premature mortality from a range of other causes.

More sophisticated methods are therefore required to better describe the impact of violence, and the burden-of-disease methodology provides

---

[3]In addition to issues of definition, regional differences between the homicide rates in Figure 1 and the murder rates in Figure 2 can be ascribed to the different geographic boundaries of the defined regions as well as the methodologies underpinning the collection of the data. This topic falls outside of the scope of this paper and hence interested readers should refer to the original manuscripts for a more informed understanding of these rather complex issues.

adjusted estimates that take into account the age of the injured and deceased through measures such as potential years of life lost (YLL) and DALYs, which includes YLL and years lived with a disability. The burden of violence in LMICs in 2000, taking these more sophisticated measures into account, is shown in Table C-1 (Mathers et al., 2002). Even DALYs underestimate the impact of violence, however, because up until this point DALYs have failed to incorporate adequate measures of the impact of nonfatal forms of violence such as child maltreatment and IPV on health.

## The Impact of Violence on Other Causes of Ill Health

In those LMICs where more detailed data and epidemiological expertise are available, the burden of disease methodology can provide valuable information about the impact of violence on health outcomes other than injury. In South Africa, for example, injuries arising from violence, road traffic collisions, and other causes present part of a quadruple disease burden, along with HIV/AIDS, persistent infectious diseases, and emerging chronic conditions. Within this mix, violence is the major contributor to the high rates of injury, accounting for 12.9 percent of premature mortality in the country (Bradshaw et al., 2004). Injuries arising from interpersonal violence were the second leading cause of all DALYs after HIV/AIDS, accounting for 6.5 percent of the total 16.2 million DALYs (Norman et al., 2007a). An age-standardized homicide rate of 64.8 per 100,000 placed South Africa among the most violent countries in the world with male and female homicide rates respectively more than 8 and 5 five times higher than global averages (Norman et al., 2007c).

Notwithstanding this considerable direct burden, the additional impact in South Africa of violence on other health outcomes is beginning to become apparent though comparative risk assessment studies. This type of research attempts to systematically evaluate changes in population health which may result from changing the distribution of exposure to specific risk factors or a group of risk factors. Preliminary data from a recent South African study estimated that although interpersonal violence accounted for 5.3 percent of deaths as an underlying cause of death, as a risk factor it accounted for 6.7 percent of deaths when its contribution to other health outcomes resulting from child sexual abuse and IPV were included (Table C-2). Similarly, for nonfatal outcomes, interpersonal violence as an underlying cause accounted for 6.5 percent of DALYs, but 8.5 percent of DALYs as a risk factor (Norman et al., 2007b). These findings imply that standard burden-of-disease measures underrepresent the impact of interpersonal violence by at least 26 percent for deaths and 30 percent for DALYs when its contribution to other health outcomes resulting from child sexual abuse and IPV are taken into account.

**TABLE C-1** Rankings for Violence-Related DALYs by Income Level and Their Contribution to the Burden of Disease, 2000

**High-Income Countries**

| Rank | Cause | Proportion of total (%) |
|---|---|---|
| DALYs | | |
| 1 | Unipolar depressive disorders | 8.8 |
| 2 | Ischemic heart disease | 6.7 |
| 3 | Alcohol use disorders | 5.4 |
| 4 | Cerebrovascular disease | 4.9 |
| 5 | Alzheimer and other dementias | 4.3 |
| 6 | Road traffic injuries | 3.1 |
| 7 | Trachea, bronchus, lung cancers | 3.0 |
| 8 | Osteoarthritis | 2.7 |
| 9 | Chronic obstructive pulmonary disease | 2.5 |
| 10 | Hearing loss, adult onset | 2.5 |
| 12 | Self-inflicted injuries | *2.0* |
| 31 | Interpersonal violence | *0.7* |
| 88 | War | *0.0* |

**Low-Income Countries**

| Rank | Cause | Proportion of total (%) |
|---|---|---|
| DALYs | | |
| 1 | Lower respiratory infections | 6.8 |
| 2 | Perinatal conditions | 6.7 |
| 3 | HIV/AIDS | 6.6 |
| 4 | Meningitis | 4.6 |
| 5 | Diarrheal diseases | 4.6 |
| 6 | Unipolar depressive disorders | 4.0 |
| 7 | Ischemic heart disease | 3.5 |
| 8 | Malaria | 3.0 |
| 9 | Cerebrovascular disease | 2.9 |
| 10 | Road traffic injuries | 2.8 |
| 19 | Self-inflicted injuries | *1.2* |
| 21 | Interpersonal violence | *1.1* |
| 31 | War | *0.8* |

NOTE: Bold, italic figures highlight deaths or disability due to violence.
SOURCE: Reprinted from the *World Report on Violence and Health* (2002) with permission of the World Health Organisation.

**TABLE C-2** Deaths Attributable to Selected Risk Factors Compared with the Underlying Causes of Death in South Africa, 2000

| Rank | Risk Factor | % Total Deaths | Rank | Disease or Injury | % Total Deaths |
|---|---|---|---|---|---|
| 1 | Unsafe sex/STIs | 26.3 | 1 | HIV/AIDS | 25.5 |
| 2 | High blood pressure | 9.0 | 2 | Ischemic heart disease | 6.6 |
| 3 | Tobacco | 8.5 | 3 | Stroke | 6.5 |
| 4 | Alcohol harm | 7.1 | 4 | Tuberculosis | 5.5 |
| 5 | High BMI | 7.0 | 5 | *Interpersonal violence* | *5.3* |
| 6 | *Interpersonal violence* | *6.7* | 6 | Lower respiratory infections | 4.4 |
| 7 | High cholesterol | 4.6 | 7 | Hypertensive disease | 3.2 |
| 8 | Diabetes | 4.3 | 8 | Diarrheal diseases | 3.1 |
| 9 | Physical inactivity | 3.3 | 9 | Road traffic accidents | 3.1 |
| 10 | Low fruit and vegetable intake | 3.2 | 10 | Diabetes mellitus | 2.6 |
| 11 | Unsafe water, sanitation, hygiene | 2.6 | 11 | Chronic obstructive pulmonary disease | 2.5 |
| 12 | Child, maternal underweight | 2.3 | 12 | Low birth weight | 2.2 |
| 13 | Urban air pollution | 0.9 | 13 | Asthma | 1.3 |
| 14 | Vitamin A deficiency | 0.6 | 14 | Trachea/bronchi/lung cancer | 1.3 |
| 15 | Indoor smoke | 0.5 | 15 | Nephritis/nephrosis | 1.3 |
| 16 | Iron deficiency anemia | 0.4 | 16 | Septicemia | 1.2 |
| 17 | Lead exposure | 0.3 | 17 | Oesophageal cancer | 1.1 |

NOTE: Bold, italic figures highlight deaths or disability due to violence.
SOURCE: Norman et al. (2007b).

The severity and range of the long-term effects of violence on children were systematically measured in a study by Felitti et al. (1998). Their study found a graded relationship between childhood exposure to violence and other adverse events and outcomes such as alcoholism, drug abuse, depression, suicide attempts, smoking, risky sexual practices, sexually transmitted disease, physical inactivity, and severe obesity. These in turn were related to the presence of adult diseases including ischemic heart disease, cancer, chronic lung disease, skeletal fractures, and liver disease. Evidence from HICs suggests an association between child sexual abuse (CSA) and a range of psychiatric disorders (Andrews et al., 2004). Investing in the prevention of violence may therefore result in a substantial yield for improved national mental health in LMICs with a high prevalence of CSA. More generally, Pinheiro (2006) reports that children exposed to violence are at greater risk than their peers of suffering from allergies, asthma, gastrointestinal problems, depression, and anxiety. Children exposed to violence also present with poor concentration and focus and are therefore likely to underperform at school. The effects of exposure to domestic violence are also intergenerational with boys growing up in violent homes being twice as likely to become violent, abusive adults. Additionally, girls who witness the abuse of their mothers are significantly more likely to accept violence in their married lives. Thus the impact of violence on the MDGs must be read alongside this growing evidence pool that clearly demonstrates the negative, enduring effects of exposure to violence in childhood.

WHO's study on the Comparative Quantification of Health Risks estimated the lifetime impact of child sexual abuse taking into account a wide range of disease outcomes including depression, panic disorder, post-traumatic stress disorder (PTSD), alcohol and drug abuse/dependence and suicide attempts. Consequently it was estimated that CSA accounted for approximately 6 percent of cases of depression, 6 percent of alcohol and drug abuse/dependence, 8 percent of suicide attempts, 10 percent of panic disorders, and 27 percent of PTSDs (Andrews et al., 2004). Although such detailed data are simply not available in most LMICs, it is not inconceivable that with a higher prevalence, the burden of CSA may be even greater.

The first study measuring the burden of disease due to IPV in Victoria, Australia, took into account a wide range of consequences include depression, suicide, anxiety, and panic disorders; alcohol, drug, and tobacco abuse; eating disorders; and high-risk sexual behavior spread throughout a person's lifetime. The study concluded that IPV contributed 9 percent to the total disease burden among women aged 15 to 44 years and 3 percent among all Victorian women (Webster, 2004). Although not indicative of all LMICs, recent estimates from South Africa suggest that the burden is considerably higher, with IPV responsible for an estimated 7 percent (95 percent CI: 5-11.2 percent) of the burden of disease among South African women (Norman et al., 2007c).

Of course the impact of violence would be shown to be even greater if it were possible to accurately and comprehensively quantify all possible health outcomes. Important categories missing from the South African study were mental health outcomes and the impact of violence on the elderly and at the community level (Norman et al., 2007b,d). The latter would include all other health outcomes resulting from physical and sexual violence affecting adults outside the home (e.g., sexual violence perpetrated by strangers, robbery and assault, gang conflicts, etc.) as well as the deleterious and chronic effects that high rates of violence have on the national psyche, the general mental health of the population, and its effect on lifestyle choices, such as the use of public transport or health-seeking behavior.

## The Economic Impact of Violence on Health

The economic cost of violence can be assessed in terms of a variety of direct and indirect costs (Table C-3). The direct costs (or impacts) include the medical costs related to the treatment of the victims of violence and nonmedical costs associated with the three levels of prevention.[4] Indirect costs include those that are tangible such as the impact of violence on the broader macro economy and those that are intangible such as those relating to quality of life (WHO and CDC, n.d.).

However, the current paucity of accurate and detailed data on even the direct costs and impacts relating to violence in LMICs makes it difficult to apply the WHO/CDC framework in its entirety. Data on the economic costs of interpersonal violence in LMICs are scarce (Bowman and Stevens, 2004). However, based on available estimates from South Africa, the Caribbean, and Latin America, it is clear that the economic costs of violence are enormous in LMICs.

Overall the WHO reports that health care expenditure related to violence consumes a significant portion of GDP in LMICs. The cost of health expenditures related to violence as a percentage of GDP was 1.9 percent in Brazil, 4.3 percent in Colombia, 4.3 percent in El Salvador, 1.3 percent

---

[4]Within the public health approach are three "levels of prevention," typically described as primary, secondary, and tertiary, which refer to the timing of the prevention response. Primary prevention attempts to prevent violence before it occurs and can target potential perpetrators by curbing tendencies toward violent behavior, or potential victims by reducing the factors and characteristics that predispose them to victimization. Secondary prevention focuses on the immediate response to violence, such as emergency medicine including prehospital care for victims, and retribution through the criminal justice system. Tertiary prevention is aimed at mitigating the long-term effects of violence-related trauma and the rehabilitation and reintegration of offenders and victims (Dahlberg and Krug, 2002).

**TABLE C-3** A Typology for Assessing the Cost of Violence

| Cost Category | Type of Cost | Components | Disaggregating Options |
|---|---|---|---|
| Direct | Medical | Inpatient costs<br>Outpatient costs<br>Ambulance fees<br>Physician fees<br>Drugs/lab tests<br>Counseling costs | By demographic group<br>By type of injury<br>By mechanism<br>By intentionality |
| | Non-Medical | Costs of policing and incarceration<br>Costs of legal services<br>Direct perpetrator control costs<br>Costs of foster care<br>Private security contracts | |
| Indirect | Tangible | Productivity losses (perpetrators and victims, earnings and time)<br>Lost investments in social capital<br>Life insurance costs<br>Indirect protection costs<br>Macro-economic costs | |
| | Intangible | Health-related quality of life (pain and suffering, psychological costs)<br>Other quality of life (reduced job opportunities, access to schools, public services, community participation) | |

SOURCE: Matzopolous (in press).

in Mexico, 1.5 percent in Peru, and 0.3 percent in Venezuela. These direct health expenditures represented less than 30 percent of the estimated costs and impacts of violence within these countries (Buvinic et al., 1999). Similarly, studies in the United States have established that the direct medical costs associated with the treatment of a gunshot wound amount to only 13 percent of the total costs related to the injury (Peden and Van der Spuy, 1998) and medical treatment accounts for less than 20 percent of the lifetime costs of injury in general when the loss of productivity is taken into account (Corso et al., 2006). In Columbia, for example, armed violence has been estimated to account for US$ 4 billion in lost productivity. In Brazil, lost productivity due to homicides has been calculated at US$ 10 billion or 0.5 percent of the annual GDP (Small Arms Survey, 2006).

For example, according to pilot studies undertaken by the Small Arms Survey, the direct medical costs of treating firearm injuries in Rio de Janeiro, Bogotá, and Cali amounted to a per-patient average of US$ 4,521, 6,804, and 11,403, respectively. When national mortality and morbidity data are included to estimate loss of future earnings in the largely male population of gunshot victims, the figures climb to US$ 10 billion per year in Brazil and US$ 4 billion in Colombia. The direct medical costs of IPV were calculated at US$454,000 in Jamaica in 2001 (Waters et al., 2005).

At the more local level of individual cities and hospitals, a number of South African studies again highlight the high economic costs of violence. One study at Groote Schuur Hospital in Cape Town found that the direct treatment costs for firearm-related violence amounted to ZAR 3,858,331 for a total of 969 patients (Peden and van der Spuy, 1998). In a more recent study conducted by Allard and Burch (2005) the minimum cost of treating an abdominal firearm-related injury for 21 patients at G.F. Jooste Hospital in Cape Town was estimated at ZAR 215,649. This figure represents an amount 13 times the per capita government expenditure on health in South Africa in 2001. Indirect costs of violence were included in Phillips' (1998) study of homicide in the city of Cape Town. She calculated total costs of homicide (excluding intangibles) to be ZAR 11.8 million for that year.

The lack of a costing culture within many public health systems in LMICs makes the generation of reliable violence costs difficult. In such countries rudimentary surveillance and reporting systems are still under development so costing is not viewed as a reporting priority at this time. Nevertheless, as the incidence of violence in LMICs is much higher, it follows that the economic costs, or at least the relative economic costs, may be higher. Further empirical research is needed that takes into account the differences in treatment costs across income contexts. Moreover, the calculation of the costs of other health burdens such as HIV has mobilized civil society to lobby for prevention. An accurate estimation of the costs of violence in LMICs is therefore imperative to the violence prevention agenda.

With respect to IPV, lost earnings and opportunity costs were extrapolated to US$ 1.73 billion in Chile and US$ 32.7 million in Nicaragua from pilot study results in both countries. IPV alone has been calculated to cost the economies of Nicaragua and Chile 1.6 and 2 percent of their GDPs, respectively. The GDP effects of suicide appear even more difficult to measure and are scarce in the literature. A study conducted in Alberta, Canada, showed that suicide significantly detracts from future GDP. The study calculated that suicide costs the equivalent of 0.3 percent of the provincial GDP.

However limited, violence costing in research has begun to clearly demonstrate the substantial economic impacts of violence in LMICs. Greater general investment in improving on and prioritizing this area of research is imperative for generating a more accurate and comprehensive profile of the costs of violence in these contexts. More specifically, such studies should disaggregate the costs of violence according to the more specific typologies of violence listed above. This would enable the identification of relative contributions of these different types to overall costs.

## The Impact of Violence on Development

Collective, interpersonal, and self-directed violence have extensive and pervasive long-term implications for development and health. Moreover, these effects are themselves multilayered and can undermine development at individual, communal, and national levels. Although the different paths by which violence exerts such economic strains remain unclear, the following section describes the available research findings on the consequences of violence for development, and how violence and underdevelopment may be linked in a vicious circle where each perpetuates the other.

### The Impact of Violence in Relation to the Millennium Development Goals

In describing the wide-ranging impacts of violence on different sectors and systems, the eight goals of the Millennium Development Plan (World Bank, 2004) provide a useful organizing framework. These eight goals are at the forefront of the global development agenda, and showing how violence impacts upon them helps to highlight its importance within this agenda.

### MDG1: Eradicating Extreme Poverty and Hunger

There is a vicious cycle between poverty and violence. On the one hand it is well established that poverty, particularly in the context of economic inequality (Nafziger, 2006; Fajnzylber et al., 1999; Unithan and Whitt, 1992), and especially when geographically concentrated, contributes to high levels of violence by weakening intergenerational family and community ties, control of peer groups, and participation in community organizations (see Box C-4; Sampson and Lauritsen, 1994; Wilson, 1987). In turn, there is also evidence that high rates of violence in a community reduce property values and undermine the growth and development of business (World Bank, 2006), thus contributing to the very inequalities and concentrations in poverty that play a role in causing violence.

Low SES has been linked to risk for interpersonal violence (GHRI, 2005). Studies of the health effects of interpersonal violence have shown that different degrees of violence can result in a number of acute and chronic health conditions that in turn imply negative influences on produc-

---

**BOX C-4**
**Socioeconomic Status, Social Inequality, and Violence:**
**Evidence from South Africa, Brazil, and Russia**


Associations between socioeconomic status (SES) and health have been relatively well documented by researchers over the last 50 years. The general gradual
relationship between these two variables is commonly referred to as the health-
wealth gradient (Deaton, 2002). Although much work in this field has focused on
the epidemiological distributions of general health outcomes by income levels
(Marmot, 1994; Link and Phelan, 1995; Feinstein, 1993), there is growing evidence to support the hypothesis that low levels of development, relative poverty,
and income inequality predict high levels of various forms of violence.

A number of studies have narrowed this general focus to assessing the relationship between development and homicide across and within nations (Unithan
and Whitt, 1992; Butchart and Engström, 2002; Neapolitan, 2003). A study by
Moniruzzaman and Andersson (2005) found a strong correlation between levels
of homicide and economic development that was especially pronounced in LMICs.
South Africa, Brazil, and Russia have been especially useful case studies for
illuminating such relationships. In South Africa, a study of the relationship between
local (community) inequality and crime found a strong positive correlation between
rates of unemployment and murder (Demombynes and Özler, 2005) and a strong
positive correlation between homicide and inequality measured by the Gini index.
In Sao Paulo, Brazil, Gawryszewski and Costa (2005) found a strong negative
correlation between homicide rates and average monthly income, with higher
homicide rates in the districts whose inhabitants had the lowest incomes. In a
study of the association between SES and overall mortality in Moscow, Russia,
Chenet, Leon, and Mckee (1998) found a strong association between homicide
and levels of education, with individuals who had received less education at
greatest risk of being killed. Another study in Russia found that negative socioeconomic changes were positively correlated with rising homicide rates (Kim and
Pridemore, 2005).

---

tivity and labor (Plichta and Falik, 2001) and exert tremendous strains on
health care systems. More generally, poor countries have higher rates of
violent crime taxing already-burdened criminal justice systems. Whether
cause or consequence, or both, countries with higher inequality have higher
murder and robbery rates (Leggett et al., 2007). Rapid urbanization has
also been associated with increases in levels of violence due in part to
pockets of concentrated poverty on the outskirts of large cities. Such problems have become formidable and often cripple the economic prospects of
entire cities (Maninger, 2000). While scenes of urban decay have become
almost synonymous with African and Asian LMICs, recent research from
Russia indicates that the transition to a more pluralistic and democratic

system of government was accompanied by a range of social problems such as unemployment, poverty, and inequality. These are conditions associated with likely increases in rates of violence, as at a micro level individual needs and values supplant those of the community, while at a macro level governments' ability to provide adequate social support is compromised. The results of the study indicated that in the face of these changes even regions with higher levels of social support were unable to contain the consequent increase in rates of violence.

Another violence-related threat to the goal of eradicating poverty and hunger are the deleterious effects of collective violence on food security. These effects are pronounced at the level of food production with global agricultural production declining by 1.5 percent during conflict periods (Teodosijevic, 2003). Total food production is usually reduced, and in some cases collapses, leading to hunger and starvation and forcing mass migration. In some cases the per-capita-per-day calorie availability plunges by an average of 7 percent as a result of conflict. According to Messer (1998), people of at least 32 countries suffered malnutrition, poverty-related inaccessibility to food stocks, and dramatic food shortages as a direct result of war in 1994. Food itself frequently becomes a weapon of war. In the Sudan, the government sold grain reserves in 1990 to help fund the war. The government and opposition forces created famine as a means to control territories and populations, and restricted access to food (Keen and Wilson, 1994). This led to widespread food poverty among the already-impoverished population (Keen, 1994). The development costs are summarized in Table C-4.

## MDG2: Achieving Universal Primary Education

Violence impacts directly on education systems by depleting LMICs of their human capital in the form of educators, undermining access to education, and hampering attempts at providing conducive learning environments. While school shootings commonly make new headlines in HICs, school violence is common within LMICs, initiating a vicious cycle of violence and limits to development. Epidemiological data has shown that girls subjected to sexual violence at schools are more likely to leave formal education (Heise et al., 1999). Unfortunately, such subjections are frequent. According to recent research undertaken in six African countries, between 16 percent and just under 50 percent of girls in primary and secondary schools report sexual abuse or harassment at the hands of either male students or teachers. In a recent study in Zimbabwe, 40 percent of girls aged between 12 and 14 indicated that they had been the victims of sexual violence (Leach et al., 2000). A sample survey of nine Caribbean countries found that 20 percent of males carried weapons to school in the last month and that 10 percent of the

**TABLE C-4** The Development Costs of War

| Category of Capital | Destruction of existing stock | Impact on new investment |
| --- | --- | --- |
| Productive capital—plant equipment and buildings. | Land mined; factories bombed. | Fall in private productive investments—foreign and local, including farmers' investments. Some new investment in new informal activities; and in arms production. |
| Economic infrastructure | Transport and communication system, power, irrigation, disrupted. | Decline in government expenditure on infrastructure. |
| Social infrastructure | Schools, hospitals, clinics damaged. | |
| Human capital | Death, migration especially of skilled workers; worsened nutrition and health or workforce. | Decline in public entitlements, reduced education in quantity and quality. Reduced private sector training. |
| Organizational capital | Government institutions, banks, agricultural extensions, science and technology organizations weakened. | No resources in formal sector; new informal organizations develop; NGOs take on new activities. |
| Social capital | Destruction of trust; work ethic; respect for property; community links. | New forms of social capital, through groups that develop links in war, NGO activity. |

SOURCE: Stewart and FitzGerald (2000).

sample had been knocked unconscious in a fight (Garber et al., 2003, cited in Leggett et al., 2007). In the Dominican Republic over half of a representative sample of students reported violence at their schools. These figures point to the manifold effects of violence on education. First, unsafe schools deter quality educators from participating in primary education in LMICs. Second, violence seems to be a characteristic of school life in developing countries, further hampering strategies aimed at achieving universal education at least at the primary level.

*MDG3: Promoting Gender Equality and Empowering Women*

The WHO Multi-country Study on Women's Health and Domestic Violence against Women suggests that this problem is pronounced in a range of

LMICs. The study collected data from over 24,000 women in Bangladesh, Brazil, Ethiopia, Japan, Namibia, Peru, Samoa, Serbia and Montenegro, Thailand, and the United Republic of Tanzania. In Ethiopia 59 percent of respondents indicated that they had ever been physically assaulted by an intimate partner. In Dhaka, Bangladesh, 40 percent of ever-married women reported having ever experienced physical violence. The health, economic, and social effects of this type of violence are far-reaching. Abused women are more likely to suffer from a range of health problems including depression, anxiety, psychosomatic symptoms, eating problems, sexual dysfunction, and many reproductive health problems, including miscarriage and stillbirth, premature delivery, HIV, and other sexually transmitted infections, leading to significantly high health care costs in those contexts in which medical institutions are consulted or available. Also, some 25 percent of women are likely to be victims of assault while pregnant, compromising the health and development of both mother and child (Heise et al., 1999). However, IPV also appears to be closely related to some development indicators. Research conducted in Chile, Egypt, India, and the Philippines showed that levels of female education and general household wealth were related to decreased levels of IPV (Bangdiwala et al., 2004). Moreover, a cross-national study by Archer (2006) found that female empowerment was associated with levels of individualism and that women were less frequently victims of violence in countries in which they were more empowered. As gender equality and individualism increased so the sex differences between victims of violence decreased. Hence there is evidence that increasing women's economic participation decreases their rate of violent victimization (Cheston and Kuhn, 2002; Shrestha, 1998).

## MDG4: Reducing Child Mortality

According to the *World Report on Violence Against Children* (Pinheiro, 2006), 2.05 children between ages 0 and 4 per 100,000 were victims of homicide in LICs in 2002. In Africa this rate was 4.16. However, the child homicide rate in Africa climbs to 5.58 per 100,000 if every person below the age of 18 is included. Although constituting a relatively small proportion of child mortality in LMICs, the long-term developmental effects of violence against children are, as shown above, far-reaching and ultimately result in a broad range of health problems.

Violence can lead to a variety of health problems for the expectant mother. These include a range of mental disorders (Patel, 2007); sexually transmitted diseases; gastrointestinal disorders; and gynecological problems, including vaginal bleeding and vaginal infections, urinary tract infections, and various chronic pain syndromes, including chronic pelvic pain (Ellsberg, 2006). Studies in Bangladesh and Latin America have also shown that IPV therefore contributes to maternal mortality (Ronsmans and Khlat, 1999; Espinoza and Camacho, 2005) in these LMICs. Maternal health also impacts the health of the child. Problems experienced in early childhood are among the numerous psychological and behavioral factors that may predispose youths and young adults to display violent and aggressive behavior (Karr-Morse and Wiley, 1997) and hence the mental health of the mother is an important factor in the formative stages of a child's life. Unwanted pregnancy, teenage motherhood, and pregnancy complications have also been shown to predict risk for violence across the lifespan of the child.

## MDG6: Combating HIV/AIDS, Malaria, and Other Diseases

Widespread violence further undermines the capacity of health care systems to provide effective programs for dealing with a host of diseases. A study of health care workers in South Africa showed that they are especially at risk for violence. The findings indicated that over 60 percent (61.1 percent) of the 176 health care practitioners working in Cape Town had been exposed to violence in its various forms (Marais et al., 2002). In a country with high levels of HIV prevalence, such figures imply direct threats on health care capacity and productivity. In addition to this violence-related effect, IPV has been shown to directly contribute to risk for HIV contraction (Dunkle et al., 2004; Petersen et al., 2005; Abrahams et al., 2004). Thus IPV needs to be addressed alongside other interventions in order to reduce HIV infection and promote safer sexual behavior (Jewkes et al., 2006). There are two examples of the apparent successes of targeting IPV in HIV interventions. A recent evaluation of the Stepping Stones HIV, communication, and relationships behavioral program, by Jewkes et al. (2006) in South Africa, showed decreased rates of reported IPV following program implementation. A recent structural intervention provides another neat demonstration of this concept and the interrelationship between violence, HIV/AIDS, and empowerment of women. The intervention took the form of a microfinance program for women in Limpopo that aimed to assist in reducing poverty, income inequality, empowering participants, and hence improve health and included a gender and HIV training curriculum. Although the focus was on improving knowledge and behavior with respect to HIV/AIDS, there was a significant decrease in reported IPV among participants (Pronyk et al., 2006).

Collective violence more than interpersonal violence fragments health care systems, as health care professionals flee war-torn areas. The food insecurity and poor sanitation resulting from various forms of collective violence have also been shown to contribute directly to diarrheal diseases, measles, acute respiratory infections, and malaria (Tool and Waldman,

1990). Areas of conflict also report higher rates of tuberculosis (Gibson et al., 1998). While some disagreement prevails as to the extent to which war-torn populations are more vulnerable to HIV, some studies have found significant evidence of such associations. Following conflict in the Ivory Coast, 90 percent of medical doctors left flashpoint areas (Betsi et al., 2006). Fleeing health care personnel along with diminishing prophylaxis stocks were all suggested to impede HIV prevention in the area.

## MDG7: Ensuring Environmental Sustainability

The most direct effect of violence on environmental sustainability is demonstrated through several sustained conflicts in LMICs that are in large part driven by competition over the extraction of high-value resources such as minerals (e.g., diamonds), narcotics, and timber. While the root causes of such conflicts are complex, they are invariably driven by economic imperatives in which the health of resident populations and environmental sustainability are marginalized. These effects may be felt long after conflicts have ceased as the means of agricultural production and basic food security is compromised. Landmines, for example, render large tracts of land unusable for agriculture, livestock, gathering firewood, and collecting water (Sethi and Krug, 2000). Consequent urbanization and increased population densities in nonafflicted rural areas strain the holding capacity of the land with devastating environmental impacts.

A broader interpretation of "environmental sustainability" includes social paradigms linked with the production of human capital and the orderly operations of government. Interpersonal violence erodes both of these prerequisites. In fact some commentators have argued that the erosion of social capital by violence is among the most significant obstacles to sustainability (Goodland, 2002). These erosions most frequently take the form of impoverishment and concentrations of high mortality in violent areas. Violence also has dramatic effects on the sectors required to maintain sustainable environments. A study of the policing sector in South Africa showed this group to be especially at risk for a range of stress-related symptoms and significant levels of suicidal ideation resulting in high suicide rates (Kopel and Friedman, 1997). High levels of stress lead to increased burnout. High levels of violence have also been shown to severely affect the productivity and efficiency of the transport (Lerer and Matzopoulos, 1996; Peltzer, 2001) and banking (Miller-Burke et al., 1999) sectors in this country. Widespread violence in many LMICs also impedes sustainable environmental development through disincentivizing direct foreign investment and tourism (Bourguignon, 1999).

*MDG8: Developing a Global Partnership for Development*

The sum total of all of the negative impacts of violence on the achievement of the above goals represents a significant obstacle to the creation of global partnerships aimed at development. As in many other sectors the *10/90 gap* is particularly pressing with regard to violence prevention. The gap refers to the fact that, of the $73 billion invested annually toward public health research worldwide, less than 10 percent is devoted to research into the health problems that account for 90 percent of the global disease burden (measured in DALYs). Despite significant advances in the recognition of this discrepancy, formulating the means to its correction has been slow. The evidence base for research and, as will become more evident in the sections that follow, rigorous and accurate surveillance systems for violence data are primarily based in HICs. Truly global partnerships must necessarily acknowledge the significant deleterious effects of violence on the potential development of LMICs and adjust resources invested in violence prevention in LMICs accordingly.

*Other Developmental Impacts of Violence*

Although the MDGs provide a useful framework within which to assess the impact of violence on some aspects of development, they also have a number of limitations. For instance, the almost exclusive focus on women and children in MDGs 3 to 5 does not accommodate the fact that male victims of homicide and suicide substantially outnumber female victims. In LMICs the male-to-female ratio for homicide is more than three times higher than in HICs and males also significantly outnumber females for suicide in these contexts (Mathers et al., 2002). This enormous differential has major socioeconomic consequences as young men are often the breadwinners in LMICs. Likewise, the MDG 4 focus on reducing child mortality emphasizes a reduction in infant mortality rates and under 5 mortality rates. While violence does impact upon both of these rates, its burden is largely concentrated in early to middle life and most prevalent in the 15-to-44-year cohort. The nonfatal health outcomes of violence have been shown to be important mediators of childhood health, with the child being defined as every human being below the age of 18 under the Convention on the Rights of the Child.

Describing the impacts of violence on early childhood development is especially useful for gauging the potentially detrimental developmental effects of violence across the human lifespan. A key review by Walker et al. (2007) identified exposure to violence as a major contributing factor to compromised human development with far-reaching intergenerational effects in developing countries. In fact, exposure to violence (alongside malaria, intrauterine growth restriction, maternal depression, and exposure to heavy metals) was identified as in urgent need of intervention. Children exposed to violence in South Africa present higher levels of PTSD (Magwaza et al., 1993), aggression (Liddel et al., 1994), attention problems, and depression (Barbarin et al., 2001). The effects of violence in Eritrea and Bosnia appeared to be mediated by levels of social cohesion and caregiver mental health—both of which are further compromised in various forms across the different typologies of violence.

## The Economic Impact of Violence on Development

As indicated in Section 3.3, the economic costs associated with violence are significant. As well as the substantial health care expenditure that violence consumes in LMICs, there are numerous costs related to development. These costs represent formidable challenges to investing in sustainable development. The most widely acknowledged relate to war and conflict, and these are succinctly encapsulated in the following excerpt from Hillier and Wood (2003, p. 4):

> The uncontrolled proliferation and misuse of arms by government forces and armed groups takes a massive human toll in lost lives, lost livelihoods, and lost opportunities to escape poverty. An average of US$22bn a year is spent on arms by countries in Africa, Asia, the Middle East, and Latin America—a sum that would otherwise enable those same countries to be on track to meet the Millennium Development Goals4 of achieving universal primary education (estimated at $10bn a year) as well as targets for reducing infant and maternal mortality (estimated at $12bn a year).

Violence in whatever form absorbs sizeable amounts of health care expenditure that could be better used to prevent other forms of health threat. A seminal study by Milanovic (2005) showed that war and civil strife alone accounted for an income loss of about 40 percent over the last 20 years in the least developed countries. National spending on collective violence in the form of "defense" budgetary allocations and investment in postconflict recovery have been shown to lead to drastic reductions in national investment in health care services. In essence this type of spending "squeezes" the resources available for development.

Although the top 15 military spenders are mostly HICs, many LMICs spend a greater proportion of their available resources on defense than these developed countries. Mainly attributable to the wars in Afghanistan and Iraq, the United States spent approximately 6 percent of its GDP on the military in 2003. Yet in 2001 Burundi and Ethiopia spent 8 and 6.2 percent, respectively (Jolly, 2004). These are both postconflict countries and so this high proportion of spending detracts from spending on schools, hospitals, and social development. Significantly, military spending as a percentage of GDP is associated with economic slowdowns across countries. This is alarming as many researchers have pointed to the changing nature of insecurity over the last couple of decades. Human security threats no longer take traditional cross-border forms but are predominantly within nations (Jolly, 2004).

In Africa, war and conflict have been shown to consume a startlingly significant portion of GDP (Table C-5). In 2005, spending on the military amounted to US$ 7.2 billion in sub-Saharan Africa in 2005 (Omitoogun, 2001). However, military expenditure does not paint a complete picture of total war costs. For example, a case study of the war in Sri Lanka showed that military spending accounted for just over half of the total costs of the war.

Studies in both Jamaica and South Africa have demonstrated that violence (in the form of violent crime) represents a substantial cost to business (NEDCOR Project, 1996; Francis et al., 2003). Global estimates suggest that crime and violence together cost approximately 14 percent of GDP in LMICs. This is almost three times more than the 0.5 percent of GDP calculated as the cost of violence in HICs (Pfizer, 2001). The multiplier effects of this disparity are significant. The Inter-American Development Bank estimated that GDP in Latin American countries would be 25 percent higher if rates of violence were equal to global rates (Londoño and Guerrero, 1999).

**TABLE C-5** The Burden of Military Expenditure as a Share of GDP in 10 Countries with the Highest Milex: GDP Ratio in Africa 1991-1999

| Countries | 1991 | 1992 | 1993 | 1994 | 1995 | 1996 | 1997 | 1998 | 1999 |
|---|---|---|---|---|---|---|---|---|---|
| Algeria | 1.2 | 2.2 | 2.6 | 3.2 | 3.0 | 3.3 | 3.7 | 4.0 | 3.8 |
| Angola | 6.8 | 12.0 | 12.5 | 19.8 | 17.6 | 19.5 | 22.3 | 11.4 | 23.5 |
| Botswana | 4.4 | 4.3 | 4.5 | 3.9 | 3.5 | 2.9 | 3.1 | 3.7 | 3.4 |
| Burundi | 3.8 | 3.6 | 3.7 | 3.9 | 4.2 | 5.7 | 6.3 | 5.9 | 6.1 |
| Djibouti | 5.9 | 6.1 | 5.6 | 5.4 | 5.1 | 4.2 | 4.5 | 4.4 | No data |
| Eritrea | No data | No data | 21.4 | 13.0 | 19.9 | 22.8 | 13.5 | 29.0 | 22.9 |
| Ethiopia | 2.0 | 2.7 | 2.9 | 2.4 | 2.0 | 1.9 | 3.4 | 5.1 | 9.0 |
| Morocco | 4.1 | 4.3 | 4.4 | 4.9 | 4.7 | 3.9 | No data | No data | No data |
| Rwanda | 5.5 | 4.4 | 4.6 | 3.4 | 3.9 | 5.2 | 4.1 | 4.3 | 4.2 |
| Zimbabwe | 3.8 | 3.7 | 3.4 | 3.3 | 3.6 | 3.2 | 3.4 | 2.7 | 3.4 |

SOURCE: Omitoogun (2001).

## The Emergence of Violence Prevention as Part of the
## Health and Development Agenda

Despite the numerous and substantial impacts as a direct and indirect result of violence, it has received limited attention on the global health agenda. Violence is mentioned only once in the World Bank's seminal publication, *The Millennium Development Goals for Health: Rising to the Challenges*, despite its extensive influence on all eight of the millennium goals, as described in Section 3 of this paper. However, there are indications of an increasing awareness among policy makers of the role that violence plays in undermining international health and development, and the potential of violence prevention as a means of reducing these destructive effects. Two recent World Bank reports consistently highlight violence as a fundamental threat to human development. A World Bank publication focused on using participatory methods to foreground the perceptions, needs, and experiences of the poor. The report emphasizes violence as a much-cited everyday reality and constant threat to the potential development of the poor (Narayan, 1999). The 2007 World Bank report on Human Development cites numerous examples of the way that violence compromises individual development (World Bank, 2006).

Many LMICs have lobbied for violence prevention to receive increased prioritization and are favorably disposed to the recommendations emanating from violence prevention agencies. South Africa, emerging from decades of apartheid rule, was initially at the forefront of the movement tabling resolution 94.5 at the end of its tenure in chairing the World Health Assembly in 1994. More recently the African Union adopted the recommendations of the *World Report on Violence and Health* in declaring 2005 the "African year of violence prevention." LMICs have also played host to two World Conferences on Injury Prevention and Safety Promotion, in India in 2000 and in South Africa in 2006. The conference will be hosted for a third time in an LMIC in Mexico in 2008.

The emergence of violence within the health and development agenda can in part be ascribed to the role played by the World Health Assembly and partner organizations in driving violence prevention and injury prevention in general, an initiative that has seen injury-related topics being the focus of two World Reports in the last 5 years: namely the *World Report on Violence and Health* and the *World Report on Road Traffic Injury Prevention*. Since the publication of the *World Report on Violence and Health* there has been a World Health Assembly resolution (WHA49.25) calling on countries to invest in violence prevention, and by 2006 three out of six WHO regional committees (Africa, the Americas, and Europe) had adopted similar resolutions.

The inclusion of violence prevention on the agenda of other multilateral agencies is also a useful indication of its emergence as a global priority. The World Bank's Disease Control Priorities, for example, includes a single chapter on all of injuries and violence in its first edition in 1993, whereas the second in 2006 had an entire chapter dedicated to interpersonal violence alongside another entire chapter that addressed unintentional injuries and a third chapter on trauma care. The United Nations General Assembly has also reviewed special reports on violence against children and violence against women, which have resulted in resolutions calling for greater investment in multisectoral efforts to address these forms of violence.

## Conclusion

This paper has demonstrated that violence is a global health issue of especial concern to LMICs, and that violence is inextricably linked with a range of other health indicators. Yet, despite current projections indicating that violence in LMICs (as a result of both interpersonal and collective violence) is set to become an increasingly important threat to health, vigorous and concerted violence prevention efforts can arrest this trend.

While there are indications that violence prevention is also gaining more prominence in LMICs, it will need to be integrated and institutionalized within government ministries if it is to be successfully implemented. An important first step would be for the improvement of data systems and research on the economic and other social costs of violence in LMICs so that violence can be better framed and understood as an issue well beyond social order and "law enforcement."

Ongoing support of intersectoral collaborative forums is one of several areas that could benefit from development aid and the involvement of international development partners, as this is an area where many LMIC governments are underskilled. Also, much of the research and evidence relating to violence prevention arises from a small number of HICs. This imbalance needs to be addressed as LMICs may require a different set of interventions. This could be facilitated by the availability of more funding and the development of mechanisms to support and sustain equitable multilateral research cooperation.

Another key requirement is the development of research capacity within research organizations and among implementing agencies in the criminal justice, policing, and social development sectors, which may require the establishment of a program or fund for research, capacity development, and exchanges and/or placements. A fund could also be established to support the education of public-sector managers in LMICs in fields related to violence prevention (public health, psychology, sociology, criminology, biostatistics, and other related disciplines) with conditions to ensure their continuing work in the public sector for a suitable period following completion of their studies.

There are certainly other important areas of synergy to explore to help shape and fast-track this agenda, such as those existing between the public health and rights-based approaches to violence prevention. It may also be worthwhile to document the recent developments in the policy and prevention environments together with some of its current challenges more comprehensively. In addition, there is a pressing need to explore opportunities to provide technical support and assistance to and within such environments, with a view to replicating some of the key studies that have successfully raised the profile of violence prevention in HICs. In the interim, efforts to consolidate and share information on key developments and successes in violence prevention research, policy, and practice in LMICs should be encouraged.

## References

Aalund, O., L. Danielsen, E. Katz, and P. Mazza. 1989. Injuries due to deliberate violence in areas of Argentina. I. The extent of violence. Copenhagen Study Group. *Forensic Science International* 42:151-163.

Abrahams, N., R. Jewkes, M. Hoffman, and R. Laubscher. 2004. Sexual violence against intimate partners in Cape Town: prevalence and risk factors reported by men. *Bulletin of the World Health Organisation.* Geneva, Switzerland: World Health Organisation, 82:330-337.

Abromowitz, S. 2005. The poor have become rich and the rich have become poor: Collective trauma in the Guinean languette, *Social Science and Medicine* 61: 2106-2118.

African Network for the Prevention and Protection Against Child Abuse and Neglect. 2000. *Awareness and views regarding child abuse and child rights in selected communities in Kenya.* Nairobi, Kenya.

Allard, D., and V. Burch. 2005. The cost of treating serious abdominal firearm-related injuries in South Africa. *South African Medical Journal* 95(8):591-594.

Andrews, G., J. Corry, T. Slade, C. Issakidis, and H. Swanston. 2004. Child sexual abuse. In *Comparative quantification of health risks: Global and regional burden of disease attributable to selected major risk factors.* Vol. 1, edited by M. Ezzati, A. D. Lopez, A. Rodgers, and C. Murray. Geneva: World Health Organisation.

Archer, J. 2006. Cross-cultural differences in physical aggression between partners: a social-role analysis. *Personality and Social Psychology Review* 10(2):133-153.

Bangdiwala, S. I., L. Ramiro, L. S. Sadowski, I. A. S. Bordin, W. Hunter, and V. Shankar. 2004. Intimate partner violence and the role of socioeconomic indicators in WorldSAFE communities in Chile, Egypt, India and the Phillipines. *Injury Control and Safety Promotion* 11:101-109.

Barbarin, O. A., L. Richter, and T. deWet. 2001. Exposure to violence, coping resources, and psychological adjustment of South African children. *American Journal of Orthopsychiatry* 71:16-25.

Bennis, P., and K. Lever. 2005. *The Iraq quagmire: The mounting costs of war and the case for bringing home the troops.* Institute for Policy Studies and Foreign Policy in Focus. Washington: IPS.

Bertolote, J., and A. Fleischmann. 2002. A global perspective in the epidemiology of suicide. *Suicidology* 7:6-8.

Betsi, N. A., B. G. Koudou, G. Cissé, A. B. Tschannen, A. M. Pignol, Y. Ouattara, Z. Madougou, M. Tanner, and J. Utzinger. 2006. Effect of an armed conflict on human resources and health systems in Côte d'Ivoire: prevention of and care for people with HIV/AIDS. *AIDS Care* 18(4):356-365.

Bezerra-Flanders, W., and J. C. Clark. 2006. Perspectives on elder abuse and neglect in Brazil. *Educational Gerontology* 32(1):63-72.

Bilmes, L., and J. E. Stiglitz. 2006. *The economic costs of the Iraq War: An appraisal three years after the beginning of the conflict.* Harvard University. John F. Kennedy School of Government (Faculty Research Working Paper, RWP06-002). http://ksgnotes1.harvard.edu/Research/wpaper.nsf/rwp/RWP06-002 (accessed February 16, 2006).

Bourguignon, F. 1999. *Crime, violence and inequitable development.* Washington, DC: The World Bank.

Bowman, B. and G. Stevens. 2004. Injury costing in South Africa: The state of the sector. In S. Suffla and A. van Niekerk (Eds.), *Crime, Violence and Injury Prevention in South Africa: Developments and Challenges.* Cape Town: MRC, pp.170-183.

Bradshaw, D., N. Nannan, R. Laubscher, P. Groenewald, J. Joubert, B. Nojilana, D. Pieterse, and M. Schneider. 2004. *South African National Burden of Disease Study 2000: Estimates of provincial mortality*, Medical Research Council, Cape Town.

Browne, K. et al. 2002. *Child abuse and neglect in Rumanian families: A national prevalence study 2000.* Copenhagen, Denmark. World Health Organisation Regional Office for Europe.

Burnham, G., R. Lafta, S. Doocy, and L. Roberts. 2006. Mortality after the 2003 invasion of Iraq: A cross-sectional cluster sample survey. *Lancet* 368(9545):1421-1428.

Butchart, A., and K. Engström. 2002. Sex and age-specific relations between economic development, economic inequality, and homicide rates in people aged 0-24 years: A cross-sectional analysis. *Bulletin of the World Health Organisation.* Geneva, Switzerland, 80:797-805.

Buvinic, M., A. Morrison, and M. Shifter. 1999. *Technical study: Violence in Latin America and the Caribbean: A framework for action.* Washington, DC: Inter-American Development Bank.

Chenet, L., D. Leon, and M. Mckee. 1998. Deaths from alcohol and violence in Moscow: Socio-economic determinants. *European Journal of Population* 14:19-37.

Cheston, S., and L. Kuhn. 2002. Empowering women through microfinance. In *Pathways out of poverty: Innovations in microfinance for the poorest families.* Edited by S. Daley-Harris. Bloomfield, CT: Kumarian Press. Pp. 167-228.

Corso, P., E. Finkelstein, T. Miller, I. Fiebelkorn, and E. Zaloshnja. 2006. Incidence and lifetime costs of injuries in the United States. *Injury Prevention* 12:212-218.

Dahlberg, L. L., and E. G. Krug. 2002. 'Violence—a global public health problem,' in E. G. Krug, L. L. Dahlberg, J. A. Mercy, A. B. Zwi and R. Lozano (eds.), *World report on violence and health.* Geneva, Switzerland: World Health Organization.

De Jong, J., Mulhern, M., Ford, N. van der Kam, S. and R. Kleber. 2000. The Trauma of War in Sierra Leone', Lancet 335 (9220): 2067-2068.

Deaton, A. 2002. Policy implications of the gradient of health and wealth. *Health Affairs* 21(2):13-30.

Demombynes, G., and B. Özler. 2005. Crime and local inequality in South Africa. *Journal of Development Economics* 76:265-292.

Derluyn, I., E. Broekaert, G. Schuyten, and E. Temmerman. 2004. Post-traumatic stress in former Ugandan child soldiers. *Lancet* 363:861-863.

Duffield, M. 2001. *Global governance and the new wars: the merger of development and security*. London: Zed Books (3rd ed. 2005).

Dunkle, K. L., R. K. Jewkes, H. C. Brown, G. E. Gray, J. A. McIntryre, and S. D. Harlow. 2004. Gender-based violence, relationship power and risk of prevalent HIV infection among women attending antenatal clinics in Soweto, South Africa. *Lancet* 363:1415-1421.

Eddleston, M., M. H. R. Sheriff, and K. Hawton. 1998. Deliberate self-harm in Sri Lanka—an overlooked tragedy in the developing world. *British Medical Journal* 317:133-135.

Ellsberg, M. 2006. Violence against women and the Millennium Development Goals: Facilitating women's access to support. *Int J Gynaecol Obstet*, 94:325-332.

Ensink, K., B. Robertson, C. Zissis, and P. Leger. 1997. Posttraumatic stress disorder in children exposed to violence. *South African Medical Journal* 87(11):1533-1537.

Espinoza, H., and V. Camacho. 2005. Maternal death due to domestic violence: Unrecognized critical component of maternal mortality. *Pan American Journal of Public Health* 17(2):123-129.

Fajnzylber, P., D. Lederman, and N. Loayza. 1999. *Inequality and violent crime*. Regional Studies Program, Office of the Chief Economist for Latin America and the Caribbean. Washington, DC: The World Bank. December.

Feinstein, J. 1993. The relationship between socio-economic status and health: a review of the literature. *Milbank Quarterly* 71(2):279-322.

Felitti, V. J., R. F. Anda, D. Nordenberg, D. F. Williamson, A. M. Spitz, V. Edwards, M. P. Koss, and J. S. Marks. 1998. Relationship of childhood abuse and household dysfunction to many of the leading causes of death in adults. The Adverse Childhood Experiences (ACE) Study. *American Journal of Preventive Medicine* 14(4): 245-258.

Fieggen, A. G., M. Wieman, C. Brown, A. B. Van As, G. H. Swingler, and J. C. Peter. 2004. Inhuman shields—children caught in the crossfire of domestic violence. *South African Medical Journal* 94(4):293-296.

Francis, A., A. Harriott, et al. 2003. *Crime and development: The Jamaican experience*. University of the West Indies (Mona Campus).

Gawryszewski, V. P., and L. S. Costa. 2005. Social inequality and homicide rates in Sào Paulo City, Brazil. *Revista de Saude Publica* 39(2):191-197.

GHRI (Global Health Research Initiative). 2005. *Global health research casebook* (2005). Ottawa, Canada: GHRI.

Gibson, N., F. Boillot, and H. Jalloh. 1998. The costs of tuberculosis to patients in Sierra Leone's war zone. *International Journal of Tuberculosis and Lung Disease* 2(9):726-731.

Goodland, R. 2002. Sustainability: Human, social, economic and environmental. In *Social and Economic Dimensions of Global Environmental Change, Encyclopaedia of Global Environmental Change*. Vol. 4, edited by P. Timmerman. New York: John Wiley and Sons.

Gorman, M. 2000. The growing problem of violence against older persons in Africa. *Southern African Journal of Gerontology* 9(2):33-36.

Heise, L., and C. Garcia-Moreno. 2002. Violence by intimate partners. In *World report on violence and health*. Edited by E. Krug, L. L. Dahlberg, J. A. Mercy, et al. Geneva, Switzerland: World Health Organisation. Pp. 87-121.

Heise, L., M. Ellsberg, and M. Gottemoeller. 1999. Ending violence against women. *Population reports*. Series L, No. 11. Baltimore, MD: Population Information Program, Johns Hopkins University School of Public Health.

Hillier, D., and B. Wood. 2003. Shattered lives: The case for tough international arms control London, England: Amnesty International and Oxfam.

Jewkes, R., C. Vundule, F. Maforah, and E. Jordaan. 2001. Relationship dynamics and adolescent pregnancy in South Africa. *Social Science and Medicine* 52(5):733-744.

Jewkes, R., M. Nduna, J. Levin, N. Jama, K. Dunkle, N. Khuzwayo, M. Koss, A. Puren, K. Wood, and N. Duvvury. 2006. A cluster randomized-controlled trial to determine the effectiveness of Stepping Stones in preventing HIV infections and promoting safer sexual behaviour amongst youth in the rural Eastern Cape, South Africa: Trial design, methods and baseline findings. *Tropical Medicine and International Health* 11(1):3-16.

Jolly, R. 2004. Military spending and development. *Insights 50*, http://www.id21.org/insights/insights50/index.html (accessed July 28, 2007).

Kaldor, M. 1999. *New and old wars. Organized violence in a global era.* Stanford, CA: Stanford University Press.

Karr-Morse, R., and M. S. Wiley. 1997. *Ghosts from the nursery: Tracing the roots of violence.* New York: Atlantic Monthly Press.

Keen, D. 1994. The functions of famine in Southwestern Sudan: Implications for relief. In *War and hunger.* Edited by J. Macrae and A. Zwi. London, England: Zed Books. Pp. 111-124.

Keen, D., and K. Wilson. 1994. Engaging with violence: A reassessment of relief in wartime. In *War and hunger: rethinking international responses to complex emergencies.* Edited by J. Macrae and A. Zwi. London, England: Zed Books. Pp. 207-221.

Keikelame, J., and M. Ferreira. 2000. *Elder abuse in black townships on the Cape Flats.* Research Report. Cape Town, South Africa: HSRC/UCT Centre for Gerontology.

Ketsela, T., and D. Kedebe. 1997. Physical punishment of elementary school children in urban and rural communities in Ethiopia. *Ethiopian Medical Journal* 35:23-33.

Kim, S., and W. Pridemore. 2005. Social support and homicide in transitional Russia. *Journal of Criminal Justice* 33:561-572.

Kinyanda, E. 2006. Deliberate self-harm in urban Uganda: A case-control study. Doctoral diss., Norway: Norwegian University of Science and Technology.

Kopel, H., and M. Friedman. 1997. Posttraumatic symptoms in South African police exposed to violence. *Journal of Traumatic Stress* 10:307-317.

Krug, E., L. Dahlberg, A. Zwi, and R. Lozano. 2002. *World report on violence and health.* Geneva: WHO.

Lachs, M., and K. Pillemer. 2004. Elder abuse. *Lancet* 364:1263-1272.

Lalor, K. 2004. Child sexual abuse in sub-Saharan Africa: A literature review. *Child Abuse and Neglect* 28:439-460.

Leach, F., P. Machakanja, and J. Mandoga. 2000. *Preliminary investigation of the abuse of girls in Zimbabwean junior secondary schools.* Education Research Paper No. 39, London, England: Department for International Development (DFID).

Leeb, R. T., L. Paulozzi, C. Melanson, T. Simon, and I. Arias. 2007. *Child maltreatment surveillance: Uniform definitions for public health and recommended data elements, version 1.0.* Atlanta, GA: Centers for Disease Control and Prevention, National Center for Injury Prevention and Control.

Leggett, T., B. Van Bronkhorst, G. Demombynes, and A. Morrison. 2007. *Crime, violence, and development: Trends, costs, and policy options in the Caribbean.* Washington, DC: United Nations Office on Drugs and Crime and the World Bank.

Lerer, L., and R. Matzopoulos. 1996. Meeting the challenge of railway injury in a South African city. *Lancet* 358:664-666.

Liddell, C., J. Kvalsvig, P. Qotyana, and A. Shabalala. 1994. Community violence and young South African children's involvement in aggression. *International Journal of Behavior* 17:613-628.

Link, B. G., and J. C. Phelan. 1995. Social conditions as fundamental causes of diseases. *Journal of Health and Social Behavior* Extra Issue 80-94.

Londoño, J. L., and R. Guerrero. 1999. *Violence in America Latina: Epidemiologia y Costos.* IDB working Document R-375. http://www.iadb.org/res/publications/pubfiles/pubr-375. pdf (accessed June 8, 2007).

Machel, G. 2001. *The impact of war on children.* London, England: Hurst and Company.

Maddaleno, M., A. Concha-Eastman, and S. Marques. 2006. Youth violence in Latin America: a framework for action. *African Safety Promotion: A Journal of Injury and Violence Prevention* 4(2):1-5.

Madu, S. N., and K. Peltzer. 2001. Prevalence and patterns of child sexual abuse and victim-perpetrator relationship among secondary school students in the Northern Province (South Africa). *Archives of Sexual Behavior* 30(3):311-321.

Magwaza, A. S., B. J. Killian, I. Petersen, and Y. Pillay. 1993. The effects of chronic violence on preschool children living in South African townships. *Child Abuse and Neglect* 17:795-803.

Maninger, S. 2000. The urbanisation of conflict. *African Security Review* 9(1), http://www.iss. co.za/pubs/ASR/9No1/UrbanisationConflict.html (accessed August 18, 2007).

Marais, S., E. Van der Spuy, and R. Röntsch. 2002. Crime and violence in the workplace—effects on health workers, part II. *Injury and Safety Monitor* 1(1):8-10.

Marmot, M. G. 1994. Social differences in health within and between populations. *Daedalus* 123(4):197-216.

Mathers, C. D., and D. Loncar. 2006. Projections of global mortality and burden of disease from 2002 to 2030. *PLoS Med* 3(11):e442, doi:10.1371/journal.pmed.0030442.

Mathers, C. D., M. Inoue, Y. Guigoz, R. Lozano, L. Tomaskovic. 2002. Statistical annex. In *World report on violence and health.* Edited by E. Krug, L. L. Dahlberg, J. A. Mercy, et al. Geneva, Switzerland: World Health Organization. Pp. 255-325.

Mathews, S., N. Abrahams, L. Martin, L. Vetten, L. van der Merwe, and R. Jewkes. 2004. *Every six hours a woman is killed by her intimate partner: a national study of female homicide in South Africa.* Medical Research Council.

Matzopoulos, R., and B. Bowman. 2006. Violence and children in South Africa. In *Handbook on paediatric trauma and child abuse.* Edited by S. van As and S. Naidoo. Cape Town, South Africa: Oxford University Press. Pp. 19-28.

Messer, E. 1998. Conflict as a cause of hunger. In *Who's hungry? And how do we know? Food, shortage, poverty and deprivation.* Edited by L. DeRose, E. Messer, and S. Millman. New York: United Nations University Press.

Milanovic, M. 2005. *Why did the poorest countries fail to catch up?* Washington, DC: Carnegie Endowment, Carnegie Paper No. 62.

Miles, S. and E. Medi. 1994. Disabled Children in Post-War Mozambique: Developing Community-Based Support, *Disasters* 18 (3).

Miller-Burke, J., M. Attridge, and P. Fass. 1999. Impact of traumatic events and organizational response. A study of bank robberies. *Journal of Occupational and Environmental Medicine* 41(2):73-83.

Minayo, M. C. 2003. Violence against the elderly: The relevance of an old health problem. *Cad Saude Publica* 19(3):783-791.

Mollica, R. 1999. Psychological effects of mass violence. In Leaning, J., S. GBriggs, and L. Chen. Eds. *Humanitarian Crises: the Medical and Public Health Response.* Cambridge, MA: Harvard University Press.

Moniruzzaman, S., and R. Andersson. 2005. Relationship between economic development and suicide mortality: a global cross-sectional analysis in an epidemiological transition perspective. *Public Health* 118(5):346-348.

MRC (Medical Research Council). 2002. *Umthente Uhlaba Usamila: The 1st South African National Youth Risk Behaviour Survey.* Cape Town, South Africa: Medical Research Council.

# 244 APPENDIX C

Muggah, R. (in press). A hard pill to swallow: The causes and consequences of collective violence on population health in Africa. In *WHO-AFRO Report on violence and Health in Africa*. Harare, Zimbabwe: WHO.

Nafziger, E. 2006. Development, inequality, and war in Africa. *The Economics of Peace and Security Journal* 1(1):14-19.

Narayan, D. (Ed.). 1999. Can anyone hear us? Voices from 47 countries. *Voices of the poor,* Vol. 1. Washington, DC: The World Bank.

Neapolitan, J. 2003. Explaining variation in crime victimization across nations and within nations. *International Criminal Justice Review* 13:76-85.

The NEDCOR Project. 1996. *The NEDCOR Project on crime, violence and investment. Main report.* Johannesburg, South Africa: NEDCOR.

Norman, R., R. Matzopoulos, P. Groenewald, and D. Bradshaw. 2007a. The high burden of injuries in South Africa. *Bulletin of the World Health Organization* 85(9):695-701.

Norman, R., D. Bradshaw, M. Schneider, J. Joubert, P. Groenewald, S. Lewin, K. Steyn, T. Vos, R. Laubscher, N. Nannan, B. Nojilana, D. Pieterse, and the South African Comparative Risk Assessment Collaborating Group. 2007b. A comparative risk assessment for South Africa in 2000: Towards promoting health and preventing disease. *South African Medical Journal* 97(8):637-641.

Norman, R., M. Schneider, D. Bradshaw, P. Groenewald, R. Laubscher, J. Joubert, N. Nannan, B. Nojilana, D. Pieterse, T. Vos, and the South African Comparative Risk Assessment Collaborating Group. 2007c. Towards promoting health and preventing disease—a comparative risk assessment for South Africa, 2000 (invited seminar). *Burden of Disease Today Conference*, Sandton Convention Centre, Johannesburg, March 15-16.

Norman, R., D. Bradshaw, M. Schneider, R. Jewkes, S. Mathews, N. Abrahams, R. Matzopoulos, T. Vos, and the South African Comparative Risk Assessment Collaborating Group. 2007d. Estimating the burden of disease attributable to interpersonal violence in South Africa in 2000. *South African Medical Journal* 97(8):653-656.

Omitoogun, W. 2001. Military expenditure and conflict in Africa in Stockholm International Peace Research Institute (SIPRI) yearbook 2005: Armaments, disarmament, and international security. Oxford, England: Oxford University Press.

PAHO (Pan American Health Organization). 2002. *Risk factors for gang involvement, 2002.* http://www.paho.org/common/Display.asp?Lang=E&RecID=4503 (accessed June 5, 2007).

PAHO. 2003. *Integrated management of adolescent needs: A comprehensive initiative to address the health and development needs of the adolescent population of the Americas.* Unpublished report. Washington, DC: Pan American Health Organization.

Patel, V. 2007. Mental health in low- and middle-income countries. *Br Med Bull*, 81-96.

Peden, M., and J. van der Spuy. 1998. The cost of treating firearm victims. *Trauma Review* 6:4-5.

Peden, M., K. McGee, and G. Sharma. 2002. *The injury chart book: A graphical overview of the global burden of injuries.* Geneva, Switzerland: World Health Organisation.

Peltzer, K. 2001. Stress and traumatic symptoms among police officers at a South African police station. *Acta Criminologica* 14(3):52-56.

Petersen, I., A. Bhana, and M. McKay. 2005. Sexual violence and youth in South Africa: the need for community-based prevention interventions. *Child Abuse andNeglect* 29(11):1233-1248.

Pfizer. 2001. Responding to the global public health challenge of violence. *The Pfizer Journal*, Global Edition, 11:1.

Phillips, R. 1998. *The economic costs of homicide to a South African city*. Unpublished masters thesis, University of Cape Town.

Pinheiro, S. (Ed.). 2006. *World report on violence against children*. United Nations, Geneva, Switzerland: Roto Presse SA.

Plichta, S. B., and M. Falik. 2001. Prevalence of violence and its implications for women's health. *Women's Health Issues* 11:244-258.

Pronyk, P. M., J. R. Hargreaves, J. C. Kim, L. A. Morison, G. Phetla, C. Watts, J. Busza, and J. D. H. Porter. 2006. Effect of a structural intervention for the prevention of intimate-partner violence and HIV in rural South Africa: A cluster randomised trial. *Lancet* 368:1973-1983.

Ronsmans, C., and M. Khlat. 1999. Adolescence and risk of violent death during pregnancy in Matlab, Bangladesh. *Lancet* 354(9188):1448.

Sampson, R. J., and J. L. Lauritsen. 1994. Violent victimization and offending: Individual-, situational-, and community-level risk factors. In *Understanding and preventing violence, volume 3, social influences*. Edited by A. J. Reiss and J. A. Roth. Washington, DC: National Academy Press. Pp. 1-114.

Sethi, D., and E. Krug (Eds.). 2000. *Guidance for surveillance of injuries due to landmines and unexploded ordnance*. Geneva, Switzerland: WHO.

Shrestha, M. 1998. *Report on self-help banking program and women's empowerment*. Asian Development Bank. Nepal.

Sidel, V. 1995. The international arms trade and its impact upon health. *British Medical Journal* 311:1677-1680.

Small Arms Survey. 2006. *Small Arms Survey: Unfinished business*. Oxford, England: Oxford University Press.

Speizer, I. S., M. Goodwin, M. E. Clyde, and J. Rogers. n.d. *Research brief: Childhood sexual abuse among women in El Salvador, Guatemala, and Honduras*. Centers for Disease Control.

Stephenson, R., P. Sheikhattari, N. Assasi, H. Eftekhar, Q. Zamani, B. Maleki, and H. Kiabayan. 2006. Child maltreatment among school children in Kurdistan Province, Iran. *Child Abuse and Neglect* 30(3):231-245.

Stewart, F., and V. Fitzgerald. 2000. *War and underdevelopment, Vol. 1. The economic and social consequences of conflict*. Oxford, England: Oxford University Press.

Swart, L., M. Seedat, G. Stevens, and I. Ricardo. 2002. Violence in adolescents' romantic relationships: findings from a survey amongst school-going youth in a South African community. *Journal of Adolescence* 25(4):385-395.

Teodosijevic, S. 2003. *Armed conflicts and food security*. ESA Working Paper 03-11. Rome, Italy: FAO.

Tool, M., and R. Waldman. 1990. Prevention of excess mortality in refugee and displaced populations in developing countries. *JAMA* 263:3296-3302.

United Nations. 1998. *The international crime victim survey in countries in transition: national reports*. Rome: United Nations Interregional Crime and Justice Research Institute.

Unithan, P., and H. Whitt. 1992. Inequality, economic development, and lethal violence: a crossnational analysis of suicide and homicide. *International Journal of Comparative Sociology* 33(4):182-196.

Van der Merwe, A., and A. Dawes. 2000. Prosocial and antisocial tendencies in children exposed to community violence. *Southern African Journal of Child and Adolescent Mental Health* 12(1):19-37.

Walker, S. P., T. D. Wachs, J. M. Gardner et al. 2007. Child development: Risk factors for adverse outcomes in developing countries. *Lancet* 369(9556):145-157.

Waters, H. R., A. A. Hyder, Y. Rajkotia, S. Basu, and A. Butchart. 2005. The costs of inter-personal violence—an international review. *Health Policy* 73:303-315.

Webster, K. (Ed.). 2004. *The health costs of violence: Measuring the burden of disease caused by intimate partner violence: A summary of findings*. Melbourne, Australia: VicHealth.

WHO (World Health Organisation). 2005. *Multi-country study on women's health and domestic violence against women: initial results on prevalence, health outcomes and women's responses.* Geneva, Switzerland: WHO.

WHO. 2007. *Violence threatens health in Iraq.* http://www.who.int/mediacentre/news/releases/2007/pr15/en/index.html (accessed May 25, 2007).

WHO. (n.d.). *Estimates by income level. Revised Global Burden of Disease (GBD) 2002 estimates.* http://www.who.int/healthinfo/bodgbd2002revised/en/index.html (accessed May 12, 2007).

WHO and CDC (Centers for Disease Control and Prevention). n.d. *Draft guidelines for estimating the economic costs of injuries due to interpersonal and self-directed violence.* Unpublished draft document. Geneva, Switzerland: WHO and CDC.

WHO and INPEA (International Network for the Prevention of Elder Abuse). 2002 Missing voices: views of older persons on elder abuse. Geneva, World Health Organisation.

WHO and IPSCAN (International Society for Prevention of Child Abuse and Neglect). 2006. *Preventing child maltreatment: a guide to taking action and generating evidence.* Geneva, Switzerland: WHO.

Wilson, W. J. 1987. *The truly disadvantaged: The inner city, the underclass, and public policy.* Chicago, IL: University of Chicago Press.

Wolf, R., L. Daichman, and G. Bennett. 2002. Abuse of the elderly. In *World report on violence and health.* Edited by E. G. Krug, L. L. Dahlberg, J. A. Mercy, A. B. Zwi, and R. Lozano. Geneva, Switzerland: World Health Organisation. Pp. 125-145.

World Bank. 2004. *The millennium development goals for health. Rising to the challenges.* Washington, DC: World Bank.

World Bank. 2006. *World development report 2007: Development and the next generation.* Washington, DC: World Bank.

Zwi, A. B., R. Garfield, and A. Loretti. 2002. Collective violence. In *World report of violence and health.* Edited by E. Krug, L. Dahlberg, J. A. Mercy, A. B. Zwi, and R. Lozano. Geneva: WHO. Pp. 213-239.

# Appendix D

# Biographies of Planning Committee Members and Workshop Speakers

## PLANNING COMMITTEE MEMBERS

**Mark L. Rosenberg, M.D., M.P.P.** (*Chair*), is the executive director at the Task Force for Child Survival and Development. Before assuming his current position, Dr. Rosenberg served the Public Health Service at the CDC for 20 years. During this time, he led CDC's work in violence prevention, and later became the first permanent director of the National Center for Injury Prevention and Control. He also held the position of the special assistant for behavioral science in the Office of the Deputy Director (HIV/AIDS). In his early work with CDC, he worked in the smallpox eradication effort and in enteric diseases. Dr. Rosenberg is a member of the boards of directors of both the American Suicide Foundation and the National Safety Council. He is a member of the editorial board of the *Journal of Suicide and Life-Threatening Behavior* and the co-editor in chief of *Injury Control and Safety Promotion*. Dr. Rosenberg is board certified in both psychiatry and internal medicine with training in public policy. He was educated at Harvard University, where he received his undergraduate degree as well as degrees in public policy and medicine. He completed a residency in internal medicine and a fellowship in infectious diseases at Massachusetts General Hospital, a residency in psychiatry at Boston Beth Israel Hospital, and a residency in preventive medicine at CDC. He is on the faculty at Morehouse Medical School, Emory Medical School, and the Rollins School of Public Health at Emory University. Dr. Rosenberg's research and programmatic interests are concentrated on injury control and violence prevention, HIV/AIDS, and child well-being with special attention to behavioral sciences, evaluation, and health communications. He has authored more than 120 publications and has received the Surgeon General's Exemplary Service Medal as well as the Meritorious Service Medal, Distinguished Service Medal, and Outstanding Service Medals from the U.S. Public Health Service. Dr. Rosenberg is a member of the Institute of Medicine.

**James A. Mercy, Ph.D.** (*Vice-Chair*), is the special adviser for strategic directions of the Division of Violence Prevention in the National Center for Injury Prevention and Control of the CDC. He received his Ph.D. in sociology from Emory University in Atlanta in 1982. After his graduation, Dr. Mercy began working at CDC in a newly formed activity to examine violence as a public health problem. Over the past two decades he has played a fundamental role in developing the public health approach to violence. He has conducted and overseen numerous studies of the epidemiology of youth suicide, family violence, homicide, and firearm injuries. He also served as a coeditor of the WHO *World Report on Violence and Health*. Most recently, he served on the editorial board of the United Nation's Secretary-General's Study of Violence Against Children.

**Sir George A.O. Alleyne, M.D.,** is a native of Barbados. He obtained his bachelor of medicine and surgery degree from the University of London in 1957 and his M.D. from the same university in 1965. He began a career in academic medicine in 1962 at the University of the West Indies and was appointed professor of medicine in 1972. Dr. Alleyne has served as a member of various bodies, including the Scientific and Technical Advisory Committee of the World Health Organization (WHO), Tropical Disease Research Program, and the Institute of Medicine Committee on Scientific Investigation in Developing Countries. From 1970 to 1981, Dr. Alleyne served as a member and chair of the Pan American Health Organization (PAHO) Advisory Committee on Medical Research. Dr. Alleyne joined the PAHO staff in 1981 as chief of research promotion and coordination. In 1983 he became director of health programs development, and in 1990 he became assistant director of the organization. In 1995, Dr. Alleyne began his first term as director of the Pan American Health Organization. Equity and Pan Americanism are principles that resonate throughout Dr. Alleyne's work and writings, and guide the execution of the PAHO's regional programming, reflecting a persistent search to achieve the goal of health for all. Her Majesty Queen Elizabeth II made him knight bachelor in 1990 for his services to medicine. In 2001, Sir George Alleyne was awarded the Order of the Caribbean Community, the highest honor that can be conferred on a Caribbean national. He ended his second four-year term as director of PAHO in 2003.

**Robert Alexander Butchart, M.A., Ph.D.,** is the prevention of violence coordinator in WHO's Department of Injuries and Violence Prevention. His main task is to implement the recommendations of the *World Report on Violence and Health*. This involves the development of technical guidelines, policy papers, and research that can be used to support applied prevention programs and advocate for increased investment in violence prevention. Specific projects include country-level violence prevention demonstration programs, the systematic documentation of violence prevention programs, and research into the economic dimensions of interpersonal violence, including the costs of its consequences and the cost-effectiveness of preventive programs. After receiving his master's degree in clinical psychology in 1986, he worked in Johannesburg, South Africa, as coordinator of a brain injury assessment and rehabilitation clinic and in 1989 helped conduct the first epidemiological study of non-fatal injuries in that city. In 1994 he was on the steering committee of the Goldstone Commission's investigation into political violence and children in South Africa. He completed his doctorate in 1995, with a focus on the sociology of public health in Africa. In 1999-2000 he was a visiting scientist in the Karolinska Institute and from 1998 to 2001 was principal investigator for the South African Violence Injury Surveillance Consortium and a founder of the Uganda-based Injury Prevention Initiative for Africa.

**Jacquelyn C. Campbell, Ph.D., R.N.,** is the Anna D. Wolf Chair at Johns Hopkins University School of Nursing. Dr. Campbell's overall research and policy initiatives are in the area of family violence and violence against women, with continuous research funding since 1984 from the National Institutes of Health (NIH; National Institute of Nursing Research, National Institute on Drug Abuse [NIDA], National Institute of Mental Health [NIMH]), the National Institute of Justice, the Centers for Disease Control and Prevention (CDC), and the Department of Defense, including being principal investigator on three NIH, two CDC, one Department of Defense, and one National Institute of Justice funded research grants on battering. Specific research areas include risk factors and assessment for intimate partner homicide, abuse during pregnancy, marital rape, physical and mental health effects of intimate partner violence, prevention of dating violence, and interventions to prevent and address domestic violence. Her research results are used as the basis of health policy recommendations to state, national, and international organizations. Dr. Campbell's awards include fellowship in the American Academy of Nursing, the Kellogg National Leadership Program, a Robert Wood Johnson Urban Health Fellowship, three honorary doctorates, and the Simon Visiting Scholar at the University of Manchester in the United Kingdom. She has authored or coauthored more than 125 articles and chapters, mainly about battered women and family violence. She is author, coauthor, or editor of five books: *Nursing Care of Survivors of Family Violence* (1993); *Sanctions and Sanctuary: Cultural Perspectives on the Beating of Wives* (1992), which has been updated and is now called *To Have & To Hit*; *Assessing Dangerousness: Violence by Sexual Offenders, Batterers and Child Abusers* (1999); *Ending Domestic Violence: Changing Public Perceptions/Halting the Epidemic* (1997); *Empowering Survivors of Abuse: Health Care for Battered Women and Their Children* (1998), and *Family Violence in Nursing Practice* (2004). Dr. Campbell has also been working with wife abuse shelters and advocacy organizations for the last 25 years, including leading support groups and serving on four shelter boards. Currently, she is on the boards of directors of the Family Violence Prevention Fund in San Francisco and the House of Ruth in Baltimore, and has served on the congressionally appointed Department of Defense (DoD) Task Force on Domestic Violence. Dr. Campbell is a member of the Institute of Medicine.

**Darnell Hawkins, Ph.D., J.D.,** is currently professor emeritus in the Department of African American Studies at the University of Illinois, Chicago. He specializes in criminology and the sociology of law and conducts research on topics that bridge the intersection between race-ethnicity and crime-justice. Dr. Hawkins is a member of the MacArthur Foundation Network on Adolescent Development and Juvenile Justice and of the Committee on Law and Justice of the National Research Council. He has been a member of the National Academies Committee on Law and Justice; Committee on Assessment of Family Violence Interventions; Panel on Juvenile Crime: Prevention, Treatment, and Control; and chair of the National Science Foundation (NSF) Minority Graduate Panel on Anthropology and Sociology.

## WORKSHOP SPEAKERS

**Carl C. Bell, M.D.,** is president and chief executive officer of Community Mental Health Council, Inc. (a $21 million comprehensive CMHC in Chicago with 360 employees), is principal investigator of "Using CHAMP to Prevent Youth HIV Risk in a South African Township," an NIMH R-01 Grant. He is director of public and community psychiatry, clinical professor of psychiatry and public health, and co-director of the Interdisciplinary Violence Prevention Research Center at the University of Illinois at Chicago. He has 350 publications, the most recent being *The Sanity of Survival: Reflections on Community Mental Health and Wellness* (2004) and *Eight Pieces of Brocade*—a 45-minute chi kung exercise DVD.

**Stephen Blount, M.D., M.P.H.,** is responsible for CDC's global health portfolio, which includes an annual budget of $900 million, 200 U.S.

government staff assigned to 50 countries, and 1,500 locally hired staff and contractors. He provides programmatic and financial oversight for the Global AIDS Program; global immunization and disease eradication activities; malaria, tuberculosis, and tobacco control efforts; and international training programs. Dr. Blount is the lead strategist for CDC's global activities and manages key partnerships with ministries of health, other U.S. government agencies, UN organizations, the World Bank, private foundations, multinational corporations, nongovernmental organizations, and academic institutions. As the first director of the Office for Global Health in 1997, Dr. Blount led the development of CDC's global health strategy, including goals, objectives, priority program areas, and performance measures. Since 2003, as part of the first agency-wide transformation of CDC's structure since 1980, Dr. Blount has led the reorganization of its international activities to better align human, technical, and financial resources with the agency's goals and priorities and to improve global business services. After training in family medicine and public health, Dr. Blount served as the director of epidemiology at the Detroit Health Department before joining CDC. From 1993 to 1997, he was assigned to the World Health Organisation and worked at the Caribbean Epidemiology Center in Trinidad, where he served as director. He received his B.S. in psychology in 1975, his M.D. in 1978 from Tufts University, and his M.P.H. in 1980 from the University of Michigan.

**Holly Burkhalter** is vice president of government relations for the International Justice Mission (IJM), an international human rights agency that assists victims of violence, sexual exploitation, slavery, and oppression. Ms. Burkhalter graduated from Iowa State University in 1978 (Phi Beta Kappa) and received the University's Outstanding Young Alumnus award in 1984. Before beginning her career with IJM, Ms. Burkhalter most recently served as the U.S. policy director of Physicians for Human Rights, a Boston-based human rights organization specializing in medical, scientific, and forensic investigations of violations of internationally recognized human rights. Prior to joining Physicians for Human Rights, Ms. Burkhalter worked with Human Rights Watch for 14 years as advocacy director and director of its Washington office. Previously, Ms. Burkhalter staffed the House Foreign Affairs Subcommittee on Human Rights and International Organizations from 1981 to 1983. From 1977 to 1981 she worked for Representative (now Senator) Tom Harkin (D.-Iowa).

**Eric D. Caine, M.D.,** joined the faculty of the University of Rochester in 1978, following medical school at Harvard, residency training at the Massachusetts Mental Health Center and the National Institute of Mental Health, and further postdoctoral research at NIMH. During college and medical school, his interests focused primarily on substance abuse treatment, suicide, and end-of-life issues. The first two were tied specifically to fundamental concerns about public health, prevention, and public policy development. As he progressed through medical school and his psychiatry residency, Dr. Caine focused on the relationships between organized brain functioning and behavioral disorders; in addition to the standard residency he pursued additional training in neuropsychology and neurology as a means of fostering interests in "neuropsychiatry." His research initially dealt with Huntington's disease and Tourette's syndrome and, to a lesser extent, Alzheimer's disease. Suicide research and prevention gradually have become the focal points during the last 15 years both for investigation and for national and international consultation. His greatest personal career rewards in medicine, in addition to those related to patient care, have come from supporting this developmental process and seeing several generations of faculty emerge in their own right as outstanding researchers, educators, and clinicians. Presently Dr. Caine directs five NIH grants—among them, "The Developing Center for Public Health and Population Interventions for the Prevention of Suicide" ("PHP-Center," NIMH/NIDA P20); "China-Rochester Suicide Research Training ICOHRTA" (NIH Fogarty International Center D43); and "China Collaborative Suicide Research Training Program" (CCSRT; NIH Fogarty International Center D43).

**Alan Court, M.A.,** is currently the director of the United Nations Children's Fund (UNICEF) Programme Division. Mr. Court joined UNICEF in 1975 where he oversees the centerpiece of UNICEF's work. In this capacity, he is at the forefront of program policy, guidance, and management intended to assist staff in the implementation and success of UNICEF programs and plays a central role in guiding UNICEF programs toward the achievement of the Millennium Development Goals. Prior to this, Mr. Court served as director of the UNICEF Supply Division in Copenhagen, where he was credited with turning the division's function into an innovative and cutting-edge one that provides essential commodities and services to governments through a mix of programs and procurement services that directly impact program implementation as well as delivery performance, especially in humanitarian emergencies. Before serving at these two headquarters locations, Mr. Court had a long and distinguished career in the field where, from August 1998 to December 2000, he was the UNICEF country representative in India. Beforehand, he served as deputy regional director of the Americas and Caribbean region in Bogotá, Colombia, after having served as UNICEF representative in Bolivia from 1993 to 1995. In 1992, he served as special representative in the former Yugoslavia. Prior to that, he was the UNICEF representative in Chad after having served as program coordinator in Nepal. In 1983, Mr. Court was the program planning officer in Ethiopia, after having managed nutrition and agricultural programs in Indonesia. His first appointment with UNICEF was in Bangladesh from 1975 to 1978. Mr. Court holds a master's degree in rural social development from the University of Reading School of Education. He is a national of the United Kingdom.

**Linda L. Dahlberg, Ph.D.,** is the associate director for science in the Division of Violence Prevention at the U.S. Centers for Disease Control and Prevention. In her current position, Dr. Dahlberg serves as one of the senior advisers on matters of science and policy to the director of the Division of Violence Prevention. She also coordinates international research and programmatic activities for the division and serves as a subject matter expert and consultant on a number of international scientific planning committees and advisory boards. Dr. Dahlberg has spent much of the past 15 years working in the area of violence prevention—specifically on the efficacy and effectiveness of interventions to reduce violence. More recently she served as the executive scientific editor of the *World Report on Violence and Health*—published by WHO in October 2002. She has authored and coauthored many publications in peer-reviewed journals, has given numerous presentations across the United States and abroad, and has received awards of excellence in both teaching and research. Dr. Dahlberg holds a B.A. degree from the University of Northern Colorado, and an M.A. and Ph.D., both in sociology, from Indiana University-Bloomington.

**John Donnelly** is a reporter in the Washington bureau of the *Boston Globe*, covering global and domestic health and the environment. From 2003 to mid-2006, he opened and ran the *Globe's* first-ever Africa bureau. Based in South Africa, he traveled widely around the continent, focusing on a wide range of health issues, including AIDS, malaria, tuberculosis, and the attempt to eradicate polio; politics; counterterrorism; development policy; and the future of oil in Africa. Before moving to Africa, he was the *Globe's* foreign affairs correspondent for five years, based in Washington. Prior to the September 11th attacks, he examined the differences between what was said in Washington and what was happening around the world, traveling to the Middle East, Europe, Africa, Latin America, and the Caribbean. After the attacks, he covered the buildup to the war in Afghanistan, the war in Afghanistan, the buildup to the Iraq war, and the war in Iraq. In addition, in 2002, he directed a year-long global health project at the *Globe* called "Lives Lost" that looked at how simple interventions could save millions of lives every year. The project won several major awards in 2004. In recent years, Donnelly has received awards from the Global Health Council, RESULTS, InterAction, and the American Society of Tropical Medicine and Hygiene. Prior to joining the *Globe*, he worked for a year in Washington for Knight Ridder Newspapers and spent four years based in Jerusalem and Cairo covering the Middle East for Knight Ridder and the *Miami Herald*. At the *Herald*, he was part of the Pulitzer Prize-winning coverage of Hurricane Andrew and was one of four reporters on its Enterprise Team, winning an award for his coverage of health issues in Haiti. He has also worked for the Associated Press in New York City and in Vermont and was a staff reporter for the *Burlington Free Press*. He attended the University of Maine and University of Vermont, majoring in English. He was a Duke University Media Fellow during the fall of 2000 and will soon begin a nine-month fellowship with the Kaiser Family Foundation to study U.S. programs designed to help orphans in Africa.

**Marco Ferroni, Ph.D.,** is deputy manager of the Sustainable Development Department at the Inter-American Development Bank (IDB) in Washington, D.C. Earlier in his career, he was the bank's principal evaluation officer, a senior adviser to the World Bank, a member of the Board of Executive Directors at the IDB, and a senior economist and manager at the Ministries of Public Economy and Foreign Affairs in Switzerland. Mr. Ferroni holds a Ph.D. from Cornell University and has published on foreign aid, debt and development finance, public expenditure reform, international public goods, and the interrelationship between trade and macroeconomic regimes and agricultural growth. He is the author, with Ashoka Mody, of *International Public Goods: Incentives, Measurement, and Financing* (Kluwer Academic Publishers and the World Bank, 2002).

**Thomas E. Feucht, Ph.D.,** is the deputy director for research and evaluation at the National Institute of Justice (NIJ), U.S. Department of Justice. A member of the Senior Executive Service, he heads NIJ's Office of Research and Evaluation, the social and behavioral science section of NIJ. Dr. Feucht received his doctorate in sociology in 1986 from the University of North Carolina-Chapel Hill, with an emphasis on quantitative research methods and statistics. From 1987 to 1994, Dr. Feucht served on the faculty at Cleveland State University (CSU), in the Sociology Department and the College of Urban Affairs. Dr. Feucht joined the staff at the National Institute of Justice in 1994. From 1996 until 1998, he served as director of the Crime Control and Prevention Division's Office of Research and Evaluation (ORE). In that position, Dr. Feucht managed NIJ's research portfolios in the areas of law enforcement, crime prevention, and substance abuse. In 1998, Dr. Feucht became ORE's deputy director; in 2005, was appointed to the federal government's Senior Executive Service and became NIJ's deputy director for research and evaluation. Dr. Feucht serves on the Social, Behavioral, and Economic Sciences (SBE) Subcommittee of the National Science and Technology Council, White House Office of Science and Technology

Policy. This interagency working group is responsible for helping to shape SBE research policy across the federal government. From 1998 to 2000, Dr. Feucht served as chief of staff to the Attorney General's Methamphetamine Interagency Task Force, established as part of the 1996 Methamphetamine Control Act. He has conducted and published research in the areas of substance abuse, intravenous drug use and HIV, prostitution, prison drug use, and school violence.

**James Garbarino, Ph.D.,** holds the Maude C. Clarke Chair in Humanistic Psychology and is director of the Center for the Human Rights of Children at Loyola University, Chicago. Previously he was Elizabeth Lee Vincent Professor of Human Development and co-director of the Family Life Development Center at Cornell University. He earned his B.A. from St. Lawrence University in 1968 and his Ph.D. in human development and family studies from Cornell University in 1973. He is a fellow of the American Psychological Association. Dr. Garbarino has served as consultant or adviser to a wide range of organizations, including the National Committee to Prevent Child Abuse, the National Institute for Mental Health, the American Medical Association, the National Black Child Development Institute, the National Science Foundation, the U.S. Advisory Board on Child Abuse and Neglect, and the Federal Bureau of Investigation. In 1991 he undertook missions for UNICEF to assess the impact of the Gulf War on children in Kuwait and Iraq, and he has served as a consultant for programs serving Vietnamese, Bosnian, and Croatian child refugees. Books he has authored or edited include *See Jane Hit: Why Girls Are Growing More Violent and What We Can Do About It* (2006) and *And Words Can Hurt Forever: How to Protect Adolescents from Bullying, Harassment, and Emotional Violence* (2002). He also serves as a scientific expert witness in criminal and civil cases involving issues of violence and children. Some of Dr. Garbarino's most recent awards and honors include the Brandt F. Steele Award from the Kempe National Center on Child Abuse and Neglect (1993); the American Psychological Association's Division on Child, Youth and Family Services' Nicholas Hobbs Award (1994); the President's Celebrating Success Award from the National Association of School Psychologists (2003), and the Outstanding Service to Children Award of the Chicago Association for the Education of Young Children (2003).

**Richard Garfield, Dr.P.H.,** is the Henrik H. Bendixen Professor of Clinical International Nursing and coordinator of a WHO-PAHO Nursing Collaborating Center at Columbia University, and a visiting professor at Karolinska Institute in Sweden. He combines the qualitative perspective of community health promotion and the quantitative approaches of epidemiology to assess morbidity and mortality changes among civilian groups in humanitarian crises around the world. He has assessed the impact of economic embargoes in Cuba, Haiti, Yugoslavia, Afghanistan, Iraq, and Liberia for national governments and UN organizations. He has visited Iraq frequently since 1996 to collaborate with UNICEF, WHO, the World Food Program, and the Iraqi Ministry of Health. He was a coauthor of WHO's *World Report on Violence and Health* and the report of the Independent Commission to Evaluate the Oil for Food Program (Volcker Commission). He is currently running household studies focused on insecurity and recovery in Katrina-affected areas in the United States and in postwar areas of southern Sudan.

**David Gartner, J.D.,** is the policy director for the Global AIDS Alliance (GAA), an advocacy organization dedicated to achieving a comprehensive response to the AIDS pandemic and to expanding educational opportunities in affected countries. Mr. Gartner previously worked as a counsel on the Senate Health, Education, Labor, and Pensions Committee. He has appeared as a commentator on CBS, CNN, and NPR and written for a wide variety of publications, including the *New York Times*, the *Philadelphia Inquirer* and the *Miami Herald*. Mr. Gartner is a graduate of Yale Law School and did graduate work in political science at the Massachusetts Institute of Technology; he was a visiting lecturer at Yale University.

**Rodrigo Guerrero, M.D.,** is currently the president of the board at Vallenpaz, a nongovernmental organization dedicated to work with peasants in rural areas of Colombia, a position he has held since 2000. Born in Cali, Colombia, he is currently emeritus at Universidad del Valle, in Cali, where he served as a professor, dean of the Division of Health Sciences (1972-1975), and president (1982-1984). He worked as the director of Universidad del Valle's hospital from 1976 to 1978 and as the secretary of health for the City of Cali (1978-1980). He was elected mayor of Cali in 1992 and served for two years. In addition, Dr. Guerrero has served as president of the Carvajal Foundation (part time 1984-1992), as regional adviser for health and violence to the Pan-American Health Organization in Washington, D.C. (1995-1997), and as a consultant to the IDB, the World Bank, and other agencies. Dr. Guerrero holds memberships to number of organizations including the National Academy of Medicine (Colombia), the Colombian Society of Epidemiology, the New York Academy of Sciences, and the Institute of Medicine. He founded and directed *Journal Colombia Médica* (1980-1994) of which he is now director emeritus. In addition, he is a member of the editorial committees of several journals: *Annals of Epidemiology*; *Cancer Epidemiology Biomarkers and Prevention*; *Injury Control and Safety Promotion*; and *Journal of Health & Population in Developing Countries*. Dr. Guerrero has authored numerous publications in scientific journals in the areas of epidemiology, physiology of reproduction, and prevention of violence.

**Rodney Hammond, Ph.D.,** is the director of the Division of Violence Prevention in the National Center for Injury Prevention and Control at the CDC in Atlanta, Georgia, a position he has held since 1996. He is responsible for CDC research and programs to prevent child maltreatment, youth violence, family and intimate partner violence, sexual assault, and suicide. The division oversees prevention research, surveillance, and programs in youth violence, family and intimate partner violence, child abuse, sexual assault, and suicide. He represents CDC in areas of violence prevention at WHO in Geneva, Switzerland, and PAHO in Washington, D.C. He was the CDC representative to the Health Working Group of the Gore-Mbecki Bilateral Commission to the Republic of South Africa. He is known for distinguished contributions in the area of youth violence prevention as a public health concern. For example, he is author and executive producer of "Dealing with Anger: A Violence Prevention Program for African American Youth," which has been nationally recognized for its application to the problems of at-risk youth. He also developed Project PACT (Positive Adolescents Choices Training), a widely disseminated program distinguished by successful violence prevention outcomes in schools and community settings. His publications appear in numerous health and science journals and books. He has received numerous awards for career contributions including the U.S. Department of Health and Human Services Secretary's Award for Distinguished Service for his efforts in public health and mental health collaboration; the National Association of School Psychologists President's Award for Mental Health; and the Society for Research on Adolescence Award for Adolescent Research and Policy Integration. Dr. Hammond is a fellow of the American Psychological Association (APA) and the APA Division of Health Psychology. He is a past chair of the APA Board of Convention Affairs and vice chair of the Board of Governors of the National College of Professional Psychology. In 2006 he was inducted into the National Academy of Practice. He completed his undergraduate degree at the University of Illinois in Champaign-Urbana and his Ph.D. in psychology at Florida State University in Tallahassee. He completed postdoctoral study at Harvard University.

**J. David Hawkins, Ph.D.,** is the Endowed Professor of Prevention and founding director of the Social Development Research Group, School of Social Work, University of Washington in Seattle. He received his B.A. in 1967 from Stanford University and his Ph.D. in sociology from Northwestern University in 1975. His research focuses on understanding and preventing child and adolescent health and behavior problems. He is principal investigator of the Seattle Social Development Project, a longitudinal study of 808 Seattle elementary school students who are now 30 years old. This project began in 1981 to test strategies for promoting successful development. He is also principal investigator of the Community Youth Development Study, a randomized field experiment involving 24 communities across seven states testing the effectiveness of the Communities That Care prevention system developed by Hawkins and Richard F. Catalano. He has authored numerous articles and several books as well as prevention programs for parents and families, including *Guiding Good Choices*, *Parents Who Care* and *Supporting School Success*. He is past president of the Society for Prevention Research and has served on a number of national and state government committees including NIDA's Epidemiology, Prevention and Services Research Review Committee; the Office for Substance Abuse Prevention's National Advisory Committee; the NIH Study Section for Community Prevention and Control; the Department of Education's Safe, Disciplined, Drug-Free Schools Expert Panel; and the Washington State Governor's Substance Abuse Prevention Committee. He is a member of the editorial board of *Prevention Science*. He is listed in *Who's Who in Science and Engineering*. He has won several awards such the Prevention Science Award from the Society for Prevention Research (1999), 1999 August Vollmer Award from the American Society of Criminology (1999), and the Paul Tappan Award from the Western Society of Criminology (2003). He is a fellow of the American Society of Criminology and the Academy of Experimental Criminology.

**Fran Henry, M.B.A.,** created and directs Global Violence Prevention Advocacy, a project of the Pan American Health and Education Foundation that advances science-based prevention of violence in low- and middle-income countries. For 13 years she founded and directed Stop It Now!, an organization that uses science-based methods of public health to prevent the sexual abuse of children. Ms. Henry's previous work includes owning a management consulting company (10 years) and directing presidential (Gerald Ford) and gubernatorial (Francis W. Sargent-Massachusetts) commissions for women. She served as staff to the National Commission on Observance of International Women's Year. Ms. Henry received her undergraduate degree from the New School for Social Research and her graduate degree from Harvard University Graduate School of Business Administration. As a volunteer, she chaired the board of the Diana, Princess of Wales Memorial Fund, U.S., from 2000 to 2004.

**Kent R. Hill, Ph.D.,** is the assistant administrator for the Bureau for Global Health, U.S. Agency for International Development (USAID). From November 2001 to October 2005, Hill served as assistant administrator for the Bureau for Europe and Eurasia at USAID. As assistant administrator of the